Progress in Inflammation Research

Series Editor

Prof. Dr. Michael J. Parnham
PLIVA
Research Institute
Prilaz baruna Filipovica 25
10000 Zagreb
Croatia

Advisory Board

G. Z. Feuerstein (Merck Research Laboratories, West Point, PA, USA
W. van Eden (Universiteit Utrecht, Utrecht, The Netherlands)

Forthcoming titles:
Mind over Matter – Regulation of Peripheral Inflammation by the CNS,
    C. Stein, M. Schaefer (Editors), 2003
Heat Shock Proteins and Inflammation, W. van Eden (Editor), 2003
Pharmacotherapy of GI Inflammation, A. Guglietta (Editor), 2003
Arachidonate Remodeling and Inflammation, A.N. Fonteh, R.L. Wykle (Editor), 2003
Inflammation and Cardiac Diseases, G.Z. Feuerstein, P. Libby, D.L. Mann (Editors), 2003
Inflammatory Processes and Cancer,
    D.W. Morgan, U. Forssmann, M. Nakada (Editors), 2003
Recent Advances in Pathophysiology of COPD, P.J. Barnes, T.T. Hansel (Editors), 2003
Anti-Inflammatory or Anti-Rheumatic Drugs,
    R.O. Day, D.E. Furst, P.L. van Riel (Editors), 2003
Cytokines and Joint Injury, P. Miossec, W.B. van den Berg (Editors), 2004
Antibiotics as Anti-Inflammatories, B. Rubin, J. Tamaoki (Editors), 2004

(Already published titles see last page.)

Inflammation and Cardiac Diseases

Giora Z. Feuerstein
Peter Libby
Douglas L. Mann

Editors

Birkhäuser Verlag
Basel · Boston · Berlin

Editors

Giora Z. Feuerstein
Pharmacology Department
WP42-209,
Merck Research Laboratories
770 Sumneytown Pike
West Point, PA 19486
USA

Peter Libby
Cardiovascular Medicine
Brigham and Women's Hospital
221 Longwood Avenue
EBRC 307
Boston, MA 02115
USA

Douglas L. Mann
Winters Center for Heart Failure Research
6565 Fannin
MS 524
Houston, TX 77030
USA

A CIP catalogue record for this book is available from the Library of Congress, Washington D.C., USA

Bibliographic information published by Die Deutsche Bibliothek
Die Deutsche Bibliothek lists this publication in the Deutsche Nationalbibliografie;
detailed bibliographic data is available in the internet at http://dnb.ddb.de

ISBN 3-7643-6725-3 Birkhäuser Verlag, Basel – Boston – Berlin

© 2003 Birkhäuser Verlag, P.O. Box 133, CH-4010 Basel, Switzerland
Member of the BertelsmannSpringer Publishing Group
Printed on acid-free paper produced from chlorine-free pulp. TCF ∞
Cover design: Markus Etterich, Basel
Cover illustration: Rat heart during the acute phase of myocarditis. Azan-Mallory staining. See chapter by
K. Watanabe et al. (With the friendly permission of K. Watanabe.)
Printed in Germany
ISBN 3-7643-6725-3

9 8 7 6 5 4 3 2 1   www.birkhauser.ch

Contents

Inflammation and myocarditis

Nuclear factors in cardiac disease

Chemokines and cardiac diseases

Neurohormonal mediators and cardiac inflammation

Cyclooxygenases and cardiac diseases

Inflammation and arrhythmias

List of contributors

Zaid Abassi, Department of Physiology & Biophysics, Faculty of Medicine, Technion Medical School, P.O. Box 9649, Haifa 31096, Israel;
e-mail: abassi@tx.technion.ac.il

Marina Afanasyeva, Immunology Research Group, Department of Physiology and Biophysics, University of Calgary Health Sciences Center, 3330 Hospital Drive, Calgary, AB T2N 4N1, Canada; e-mail: afanasym@ucalgary.ca

Yoshifusa Aizawa, First Department of Medicine, Niigata University School of Medicine, Asahimachi, Niigata 951-8510, Japan; e-mail: aizaways@niigata-u.ac.jp

Farhad Amiri, University of Montreal, CIHR Multidisciplinary Research Group on Hypertension, Clinical Research of Montreal, 110 avenue des Pins ouest, Montreal, PQ Canada H2W 1R7; e-mail: amirif@ircm.qc.ca

Gary F. Baxter, Infection, Inflammation and Vascular Biology Research Group, Department of Basic Sciences, The Royal Veterinary College, University of London, Royal College Street, London NW1 0TU, UK; e-mail: gfbaxter@rvc.ac.uk

Thomas M. Behr, Department of Cardiology, Medizinische Poliklinik, University of Würzburg, Klinikstrasse 6, 97084 Würzburg, Germany;
e-mail: Behr_T@medizin.uni-wuerzburg.de

Todd Bourcier, Cardiovascular Division, Brigham and Women's Hospital, 75 Francis Street, Boston, MA 02115, USA; e-mail: tbourcier@rics.bwh.harvard.edu

Biykem Bozkurt, Winters Center for Heart Failure Research, the Cardiology Section, Department of Medicine, Veterans Administration Medical Center and Baylor College of Medicine, 6565 Fannin, Houston, TX 77030, USA

Antoine Bril, Institut de Recherches Servier, 11 rue des Moulineaux, F-92150 Suresnes, France; e-mail: antoine.bril@fr.netgrs.com

Allen P. Burke, Department of Cardiovascular Pathology, Armed Forces Institute of Pathology, 6825 16th St. NW, Washington, DC 20306-6000, USA; e-mail: burke@afip.osd.mil

Gaelle Clermont, Biomatech, ZI de l'Islon, Rue Pasteur, 38670 Chasse-Sur-Rhone, France; e-mail: g.clermont@biomatech.fr

Jack P. M. Cleutjens, Department of Pathology, Cardiovascular Research Institute Maastricht (CARIM), University of Maastricht, PO Box 616, 6200 MD Maastricht, The Netherlands

Wilson S. Colucci, Cardiovascular Medicine, Boston University Medical Center, 88 East Newton St., D-8, Boston MA 02118, USA; e-mail: wilson.colucci@bmc.org

Esther E. J. M. Creemers, Department of Pathology, Cardiovascular Research Institute Maastricht (CARIM), University of Maastricht, PO Box 616, 6200 MD Maastricht, The Netherlands; e-mail: ecre@lpat.azm.nl

Mat J.A.P. Daemen, Department of Pathology, University of Maastricht, Cardiovascular Research Institute Maastricht (CARIM), University of Maastricht, PO Box 616, 6200 MD Maastricht, The Netherlands; e-mail: mda@lpat.azm.nl

Anita Deswal, Cardiology Research (151C), Winters Center for Heart Failure Research, VA Medical Center, 2002 Holocombe Blvd, Houston, TX 77030, USA

Quy N. Diep, University of Montreal, CIHR Multidisciplinary Research Group on Hypertension, Clinical Research of Montreal, 110 avenue des Pins Ouest, Montreal, PQ Canada H2W 1R7; e-mail: quy.diep@bioaxone.com

Christopher P. Doe, Department of Investigative and Cardiac Biology, GlaxoSmithKline, 709 Swedeland Rd, King of Prussia, PA 19406-0939, USA; e-mail: chris_p_doe@gsk.com

Andrew Farb, Department of Cardiovascular Pathology, Armed Forces Institute of Pathology, 6825 16th St. NW, Washington, DC 20306-6000, USA; e-mail: farb@afip.osd.mil

Giora Z. Feuerstein, Pharmacology Department, WP42-209, Merck Research Laboratories, 770 Sumneytown Pike, West Point, PA 19486, USA; e-mail: giora_feuerstein@merck.com

Aloke V. Finn, Massachusetts General Hospital, Bigalow 800, 55 Fruit Street, Boston, MA 02114, USA; afinn@partners.org

Stefan Frantz, Medizinische Universitätsklinik Würzburg, Josef-Schneider-Str. 2, 97080 Würzburg, Germany; e-mail: frantz_s@klinik.uni-wuerzburg.de

Herman K. Gold, Massachusetts General Hospital, Bigalow 800, 55 Fruit Street, Boston, MA 02114, USA; hgold@partners.org

Mansoor Husain, Heart and Stroke Richard Lewar Centre of Excellence, University of Toronto, Ontario, Canada; e-mail: mansoor.husain@utoronto.ca

Haisong Ju, Department of Investigative and Cardiac Biology, GlaxoSmithKline, 709 Swedeland Rd, King of Prussia, PA 19406, USA; e-mail: haisong.2.ju@gsk.com

Ralph Kelly, Genzyme Corporation, 15 Pleasant St, Connector, P.O. Box 9322, Framingham, MA 01701-9322, USA; e-mail: ralph.kelly@genzyme.com

Makoto Kodama, First Department of Medicine, Niigata University of School of Medicine, Asahimachi, Niigata 951-8510, Japan; e-mail: kodamama@med.niigata-u.ac.jp

Frank D. Kolodgie, Department of Cardiovascular Pathology, Armed Forces Institute of Pathology, 6825 16th St. NW, Washington, DC 20306-6000, USA; e-mail: kolodgie@afip.osd.mil

Sandrine Lecour, Laboratoire de Physiopathologie et Pharmacologie Cardiovasculaires Expérimentales, IFR 100, Facultés de Médecine et Pharmacie, Université de Bourgogne, 7 Bd. Jeanne d'Arc-BP 87900, 21079 Dijon, France, and Hatter Institute for Cardiology Research, UCT Medical School, Cape Town, 7925, South Africa; e-mail: sandrine@capeheart.uct.ac.za

Peter Libby, Cardiovascular Medicine, Brigham and Women's Hospital, Professor of Medicine, Harvard Medical School, Brigham and Women's Hospital, 221 Longwood Avenue, EBRC 307, Boston, MA 02115; e-mail: plibby@rics.bwh.harvard.edu

Benedict Lucchesi, University of Michigan Medical School, Department of Pharmacology, 1301C Medical Sciences Research Building III, 1150 W. Medical Center Drive, Ann Arbor MI 48109-0632, USA; e-mail: benluc@umich.edu

Douglas L. Mann, Department of Medicine, Winters Center for Heart Failure Research, MS 524, 6565 Fannin, Houston, TX 77030, USA; e-mail: dmann@bcm.tmc.edu

Jay W. Mason, Cardiovascular Sciences, Covance Central Diagnostics, Reno, NY 89502, USA; e-mail: jay.mason@covance.com

Michael Marber, Department of Cardiology, KCL, The Rayne Institute, St Thomas' Hospital, London SE1 7EH, UK; e-mail: mike.marber@kcl.ac.uk

Luc Rochette, Laboratoire de Physiopathologie et Pharmacologie Cardiovasculaires Expérimentales, IFR 100, Facultés de Médecine et Pharmacie, Université de Bourgogne, 7 Bd Jeanne d'Arc, BP 87900, 21079 Dijon cedex, France; e-mail: rochette@u-bourgogne.fr

Noel R. Rose, Department of Pathology and W. Harry Feinstone Department of Molecular Microbiology and Immunology, Bloomberg School of Public Health, 615 600 North Wolfe Street, Baltimore, MD 21205, USA; e-mail: nrrose@jhsph.edu

Hani N. Sabbah, Division of Cardiovascular Medicine, Henry Ford Hospital, 2799 West Grand Boulevard, Detroit, MI 48202, USA; e-mail: HSABBAH1@hfhs.org

Michael N. Sack, Hatter Institute for Cardiology Research, UCT Medical School, Cape Town, 7925, South Africa; e-mail: sack@capeheart.uct.ac.za

Flora Sam, Myocardial Biology Unit, Boston University School of Medicine, Cardiovascular Division, Boston UMedical School, 88 East Newton St., D-8, Boston, MA 02118, USA

Shigetake Sasayama, Hamamatsu Rosai Hospital, 25 Shogen-cho, Hamamatsu, Shizuoka 430-8525, Japan; e-mail: sh-sasayama@hamamatsuh.rofuku.go.jp / sasayama@wonder.ocn.ne.jp

Douglas B. Sawyer, Myocardial Biology Unit, Boston University School of Medicine, Cardiovascular Division, Boston University Medical School, 88 East Newton St., D-8, Boston, MA 02118, USA

Ernesto L. Schiffrin, University of Montreal, CIHR Multidisciplinary Research Group on Hypertension, Clinical Research of Montreal, 110 avenue des Pins ouest, Montreal, PQ Canada H2W 1R7; e-mail: ernesto.schiffrin@ircm.qc.ca

Robert M. Smith, Hatter Institute for Cardiology Research, UCT Medical School, Cape Town, 7925, South Africa

Jos F.M. Smits, Department of Pharmacology, Cardiovascular Research Institute Maastricht (CARIM), University of Maastricht, PO Box 616, 6200 MD Maastricht, The Netherlands

Francis G. Spinale, Cardiothoracic Surgery, Room 625, Strom Thurmond Research Building, 770 MUSC Complex, Medical University of South Carolina, 114 Doughty St., Charleston, SC 29425, USA; e-mail: wilburnm@musc.edu

Duncan J. Stewart, St. Michael's Hospital, Q7-810, 30 Bond Street, Toronto, Ontario, Canada, M5G 2C4; e-mail: stewartd@smh.toronto.on.ca

Elaine J. Tanhehco, Division of Cardiovascular Medicine, Henry Ford Hospital, 2799 West Grand Boulevard, Detroit, MI 48202, USA

Masaya Tanno, Department of Cardiology, KCL, The Rayne Institute, St Thomas' Hospital, London SE1 7EH, UK; e-mail: masaya.tanno@kcl.ac.uk

David van Wagoner, Basic and Cardiac Electrophyiology Laboratories, The Cleveland Clinic Foundation, Department of Cardiology FF10, 9500 Euclid Avenue, Cleveland, OH 44195, USA; e-mail: vanwagd@ccf.org

Catherine Vergely, Laboratoire de Physiopathologie et Pharmacologie Cardiovasculaires Expérimentales, IFR 100, Facultés de Médecine et Pharmacie, Université de Bourgogne, 7 Bd Jeanne d'Arc, BP 87900, 21079 Dijon cedex, France; e-mail: cvergely@u-bourgogne.fr

Renu Virmani, Department of Cardiovascular Pathology, Armed Forces Institute of Pathology, 6825 16th St. NW, Washington, DC 20306-6000, USA; e-mail: virmani@afip.osd.mil

Kenichi Watanabe, Department of Clinical Pharmacology, Niigata University of Pharmacy and Applied Life Sciences, Kamisin- ei-cho, Niigata 950-2081, Japan; e-mail: watanabe@niigata-pharm.ac.jp

Caroline P.D. Wheeler-Jones, Infection, Inflammation and Vascular Biology Research Group, Department of Basic Sciences, The Royal Veterinary College, University of London, Royal College Street, London NW1 0TU, UK

Robert N. Willette, Department of Investigative and Cardiac Biology, Glaxo-SmithKline, 709 Swedeland, King of Prussia, PA 19406, USA;
e-mail: robert_n_willette@gsk.com

Joseph Winaver, Department of Physiology & Biophysics, Faculty of Medicine, Technion Medical School, P.O. Box 9649, Haifa 31096, Israel;
e-mail: winaver@techunix.technion.ac.il

Liz L.Yang, Heart and Stroke Richard Lewar Centre of Excellence, University of Toronto, Ontario, Canada; e-mail: liz.yang@utoronto.ca

Introduction

Inflammation – A new frontier in cardiac disease and therapeutics

Giora Z. Feuerstein, Peter Libby and Douglas L. Mann

Pharmacology Department, WP42-209, Merck Research Laboratories, 770 Sumneytown Pike, West Point, PA 19486, USA

Modern perspectives on inflammation

General considerations

Inflammation is now well recognized as a reaction that bears on diverse human diseases of non-pathogenic origin. The inflammatory reaction is fundamentally an interlinked array of host defense mechanism that features:

"… localized protective response elicited by injury or destruction of tissue, which serves to destroy, dilute, to wall off (sequester) both the injurious agent and the injured tissue." [1, 2].

Histologically, the inflammatory reaction involves specialized cells and mediators (pre-formed and synthesized *de novo*) that interact with the microcirculation and tissue elements in a process that leads to one of three outcomes:

1. Complete resolution of the injury to full resumption of tissue structure and function;
2. Partial resolution with residual structural and functional damage after complete cessation of the inflammatory reaction;
3. Chronic, inflammation marked by ongoing tissue damage and remodeling of the inflammatory process.

This perspective points to the hallmark of the "Janus Face" of the inflammatory reaction – that is, the capacity of the inflammatory system to heal as well as produce damage. Furthermore, the relationships between these two dimensions of inflammation – healing and destruction – are complex. The two processes may appear to be sequential as well as co-existent. Cellular elements that can release injurious mediators may also elaborate mediators that have salutary capacity. Finally, temporal, contextual, and quantitative aspects of the mediators involved may culminate in diverse effects that are not predictable from an anticipated action of a mediator in isolation.

Examples that support these principles have been reported in many disease processes. Mediators of cytotoxic reputation such as tumor necrosis factor alpha (TNFα) may function in entirely opposite manners in different context. For example, in acute brain ischemia (stroke) an inflammatory reaction evolves in and around the ischemic zone with *de novo* synthesis and release of TNF and other cytokines [3]. TNF antagonists administered acutely at the time of the ischemic insult reduce histological damage and improve recovery, suggesting a detrimental role of this cytokine in acute stroke [4]. However, TNF administration to normal brain tissue renders the brain tolerant to ischemic insult, suggesting a role for this cytokine as a neuronal survival factor [3]. Bacterial endotoxins, such as lipopolysaccharides (LPS) have similar properties. When administered acutely, LPS is a pro-inflammatory agent par excellence. In contrast, low levels of exposure to LPS over time induce a state of resistance in animals to withstand lethal endotoxemia. Thus, low levels of activation of inflammatory cells can lead to desensitization, which in turn can prevent and/or attenuate robust inflammatory reactions, and thereby avoid severe systemic consequences and/or death.

Studies on traumatic injury to optic nerves that result in retinal degeneration highlight the therapeutic potential of inflammatory cells. In such models, benefit from application of activated macrophages onto the injury site is just contrary to expectations [5]. Data of this kind point to the capacity of activated macrophages to confer regenerative potential upon injured cells. In this vein, in models of spinal cord injury induced by mechanical trauma, treatment with myelin basic protein activated T-cells (which in normal CNS tissue are believed to induce the pathology of multiple sclerosis) result in therapeutic effects with improved functions and tissue integrity [6]. These examples clearly demonstrate the complexity of the cell biology of inflammation and its pathophysiology which harness survival as well as death factors in a contextual manner.

An important perspective on the role of inflammation in non-pathogenic diseases as associated to "response to injury" is our recognition that sentinel cells, within each and every tissue, can elicit and participate in the inflammatory reaction along with the traditional circulating leukocytes and lymphoid organs. Such cells include mast cells (of which the heart is in particularly rich in), fibroblasts, cardiac myocytes and all endothelial cells. The endothelium in particular occupies a strategic position to initiate and propagate the inflammatory reactions by regulation of inflammatory cell migration, activation and thrombosis. Endothelium is now well known for its ability to change from an anti-inflammatory, anti-adhesive and anti-coagulant cell into a phenotype that promotes leukocyte migration (by expression of adhesion molecules), secreting chemotactic factors (chemokines and lipid mediators) and promoting blood coagulation and limiting fibrinolysis [7]. Thus, in any consideration of the role of inflammation in disease, including the heart, the role of the endothelium will figure prominently.

In any inflammatory process, regardless of the organ, the site of injury plays an active role in regulation of the external inflammatory process. It is likely that fundamental stop signals as well as amplification signals are produced in varying capacities during the inflammatory process, and that certain tissue-specific factors, such as the predominant cellular composition of the organ, the matrix and mediators released by the specialized cells in each organ, govern the inflammatory reaction at large. These particular considerations require elucidation for each tissue and organ. For example, large amounts of the ligand to the toll-like receptor 4 could influence cardiac function in a way that would prevail under normal tone of the this signaling pathway [8]; or neutrophils derived arachidonate products of the 5-lipoxygenase pathway, leukotriene B4 (a pro-inflammatory mediator) may not exert the expected action in tissues where cells are rich with 15-lipoxygenase, a product of which, lipoxins, inhibits neutrophil influx [9]. Obviously, understanding the tissue-specific pathways that might amplify or dampen inflammatory reaction is important in formulating strategies for pharmacological interventions in inflammatory conditions of a particular organ.

Finally, the inflammatory system is tightly linked with the immune system at large. In fact, immune factors (e.g., complement) can initiate and propagate components of the inflammatory reaction as well as dominate its chronic state (e.g., granuloma). Thus, any discussions and considerations on the role of inflammation in diseases must include detailed understanding of the components of the system as well. Indeed, the pathway of innate immunity encompasses much of the inflammatory response.

In summary, inflammation is a fundamental reaction to all forms of injury and therefore, it comes as no surprise that many forms of cardiac diseases involve inflammatory cells and mediators. Considering the significance of the inflammatory/immune aspects of cardiac disease requires recognition that inflammation might play an important role in cardiac cells function, survival and death. Research on the role of inflammation in various cardiac disease conditions should distinguish those elements essential for repair and regeneration from those that are detrimental to such processes.

Inflammation and the heart

In this book we have attempted to present selected topics on the specific role of inflammation and immune reactions in heart diseases. Inflammation and immune factors affect the heart in two ways:

1. The role inflammation in atherosclerosis and other vascular diseases. Authoritative recent reviews have considered the role of inflammation in atherosclerosis [10–12];

2. Direct inflammatory and immune reactions in the heart.

The book focuses on immune and inflammatory processes that are more specifically and directly associated with cardiac pathological conditions such as: Ischemia; reperfusion injury; heart failure; cardiac remodeling. These elements of cardiac injury have been presented in various perspectives that address the continuum of the inflammatory reaction in all stages of cardiac pathology.

Acute cardiac injury such as myocardial infarction results in an inflammatory reaction, which is modified by reperfusion of the ischemic heart (either spontaneously or following pharmacological or instrumental intervention). As cardiac remodeling invariably evolves following cardiac tissue loss, so also does the inflammatory reaction to this tissue injury. Cells associated with repair and remodeling replace the inflammatory cells and inflammatory mediators that dominate the acute phase of the response to injury. Throughout the compensatory stages and further on to de-compensation and heart failure, both immune and inflammatory cells and mediators persistently influence the process and its final outcome. These aspects constitute the core of this book.

Naturally, due to space limitations, the book cannot claim to cover all subjects. Yet conceptual frameworks, mechanisms of actions and therapeutic possibilities considered in most chapters can be extrapolated to any other form of cardiac injury, including infective, arrhythmogenic, and mechanical malformation. In all consideration, one must always keep in mind the "Janus Face" of inflammation as a system aims to heal.

References

1 *Dorland's Illustrated Medical Dictionary*, 29th edition (2000) W.B. Saunders Co, Philadelphia, p. 897

2 *Stedman's Medical Dictionary*, 26th Edition (1995) Williams and Wilkins, Baltimore, Maryland, USA.

3 Feuerstein GZ (ed) (2001) *Inflammation and stroke*. Birkhäuser Verlag, Basel, Switzerland

4 Barone FC, Feuerstein GZ (1999) Inflammatory cells and mediators in stroke. *J Cerebral Blood Flow Metabolism* 19: 835–842

5 Rapalino O, Lazarove-Spiegler O, Agranov E, Velan GJ, Yoles E, Fraidkis M, Solomon A, Gepstein R, Katz A, Belkin M et al (1998) Implantation of stimulated macrophages results in partial recovery of paraplegic rats. *Nature Medicine* 4: 814–821

6 Moalem G, Leibowitz-Amit R, Yoles E, Mor F, Cohen IR, Schwartz M (1999) Autoimmune T-cells protect neurons from secondary degeneration cerebral nervous system axotomy. *Nature Medicine* 5: 49–63

7 Ruetzler CA, Hallenbeck JM (2001) Cyclic activation and inactivation of brain vessels

involving inflammatory mediators – implications for stroke. In: G Feuerstein (ed): *Inflammation and stroke*. Birkhäuser Verlag, Basel, 61–76

8   Nathan C (2003) Points of control in inflammation. *Nature* 420: 846

9   Levy BD, Clish CB, Schmidt B, Gronert K, Serhan CN (2001) Lipid mediators class switching during acute inflammation: Signals in resolution. *Nature Immunology* 12: 612–619

10   Ross R (1999) Atherosclerosis: An inflammatory disease. *N Engl J Med* 340: 115–126

11   Libby P (2003) Inflammation and atherosclerosis. *Nature* 420: 868–874

12   Libby P, Ross R (1996) Cytokines and growth regulatory molecules. In: V Fuster, R Ross, EJ Topol (eds): *Atherosclerosis and coronary artery disease*. Lippincott Raven Publishers, Philadelphia, 585–594

Pathological aspects and inflammation biomarkers in cardiac disease

A biomarker of inflammation in cardiovascular disease

Giora Z. Feuerstein[1], Ron Firestein[2], Douglas L. Mann[3] and Peter Libby[2]

[1]Pharmacology Department, WP42-209, Merck Research Laboratories, 770 Sumneytown Pike, West Point, PA 19486, USA; [2]Brigham and Women's Hospital, 221 Longwood Avenue, EBRC 307, Boston, MA 02115, USA; [3]Winters Center for Heart Failure Research, 6565 Fannin, MS 524, Houston, TX 77030, USA

Introduction

First discovered in 1929 by Oswald Avery, C-reactive protein (CRP) is produced and released primarily by the liver and normally circulates at very low levels [1]. However, levels of CRP increase markedly in response to trauma or disease and closely track the inflammatory burden of disease. Synthesis and release of CRP appears to be largely controlled by the cytokine IL-6. As the role of inflammation in cardiac disease gains greater acceptance, the significance of biomarkers of the inflammatory burden gains recognition as well. In the past, scientists studied the potential role of CRP as a biomarker in conjunction with clinical and other diagnostic measures to assess cardiovascular disease severity. More recent data point to a role for CRP as a prospective marker of cardiovascular risk. These data have now generated the intriguing hypothesis that CRP reductions may serve as a surrogate marker of therapeutic efficacy of interventions aimed to reduce cardiovascular morbidity and mortality. Indeed, the efficacy of cholesterol-lowering drugs such as statins in lowering cardiovascular events may depend in part on anti-inflammatory effects reflected by reduced CRP due to either direct or low density lipoprotein (LDL)-lowering effects of these drugs. Using robust correlation analyses of multiple inflammatory markers, CRP correlates excellently with heart diseases, exceeding other inflammatory markers such as IL-6 or adhesion molecules. Furthermore, CRP seems to predict risk for heart attacks and stroke in individuals with normal or low cholesterol levels as well as in apparently healthy women. This finding may help identify individuals not currently designated for preventive therapies indicated by existing guidelines. Thus, CRP may serve as an important adjunct to cholesterol, a mainstay of assessment of cardiovascular risk, and aid our rational deployment of preventive treatment for cardiovascular diseases.

Inflammation and Cardiac Diseases, edited by Giora Z. Feuerstein, Peter Libby and Douglas L. Mann
© 2003 Birkhäuser Verlag Basel/Switzerland

The biology of CRP

CRP belongs to the protein family termed pentraxins, pentamers of five non-cova-lently binding units arranged in a cyclic array [2]. Crystal structures of CRP and phosphorylcholine (PC), one of its ligands, reveal that each monomer binds two molecules Ca^{2+} to which the negatively charged PC binds. This arrangement explains the high avidity of ligands that contain tandem repeats of negative charges, including the pneumococcal capsular C polysaccharide from which the term CRP is derived. In humans during the acute phase response, blood concentrations of CRP rise markedly, while the related pentraxin, serum amyloid P (SAP), is a constitutive plasma protein (Fig. 1). The high concentration of PC exposed on injured human cell membranes can also mediate binding of CRP to injured but not normal cells. Thus, the ability of CRP to recognize injured cells provides a target on injured cells for other mediators, such as complement and macrophages bearing the Fc receptors. CRP also interacts with apoptotic cells possibly due to exposure of PC or nuclear antigens that are exposed during the apoptotic process. The precise role of CRP in apoptosis, or programmed cell death, is unclear. CRP also localizes to sites of acute inflammation and tissue damage by still undetermined mechanisms. CRP accumu-lates in the lesions of vasculitis, myocardial infarction, or experimental allergic encephalitis, although the specific ligands and mechanism of interactions are not well understood. In many cases, CRP localizes with neutrophils, but whether com-mon mechanisms recruit neutrophils and cause CRP accumulation is unclear.

CRP, the complement system, and leukocyte Fcγ receptors

In additions to the interactions of CRP with foreign macromolecules such as bacte-rial polysaccharides, recent data suggest that CRP also interacts with self antigens in the nucleus. Such evidence includes the presence of CRP in the nuclei of cells obtained from the synovium of rheumatoid arthritis patients. CRP binds to small nuclear ribonuclear protein (snRNP) particles that are uridine-rich RNA and pro-tein complexes associated with RNA splicing. A specific transport mechanism aided by the nuclear localization sequence (NLS) region present in CRP appears to facili-tate the entry of CRP into nuclei. In this manner CRP (and SAP) may help sequester nuclear materials in injured cells.

Complement binding is another important property of CRP [3]. CRP interacts directly with complement factor C1q, at a discrete binding site. The interaction between CRP and C1q leads to activation of the complement cascade *via* C3 and hence binding to complement receptors (C3a, C5a and the membrane attack com-plex) on phagocytes, facilitating phagocytosis without eliciting a strong inflamma-tory reaction. Thus, CRP-mediated phagocytosis may serve as a mechanism for

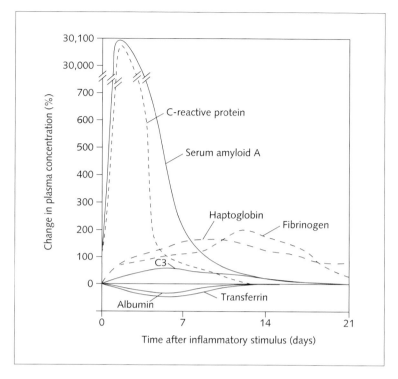

Figure 1
Time course of CRP and other pro-inflammatory proteins in the circulation. Printed with permission from the N Engl J Med *340: 448–454 (1999).*

removal of potentially harmful substances while it also preserves unharmed tissue from the damage associated with acute inflammation.

CRP may also facilitate phagocytosis by mechanisms other than complement activation. High-affinity FcγRI also binds CRP as does FcγRII [4]. Hence, macrophages from mice deficient in the Fcg receptor exhibit a defect in CRP-mediated phagocytosis.

The relevance of these biological functions to the "net pro or anti-inflammatory" properties of CRP remain unresolved. *In vitro* experiments suggest that because it stimulates the release of IL-1 and TNF-α from human monocytes, high concentrations of CRP exert a direct pro-inflammatory effect [5–7]. CRP increases the expression of adhesion molecules in endothelial cells as well as the expression of chemokines, thereby enhancing chemotaxis of inflammatory cells [8, 9]. Furthermore, CRP at high concentrations can enhance the pro-coagulant properties of monocytes by augmenting the expression of tissue factor and limiting the anti-fibrinolytic properties of endothelial cells by enhancing the expression of plasminogen activator inhibitor (PAI)-1 [10, 11]. Moreover, CRP may further compromise endogenous anti-inflammatory pathways in the vascular wall by attenuating NO release through suppression of eNOS expression [12, 13]. However, CRP also contributes to host defenses, e.g., by protecting mice injected with CRP from lethal bacterial challenge. The role of CRP in human infections is less clear as human CRP deficiency states are not known. Furthermore, CRP participates in adaptive immunity by mechanisms involved in antigen presentation. CRP may also play a role in autoimmunity, as evidenced by enhanced susceptibility of mice deficient in SAP (the mouse CRP counterpart) to lupus-like syndromes and the protective effect of CRP against chromatin-induced accelerated systemic lupus erythematosus (SLE) in mice.

CRP and human diseases

The association of elevated CRP levels in blood and tissues with inflammation in humans has been recognized since the 1930s. In diseases such as rheumatoid arthritis, deposits of CRP in synovial cell nuclei correlate with the degree of complement activation in the synovial fluid. These data suggest that CRP may aid clearance of damaged cells by enhancing C3 activation by and phagocytosis of the injured or dead cells. However, as CRP also binds to and activates the FcgRI/II receptors, a pro-inflammatory action cannot be ruled out. Additionally, CRP levels prospectively correlate with a number of important manifestations of atherosclerotic cardiovascular disease (for review see [14–16]). These studies showed that levels of CRP within the "normal" range predict increased risk of future coronary and other important cardiovascular events. We will elaborate these aspects of CRP in the following paragraphs.

Clinical aspects of CRP as an inflammatory biomarker in heart diseases

Multiple data sets have established the role for CRP as a biomarker risk factor for heart disease [17]. Elevated levels of plasma CRP predict subsequent cardiovascular events in healthy men [18, 19] and women [20] and patients with unstable angina [21–23] or history of myocardial infarction [24]. In addition, CRP identifies patients with increased risk of coronary artery disease and graft failure [25]. This latter study carries additional significance since graft atherosclerosis affects both the smaller intramural arteries of transplanted hearts in addition to the larger epicardial arteries typically involved in usual atherosclerosis [26, 27]. Indeed, raised levels of CRP correlate with arterial intercellular adhesion molecule (ICAM)-1 expression in endomyocardial biopsy specimens of transplanted hearts. In addition, CRP correlates with soluble ICAM-1 concentrations soon after transplantation and an early increase of CRP correlates (significantly) with the development, severity, and enhanced progression of coronary artery disease, heightened ischemic events, and graft failure [25]. Since CRP may at high concentrations directly induce ICAM-1 (and other cell adhesion molecules, CAMs [7]), CRP may serve as a mediator as well as a marker in inflammation associated with cardiovascular diseases (Fig. 2). However, soluble forms of adhesion molecules predict future coronary heart disease events less robustly than CRP in apparently well populations [28, 29]. A recent analysis of plasma samples obtained from patients with established coronary heart disease measured several soluble forms of adhesion molecules including ICAM-1, vascular cell adhesion molecule (VCAM)-1, E-selectin, and P-selectin. Following adjustments for age and classical risk factors, risk associated with all these markers carried little predictive significance [30, 31]. However, the marginal prognostic value reported by Malik et al. [28] should not diminish interest in the pathophysiological role of CAMs in atherosclerotic coronary artery disease. This position is justified since the mechanism of release of soluble CAMs into the circulation from the vascular inflammatory cells is not clear and may not represent the extent to which CAMs contribute to the vascular milieu [31]. Thus, poor correlation of systemic soluble CAMs with coronary heart disease (CHD) risk may not genuinely represent their role in coronary inflammation and coronary event risk. Moreover, even though the British Regional Heart Study, the source of samples used in Malik's analyses [30], provided a large sample size, technical issues concerning sample accrual, preservation, and processing may diminish the overall sensitivity of the results. In any case, caution is necessary when extrapolating the results from studies of CAMs as biomarkers to other candidates, for example cytokines. Yamashita et al. assayed the plasma levels of IL-6, IL-10, IL-12, IL-18, IFN-γ, and high-sensitivity CRP (hsCRP) [32] in patients with stable and unstable CHD. In this latter study, significantly higher concentrations of hsCRP and IL-6 in patients with unstable angina compared to those in the control or stable angina groups were found. Additionally, hsCRP levels significantly and positively correlated with IL-6 and IL-12 in those patients. Interestingly, hsCRP and the latter cytokines correlated negatively with IL-10, a T-helper-2 anti-inflammatory cytokine. Thus, other markers beyond inflammatory CRP may correlate with risk for developing exacerbations of CHD.

CRP and cardiovascular risk modifying interventions

Physical activity

In addition to serving as a marker for heart disease CRP interventions proven to reduce risk for heart (and cardiovascular) events may modify its levels. For example, physical activity, a non-pharmacologic intervention, influences the occurrence

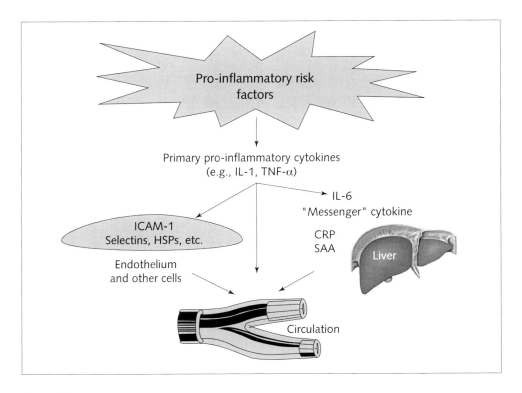

Figure 2

Inflammatory pathways in atherogenesis. The inflammatory cascade during atherogenesis begins with pro-inflammatory risk factors. Modified low density lipoprotein is but one such putative pro-inflammatory trigger. Others include advanced glycation endproducts (AGE) that accumulate during sustained hyperglycemia or with age, infectious agents and their products, cytokines produced in response to other stimuli, and mediators such as angiotensin II now known to possess pro-inflammatory properties. These primary triggers to inflammation beget a first wave of pro-inflammatory cytokines such as IL-1 or TNF. These primary pro-inflammatory cytokines will in turn stimulate the production of the messenger cytokine IL-6, providing an amplification loop for the inflammatory stimulus. IL-6 changes the program of protein synthesis by the hepatocyte. Instead of "housekeeping" proteins such as albumin, the hepatocyte exposed to IL-6 increases transcription of a series of proteins known as the acute phase reactants (see Fig. 1). Chief among these is the pentraxin C-reactive protein (CRP). The acute phase reactants can be sampled in peripheral blood. Because it has a long half-life and varies little during the day or from day to day in a healthy individual, CRP serves as a useful gauge of the inflammatory status of individuals, even those that are apparently well. As shown on the left side of the diagram, the primary pro-inflammatory cytokines can also elicit the expression on endothelial and other cells of adhesion molecules for leukocytes. These adhesion molecules can be shed from the surface of cells and sampled in periph-

of heart disease [33, 34]. In a subset of patients from the ATTICA study, a Health and Nutrition study conducted on apparently healthy people, the physical activity correlated with inflammation as monitored by several biomarkers. Physical activity was assessed by questionnaire and compared to plasma levels of hsCRP, fibrinogen amyloid A, and white blood cell (WBC) count. The study showed that leisure physical activity associated with markedly lower levels of hsCRP (and modestly reduced WBC counts) compared to sedentary life style [35]. This study corroborates several studies conducted in diverse populations [36–38]. However, such observational studies may be confounded by clustering of other health-promoting practices in addition to physical activity.

Weight loss and CRP

Weight loss also modifies disease. In a study conducted by Heilbronn et al., weight reduction in women was associated with 26% reduction of hsCRP [39], and a study by Tschernof et al. associated weight loss in women with 32% reduction in hsCRP [40]. The association of CRP with weight loss in men remains undetermined.

Aspirin (ASA) and CRP

In the Physicians' Health Study, ASA (325 mg/day) resulted in 44% reduction in risk for myocardial infarction; the greatest benefits occurred in patients with hsCRP levels in the highest quartile as compared to the lower quartile [18]. However, studies that examined the effect of ASA on CRP levels more directly yielded conflicting results [41, 42], possibly due to variation in dosing and duration of study. It is clear that more studies of high dose ASA are needed, especially in patients at high risk for cardiac events.

Statins and CRP

In the Cholesterol And Recurrent Events (CARE) trial, which tested the effect of pravastatin in CAD patients with total cholesterol above 240 mg/dl, the greatest

Figure 2 - continued
eral blood, providing yet another indirect window on the inflammatory status of the individual. Thus by sampling peripheral blood one can gain information about the proximal pro-inflammatory stimuli that initiate and perpetuate the atherogenic process. After Libby & Ridker, Circulation *100: 1148–1150 (1999).*

benefits were achieved in the group with the highest hsCRP levels [43]. The Air Force /Coronary Atherosclerosis Prevention Study (AFCAPS/TeXCAPS), a primary prevention trial with lovastatin in patients with normal lipid levels, showed that the rate of coronary events increased significantly with increased baseline CRP, and that lovastatin decreased CRP levels along with reduction of coronary events [44]. Retrospective analysis of AFCAPS/TeXCAPS yielded the remarkable observation that the statin conveyed no benefits for patients with CRP and cholesterol levels both below the median levels. More recently, a prospective, randomized, double-blind, cross-over study of several statins (atorvastatin, simvastatin, pravastatin) showed that relatively short (6 week) therapy significantly reduced hsCRP, with no substantial differences among the statins [45, 46]. Interestingly, the lack of correlation between the reduction in hsCRP levels and cholesterol suggested dissociation between these two biochemical variables. It is also noteworthy that the relationships between the cholesterol-lowering effects of statins and CRP levels encompass all forms of dyslipidemias (primary and combined dyslipidemias), as shown in studies with simvastatin ([47], combined dyslipidemias) and cerivastatin ([48], primary dyslipidemias) where CRP was significantly reduced along with LDL cholesterol. However, no clear dose-response relationships were noted in these studies which might be in part due to the small cohorts and treatment time.

Additionally, lipid-lowering interventions other than statin administration can reduce CRP levels. The recent American College of Cardiology conference (Chicago, March 2003, communicated by Michael Davidson) reported that ezetimibe, a cholesterol-lowering agent believed to act by reducing cholesterol absorption in the gut, augmented the reduction in CRP levels due to simvastatin treatment, but did not itself lower CRP levels. Future studies may determine whether the effect of statins (and possibly other lipid-lowering agents) reduces CRP levels by direct anti-inflammatory actions, improved endothelium function [49] and/or by LDL-lowering *per se*.

Anti-oxidants and CRP

Endpoint studies have cast doubt on the role of anti-oxidant vitamins in the prevention of cardiac events in higher risk individuals. In normal and diabetic patients, high doses of α-tocopherol > 800 IU/day) reduced CRP levels [50, 51].

Summary

CRP, a marker of inflammation, can aid prediction of risk for coronary heart disease. In 2003, a joint scientific statement by the American Heart Association and the

Center for Disease Control recognized hsCRP as a potentially valuable adjunct to established risk factors for assessment of coronary artery disease in patients at moderate/high risk (10–20% 10-year risk of a coronary heart disease event). The accumulating data on potential roles of CRP beyond prospective risk assessment raises a number of key questions for future investigation:

1. To what extent does CRP mediate as well as mark cardiovascular risk?
2. Could lowering of CRP serve as a target of therapy?
3. Can hsCRP levels guide therapy in individuals without traditional risk markers?
4. Could hsCRP screening aid the identification of individuals meriting intervention in populations gauged at low risk by traditional algorithms?

Until substantiated by clinical trial evidence, we do not advocate the clinical application of these new potential uses of this interesting biomarker.

References

1   Du Clos TW (2002) C-reactive protein and the immune response. *Science and Medicine* May/June, 106–117

2   Volanakis JE (2001) Human C-reactive protein: expression, structure and function. *Mol Immunol* 38: 189–197

3   Agrawal A, Shrive AK, Greenhough TJ, Volanakis JE (2001) Topology and structure of the C1q-binding site on C-reactive protein. *J Immunol* 166: 3998–4004

4   Bharadwaj D, Stein M-P, Volzer M et al (1999) The major receptor for C-reactive protein on leukocytes is the Fcg receptor II. *J Exp Med* 190: 585–590

5   Torzewski M, Rist C, Mortensen RF et al (2000) C-reactive protein in the arterial intima. role of C-reactive protein receptor-dependent monocyte recruitment in atherosclerosis. *Arterioscler Thromb Vasc Biol* 20: 2094–2099

6   Ballou CP, Lozanski G (1992) Induction of inflammatory cytokines release from cultured human monocytes by C-reactive protein. *Cytokine* 4: 361–368

7   Pasceri V, Willerson JT, Yeh ETH (2000) Direct pro-inflammatory effects of C-reactive protein on human endothelial cells. *Circulation* 102: 2165–2168

8   Pasceri V, Cheng JS, Willerson JT et al (2001) Modulation of C-reactive protein mediated monocyte chemoattractant protein-1 induction in human endothelial cells by anti-atherosclerotic drugs. *Circulation* 103: 2531–2534

9   Verma S, Li SH, Badiwala MV et al (2002) Endothelin antagonism and interleukin-6 inhibition attenuate the pro-atherogenic effects of c-reactive protein. *Circulation* 105: 1890–1896

10 Cermak J, Key NS, Bach RR et al (1993) C-reactive protein induces human peripheral monocytes to synthesize tissue factor. *Blood* 82: 513–520

11 Devaraj S, Xu DY, Jialal I (2003) C-Reactive protein increases plasminogen activator

inhibitor-1 expression and activity in human aortic endothelial cells. *Circulation* 107: 398–411

12 Verma S, Wang CH, Li SH et al (2002) A self-fulfilling prophecy: C-reactive protein attenuates nitric oxide production and inhibits angiogenesis. *Circulation* 106: 913–919

13 Venugopal SK, Devaraj S, Yuhanna I et al. (2002) Demonstration that C-reactive protein decreases eNOS expression and bioactivity in human aortic endothelial cells. *Circulation* 106: 1439–1441

14 Taubes G (2002) Does inflammation cut to the heart of the matter? *Science* 296: 242–245

15 Rossi E (2002) C-reactive protein and progressive atherosclerosis. *Lancet* 360: 1436–1437

16 Libby P, Ridker PM, Maseri A (2002) Inflammation and atherosclerosis. *Circulation* 105: 1135–1143

17 Shah PK (2000) Circulating biomarkers of inflammation for vascular risk prediction: are they ready for prime time. *Circulation* 101: 1758–1759

18 Ridker PM, Cushman M, Stampfer MJ, Tracy RP, Hennekens CH (1997) Inflammation, aspirin and the risk of cardiovascular diseases in apparently healthy men. *N Eng J Med* 336: 973–970

19 Koenig W, Sund M, Frohlich M et al (1999) C-reactive protein a sensitive marker of inflammation, predicts future risk of coronary heart disease in initially healthy middle aged men: results from the MONICA Augsburg Cohort study. *Circulation* 99: 237–242

20 Ridker PM, Buring JE, Shih J, Matias M, Hennekens CH (1998) Prospective study of C-reactive protein and the risk for future cardiovascular events among apparently healthy women. *Circulation* 98: 731–733

21 Haverkate F, Thompson SG, Pyke SD, Gallimore JR, Pepys MB (1997) Production of C-reactive protein and risk of coronary events in stable and unstable angina: European concerted action on thrombosis and disabilities angina pectoris study group. *Lancet* 349: 462–466

22 Rebuzzi AG, Quaranta G, Liuzzo G et al (1998) Incremental prognostic value of serum levels of troponin T and C-reactive protein on admission in patients with unstable angina pectoris. *Am J Cardiol* 82: 715–719

23 Biassucci LM, Liuzzo G, Grillo RL et al (1999) Elevated levels of C-reactive protein at discharge in patients with unstable angina predict recurrent instability. *Circulation* 99: 855–860

24 Ridker PM, Rifai N, Pfeffer MA, Sacks F, Braunwald E (1998) Inflammation, pravastatin and the risk of coronary events after myocardial infarction in patients with average cholesterol levels: Cholesterol and Recurrent Events (CARE) Investigation. *Circulation* 98: 839–844

25 Labarrere CA, Lee JB, Nelson DR, Al-Hassani M, Miller SJ, Pitts DE (2002) C-reactive protein, arterial endothelial activation and development of transplant coronary artery disease: a prospective study. *Lancet* 360: 1462–1467

26 Labarrere CA, Nelson DR, Faulk WP (1998) Endothelial activation and development of coronary artery disease risk factors and course. *JAMA* 278: 1169–1175

27 Labarrere CA, Nelson DR, Miller SJ et al. (2000) Value of serum soluble intercellular adhesion molecule-1 for the non-invasive risk assessment of transplant coronary artery disease, post-transplant coronary events and cardiac graft failure. *Circulation* 102: 1549–1555

28 Malik I, Danesh J, Whincup P, Bhatia V, Papacosta O, Walker M, Lennon L, Thomson A (2001) Soluble adhesion molecule and prediction of coronary heart disease: a prospective study and meta-analysis. *Lancet* 358: 971–975

29 Ridker PM, Hennekens CH, Roitman-Johnson B, Stampfer MJ, Allen J (1998) Plasma concentration of soluble intercellular adhesion molecule 1 and risks of future myocardial infarction in apparently healthy men. *Lancet* 351: 88–92

30 Ridker PM (1998) Intercellular adhesion molecule 1 and the risks of developing atherosclerotic disease. *Eur Heart J* 19: 1119–1121

31 Ridker PM (2001) Role of inflammatory biomarkers in prediction of coronary heart disease. *Lancet* 358: 946–947

32 Yamashita H, Shimada K, Seki E, Mokuno H, Daida H (2003) Concentrations of interleukins, interferon and C-reactive protein in stable and unstable angina pectoris. *Am J Cardiol* 91: 133–136

33 Sesso H, Paffenbarger R, Lee IM et al (2000) Physical activity and coronary heart disease in men. The Harvard Alumni Health Study. *Circulation* 102: 975–980

34 US Department of Health and Human Services (1996) Physical activity and health. A Report of the Surgeon General. Atlanta, GA. USDHHS, CDC and prevention, NCCDP and Health Promotion 35

35 Pitsavos C, Chrysohoou C, Panagiotakos DB, Skoumas J, Zeimbekis A, Kokkinos P, Stefanadis C, Toutouzas PK (2003) Association of leisure-time physical activity on inflammation markers (C-reactive protein, white cell blood count, serum amyloid A, and fibrinogen) in healthy subjects (from the ATTICA study). *Am J Cardiol* 91: 368–370

36 Abramson JL, Vaccarino V (2002) Relationships between physical activity and inflammation among apparently healthy middle-aged and older US adults. *Arch Intern Med* 162: 1286–1292

37 Ainsworth BE (2002) Cardiorespiratory fitness and C-reactive protein among a triethnic sample of women. *Circulation* 106: 403–406

38 Geffken D, Cushman M, Burke G, Polak J, Sakkinen P, Tracy R (2001) Association between physical activity and markers of inflammation in a healthy elderly population. *Am J Epidemiol* 153: 242–250

39 Heilbronn LK, Noakes M, Clifton PM (2001) Energy restriction and weight loss on very-low fat diets reduce C-reactive protein concentrations in obese healthy women. *Arterioscler Thromb Vasc Biol* 21: 968–970

40 Tchernof A, Nolan A, Sites CK, Ades PA, Poehlman ET (2002) Weight loss reduces C-reactive protein levels in obese postmenopausal women. *Circulation* 105: 564–569

41 Feng D, Tracy RP, Lipinska I, Murillo J, McKenna C, Tofler GH (2000) Effect of short-term aspirin use on C-reactive protein. *J Thrombosis Thrombolysis* 9: 37–41

42 Feldman M, Jialal I, Devaraj S, Cryer B (2001) Effect of low dose aspirin on serum C-reactive protein and thromboxane B2 concentrations: a placebo controlled study using a high sensitive C-reactive protein assay. *J Am Coll Cardiol* 37: 2036–2041

43 Ridker PM, Rifai N, Pfeffer MA, Sacks F, Braunwald E (1999) Long term effect of pravastatin on plasma concentration of C-reactive protein. *Circulation* 100: 230–235

44 Ridker PM, Rifai N, Clearfield M, Downs JR, Weis SE, Miles JS, Gotto AM Jr (2001) Measurement of C-reactive protein for the targeting of statin therapy in primary prevention of acute coronary events. *N Engl J Med* 344: 1959–1965

45 Jialal I, Stein D, Balis D, Grundy SM, Adams-Huet B, Devaraj S (2001) Effect of hydroxy-methyl glutaryl coenzyme A reductase inhibitor therapy on high sensitive C-reactive protein levels. *Circulation* 103: 1933–1935

46 Reisen WF, Engler H, Risch M, Korte W, Noseda G (2002) Short term effect of atorvastatin on C-reactive protein. *Eur Heart J* 23: 794–799

47 Miller M, Jialal I (2002) Effect of simvastatin (40 and 80 mg) on highly sensitive C-reactive protein in patients with combined hyperlipidemia. *Am J Cardiol* 89: 468–469

48 Ridker PM, Rifai N, Lowenthal S (2001) Rapid reduction in C-reactive protein with cerivastatin among 785 patients with primary hypercholesterolemia. *Circulation* 103: 1191–1193

49 Tan KCB, Chow WS, Tam SCF, Ai VHG, Lam KSL (2002) Atorvastatin lowers C-reactive protein and improves endothelium-dependent vasodilation in type 2 diabetes mellitus. *J Clin Endocrinol Metab* 87: 563–568

50 Upritchard JE, Sutherland WH, Mann JI (2000) Effect of supplementation with tomato juice, vitamin E, and vitamin C on low density lipoprotein oxidation and products of inflammatory activity in type-two diabetes. *Diabetes Care* 23: 733–738

51 Devaraj S, Jialal I (2000) Alpha tocopherol supplementation decreases C-reactive protein and monocyte interleukin-6 levels in type two diabetes patients. *Free Radic Biol Med* 29: 790–792

Inflammation and coronary artery disease

Renu Virmani[1], Frank D. Kolodgie[1], Allen P. Burke[1], Andrew Farb[1], Herman K. Gold[2] and Aloke V. Finn[2]

[1]Department of Cardiovascular Pathology, Armed Forces Institute of Pathology, 6825, 16th Street NW, Washington, DC 20306-6000, USA; [2]Massachusetts General Hospital, 55 Fruit Street, Boston, MA 02114, USA

Introduction

The complications of atherosclerosis are associated with a high incidence of morbidity and mortality in Western societies [1]. Coronary atherosclerosis is now considered a complex inflammatory process in response to the retention of specific atherogenic lipoproteins in the arterial wall. In addition to the localized immune response, there is emerging evidence that systemic inflammatory markers may have a diagnostic value in predicting acute cardiac events. Among the many risk factors for atherosclerosis, hyperlipidemia is thought the most influential on inflammatory processes along with specific immunological factors. Recent animal studies suggest that the induction of atherosclerosis is closely linked to lipoprotein abnormalities since genetic derangements of systemic or localized immunity alone do not initiate the disease. Although genetically engineered animals have furthered the understanding of the role of inflammation in atherosclerosis, the relevance of these findings to disease progression in humans are not as clear. This chapter will discuss the role of inflammation in the evolution of varying coronary lesions, particularly those associated with acute coronary syndromes. In addition, potential systemic factors that may influence inflammation in the vessel wall in relation to plaque instability will also be addressed.

Lesions types identified in coronary arteries of patients with sudden coronary death

Intimal mass lesions

While some atherosclerotic lesions may begin as intimal xanthomas (fatty streaks), there is substantial evidence that most adult human lesions originate from pre-existing intimal masses composed predominantly of SMCs and proteoglycans [2]. Because these lesions in children occur in similar locations as obstructive lesions in adults, intimal masses are thought to be a precursor of the majority of obstructive lesions. Unlike intimal xanthomas, there is little evidence that the intimal mass lesion may regress, and atherosclerotic lesions in the hyperlipidemic swine model arise almost exclusively from the intimal mass lesion [3]. There is very little known about the initiation of the intimal mass lesion, other than that the process is clonal [3, 4]. The stimulus for the monoclonal proliferation of SMCs is likely related to endothelial injury and accumulation of lipid within the intima [5]. The nature of endothelial injury is most likely multifactorial, although contradictory to early studies it does not involve simple desquamation but for the most part, the endothelium becomes dysfunctional. Significant numbers of inflammatory cells associated with pre-existing intimal cell masses are uncommon and the relationship between the development and progression of this lesion and inflammation is unclear.

Intimal xanthomas

Until recently, it was believed that the intimal xanthoma is the precursor lesion to the more advanced fibroatheroma. The lesion consists of lipid accumulation both in the interstitial spaces and within SMCs along with infiltration by inflammatory macrophages (Fig. 1).

Although this lesion is common in young individuals dying of non-cardiac causes and in all populations, there is no conclusive evidence that this plaque represents a progressive lesion [6]. These lesions fail to show significant SMC proliferation, calcification, accumulation of lipid pools, or necrotic core formation and although T-cells are also present, they are not as prominent as macrophages. Intimal xanthomas are known to develop focally at "lesion prone" sites where more advanced plaques appear. For example, the first 2 cm of the right coronary artery is where fibroatheromas form. It is this area of high-lesion susceptibility where fatty streaks commonly extend into the proximal one-half to two-thirds of the vessel. However, there are vascular sites where fatty streak lesions will eventually disappear with advancing age, which are referred to as areas of "lesion-resistance". In humans, sites of lesion regression are common in the thoracic aorta [7, 8].

Leukocyte attachment to flow surfaces

The binding and recruitment of circulating leukocytes to luminal surface endothelium is considered a fundamental step in the developing atherosclerotic lesion. Endothelial cells are typically resistant to leukocyte adherence but in conditions of hyperlipidemia as simulated in animal models and underlying many forms of human atherosclerosis, the focal attachment of circulating monocytes and lymphocytes to endothelial cells is preceded by the expression of specific adhesion molecules. Sev-

x20   x100

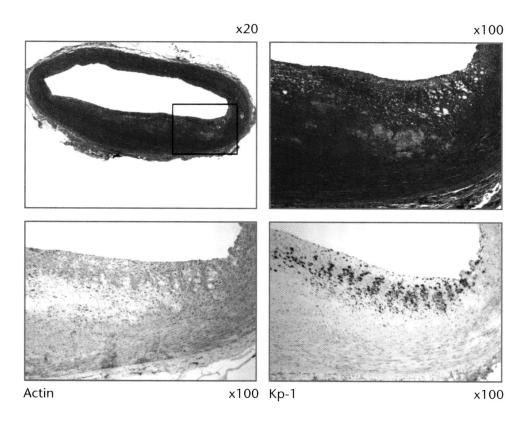

Actin   x100   Kp-1   x100

Figure 1

Intimal xanthoma. A and B are low and high power photomicrographs from the coronary artery of an asymptomatic patient showing an intimal xanthoma. B – Note presence of vacuolated cells close to the lumen and a small acellular area of lipid pool close to the media. C and D identify α-actin and CD68 positive SMCs and macrophages, respectively. There is a generalized absence of α-actin staining in macrophage-rich areas positive for the CD68 antibody.

eral protein families have a distinct functional role and provide the signals for leukocyte attachment and migration to the endothelium. These proteins include selectins, chemokines, monocyte chemo-attractant protein (MCP-1), interleukin-8 (IL-8), and intercellular adhesion molecule-1 (ICAM-1) and vascular adhesion molecule-1 (VCAM-1) which recognize specific integrins on the surface of circulating leukocytes [9]. The selectins (E and P) mediate the initial tethering of the circulating leukocytes over the endothelium to the point where the cells roll and slow their speed. P-selectin deficient mice show an absence of leukocyte rolling and are known to develop smaller atherosclerotic lesions compared with their wild type littermates

[10, 11]. The final attachment of leukocytes requires the interaction of integrin ligands on leukocyte surfaces with the immunoglobulin super-family members ICAM-1, ICAM-2 and VCAM-1, expressed on the endothelial cells [12–14].

Unlike other forms of vascular diseases, monocyte recruitment into the intima is specific to atherosclerosis and therefore the focal accumulation of monocytes reflects the expression of selective molecules in the endothelium referred to as endothelium-leukocyte adhesion molecules, or athero-ELAMs. The first of these proteins identified in the hypercholesterolemic rabbit model is VCAM-1. The expression of VCAM-1 on endothelial cells recognizes the heterodimeric integrin, very-late-antigen 4 (VLA-4) with leukocyte exclusivity on monocytes and lymphocytes and not neutrophils [15]. Other possible ligand interactions involved in monocyte recruitment are between the constitutively expressed endothelial molecule ICAM-1 and the integrin ligands LFA-1 and CD11b/CD18 (MAC-1) [16]. Both endothelial cells and macrophages produce ICAM-1 in response to inflammatory cytokines such as IL-1, TNF-α, and interferon-γ (IFN-γ). Further, different adhesion molecules are expressed in response to other inducible endothelial gene products such as MCP-1, IL-6 and IL-8 following exposure to bacterial endotoxins and specific cytokines such as IL-1 and tumor necrosis factor α (TNF-α). Thus, activation of one or more transcription factors including the early-response genes (*c-jun*, *c-fos*) and nuclear factor κB promotes the co-ordinated activation of several gene products. In particular, the NF-κB system has been causally linked to adhesion molecule expression [17].

NF-κB activation and atherosclerosis

The synthesis of adhesion molecules and pro-inflammatory cytokines is mediated in large part by the nuclear transcription factor, NF-κB. This factor is activated by diverse stimuli, such as cytokines, viruses, mitogens, pathogenic micro-organisms, modified LDL, and oxidative stress [18]. Activated NF-κB has been detected in macrophages, endothelial cells, and SMCs of atherosclerotic plaques [19, 20]. Recent evidence suggests that activation of NF-κB may be inhibited by statins [21] or low dose aspirin [22] NF-κB exists as an inactive heterodimeric complex in the cytosol bound to several protein inhibitors denoted as I-κB [23]. The heterodimer consists of p50/p65subunits and upon cell activation, I-κB becomes phosphorylated and is enzymatically degraded. The liberated p50/65 dimers then relocate to the nucleus and activate the transcription of target genes that induce the expression of cytokines (TNF-α), interleukins (IL-1, IL-2, IL-6 and IL-8), growth factors (MCSF, GM-CSF, G-CSF), chemo-attractant substances (MCP-1), adhesion molecules (ICAM-1, VCAM-1, E-selectin), and enzymes (MMP, iNOS, COX-2), that enable the local inflammatory response within the atherosclerotic plaque [24]. Finally, NF-κB target genes such as the inhibitor of apoptosis proteins (IAPs) have been shown to be critical signals, which promote cell survival [25].

Macrophage infiltration of the arterial wall

Once monocytes infiltrate the vascular wall, they transform into lipid-laden foam cells, which is a characteristic of early atherosclerosis. Two growth factors that enhance monocyte migration and lesion progression include monocyte chemotactic protein-1 (MCP-1) and macrophage colony-stimulating factor (M-CSF). These factors are known to induce the proliferation and differentiation of monocytes. Both IL-1α and TNF-α promote mRNA expression of MCP-1 and MCS-F in endothelial and SMCs in a concentration-dependent manner [26]. Evidence for the role of growth factors in early lesion formation comes from the finding of reduced fatty streaks development following blockade of MCS-F function by specific antibodies or genetic deletion studies in apo-E or LDL MCS-F-receptor deficient mice [27–29].

Pathologic intimal thickening: A precursor lesion to the fibroatheroma

The plaque most commonly observed in individuals with symptomatic coronary disease is pathologic intimal thickening, which others and we believe is the major precursor lesion to the fibroatheroma [6]. This plaque is characterized by the presence of extracellular lipid pools, which form between layers of SMCs at sites of adaptive intimal thickening (Fig. 2).

The lipid pools lie below the macrophage foam-cell layers and are located in a proteoglycan-rich matrix with collagen fibers. No established necrotic core, however, is identified in these lesions. There are large numbers of fine lipid droplets with or without peripheral laminated membranes and remnants of extracellular matrix components. The SMCs show lipid droplets in the cytoplasm along with free cholesterol, fatty acids, sphingomyelin, lysolecithin, and triglycerides.

The retention of lipoproteins by extracellular matrix molecules in the arterial intima sets the stage for the development of atherosclerotic cardiovascular disease. Atherogenic lipoproteins entering the sub-endothelial space are bound and retained through ionic interactions between the positively charged residues of apolipoproteins (apo) B and E, and negatively-charged sulfate and carboxylic acid residues on the glycosaminoglycan side chains of extracellular- or cell-associated proteoglycans. The glycosaminoglycans with the highest affinity for plasma LDL are thought to contain dermatan sulfate residues, which consist of biglycan and decorin [30]. In fact, glycosaminoglycan synthesis, in particular that of biglycan, and decorin have been shown to increase in response to oxidized lipoproteins in primate SMCs. Thus, Ox-LDL may influence lipoprotein retention by regulating glycosaminoglycan synthesis of vascular proteoglycans so as to enhance lipoprotein binding. The prolonged residual time of lipoproteins may lead to specific modifications, such as oxidation which can modulate many biological processes that promote atherogenesis some of which include the expression of monocyte adhesion molecules, chemotac-

x20   x100   Actin

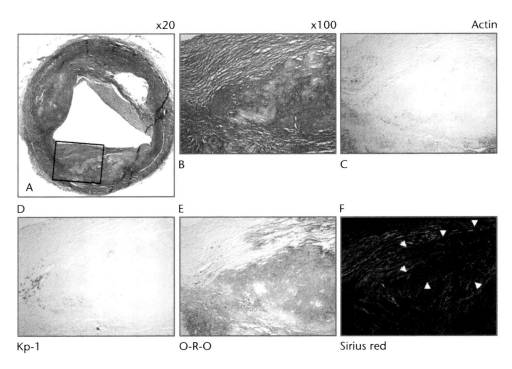

Kp-1   O-R-O   Sirius red

Figure 2
Pathological intimal thickening demonstrating lipid pools. A is Movat stained section show-
ing lipid pool represented by the black box. B–F are higher power views of the lipid pool
area stained with H&E (B), α-actin (C), CD68 (D), Oil Red O (E), and picrosirius red under
polarized light (F). Although the lipid pool shows few SMCs, it contains proteoglycan, and
collagen III matrix represent by the green birefringence. Most of the intima consists of Type
I collagen matrix (red birefringence). The area is also devoid of macrophages as demonstrat-
ed by CD68 staining (D) but shows finely dispersed lipid droplets, which stain positive with
O R O (E).

tic, and colony stimulation factors, which promote the adherence of circulating monocytes to vascular endothelial cells and deep intima [31].

The functional role of proteoglycans in the retention of atherogenic lipoproteins was recently exemplified in an elegant *in vivo* study by Skalen et al. [32]. Mice expressing proteoglycan-binding defective LDL developed significantly less atherosclerosis than mice expressing wild-type control LDL suggesting that sub-endothelial retention of apoB100-containing lipoprotein is an early step in atherogenesis, which precedes inflammatory processes. This concept of lipoprotein accumulation in the absence of inflammation was further characterized in lesions of diffuse intimal thickening (DIT) in human coronary arteries [33]. Immunohistochemical identification for apolipoprotein B 100 and 8-iso-prostaglandin $F_{2\alpha}$ (an oxidative product of LDL) showed substantial accumulation of oxidized LDL relative to normal LDL in the deep layers of DIT, which coincided with fibrillar collagen and elastin but rarely with sulfated proteoglycans. Interestingly, lipid accumulation was found only in sites with DIT of more than 200 μm and was independent of inflammatory or apoptotic processes. These data suggest that DIT rather than fatty streaks may represent a lesion in waiting, which under the appropriate conditions may rapidly become a symptomatic plaque. In another study of carotid endarterectomy specimens, Kockx et al., found lesions of pathologic intimal thickening characterized by collections of lipid pools in areas where there was a loss of SMCs. A large number of these cells however, did not stain using conventional markers of SMCs (α-actin) or macrophages (CD68), reflecting a loss of specific antigenicity perhaps associated with apoptotic cell death [34]. It is speculated however, that these cells truly represent SMCs as they are surrounded by a thickened basement membrane identified by periodic acid-Shiff (PAS) staining. By combining the terminal deoxynucleotidyl-transferase nick-end labeling (TUNEL) method, PAS stain, and immunohistochemistry for the pro-apoptotic molecule BAX, these cells were determined to be apoptotic SMCs. Transmission electron microscopy further confirmed membrane-bound vesicles of SMC origin within prominent basal lamina along with early calcification [34].

There is little known of how lesions progress from pathological intimal thickening to more advanced plaques. A recent study in C3-deficient mice, however, suggest that complement activation may play an important role [35]. Interestingly, mice deficient in C3 and low-density receptors showed increased foam cell formation, decreased SMCs, and collagen content relative to ldlr-null C3-competent control mice. Thus, suggesting that an intact complement system appears to be required in the maturation of atherosclerotic plaques beyond the foam cell stage.

Negative modulators of inflammation in atherosclerotic plaques

Transforming growth factor-β

Several lines of evidence suggest that transforming growth factor-β (TGF-β1), a well-known suppressor of growth and function in many human cell lines, is a potent inhibitor of human atherogenesis. In a study of human aorta, the expression of mRNA for TGF-β1 was found to be greater in areas prone to high-risk lesions development than those of lower risk [36]. Studies in apoE-deficient murine models provide strong evidence that eliminating TGF or disrupting its downstream signaling cascade leads to increased inflammation within plaques. Recently, Mallat et al. treated apoE-deficient mice with a neutralizing antibody against TGF-β1, β2, and β3 from weeks 6–15 [37]. These authors observed that atherosclerotic lesions con-

Table 1 - Mediators of pro- and anti-inflammatory signals in the vessel wall (modified from [138]

Mediators	Pro-inflammatory signals	Anti-inflammatory signals
Adhesion molecules	ICAM, VCAM, Selectins E and P	
Cytokines	TNF-α, IL-1, IL-8, IFN-γ, Oncostatin M, IL-4, IL-13, MCP-1	TGF-β, IL-10, IL-1ra, IL-13
Growth factors	PDGF, M-CSF	FGF-1, FGF-2
Vasoactive agents	Angiotensin II, endothelin	NO
Nuclear receptors		PPARs
Protective genes		Bcl-2, Bcl-x$_L$, A1, serpine proteinase, inhibitor 9, HO-1, Fas ligand
Mechanical forces	Stretch	Shear stress
Others	LDL, thrombin	HDL, n3-fatty acids

Abbreviations: ICAM, intracellular adhesion molecule; VCAM, vascular cell adhesion molecule; TNF, tumor necrosis factor; IL, interleukin; PDGF, platelet-derived growth factor; LDL, low-density lipoprotein; TGF, transforming growth factor; FGF, fibroblast growth factor; NO, nitric oxide; PPAR, peroxisome proliferator-activated receptors; HO, heme oxygenase; HDL, high-density lipoprotein; MCP-1, monocyte–chemo-attractant protein-1; M-CSF, macrophage colony stimulating factor

tained a high inflammatory cell content and a decreased amount of collagen. In a subsequent study by Lutgens et al., inhibition of the TGF-β pathway with a soluble recombinant TGF-β receptor II (TGFβrII:Fc) in apoE null mice treated over a prolonged period, resulted in increased inflammation, larger necrotic core formation, and decreased plaque fibrosis associated with intraplaque hemorrhages and iron and fibrin deposition [38]. Taken together, these murine studies suggest a pivotal role for TGF-β in the maintenance and balance between inflammation and fibrosis in atherosclerotic plaques. Clinical studies have shown decreased circulating plasma levels of TGF-β in unstable angina patients.

Interleukin-10

Interleukin-10 is considered a potent anti-inflammatory cytokine produced by Th2-type T-cells, B-cells, monocytes, and macrophages [39]. Various mechanisms have been proposed for the manner in which IL-10 inhibits the synthesis of pro-inflammatory cytokines. One of the most studied is the inhibition of the NF-κB by IL-10 in monocytes and T-cells by intervention of secondary oxygen-free radical messengers [40]. This results in a reduction in the synthesis of pro-inflammatory interleukins, adhesion molecules, growth factors, and chemo-attractants of immune cells that limit the local inflammatory response in the plaque. In addition, it has been shown that IL-10 is capable of inhibiting monocyte responses mediated by CD40-CD40L interactions, which appear to play a central role in the pathogenesis of atherosclerosis [41]. IL-10 has been identified in human plaques and is shown to co-localize mainly in macrophages and SMCs; high levels of IL-10 were associated with a significant decrease in local nitric oxide synthase, and cell death [42]. Further, serum levels of IL-10 are decreased in patients with unstable angina [43]. A protective effect of IL-10 against the development of diet-induced atherosclerosis has been shown in several murine models defective [44, 45] or overproducing [46] IL-10. These studies raise the possibility that IL-10 may have a therapeutic benefit in plaque stabilization.

Fibroatheromas (fibrous cap atheroma)

The fibrous cap atheroma, known as the AHA Type IV lesion, is the first of the advanced plaques of coronary atherosclerosis [47]. Virchow likened this lesion to a dermal cyst (a sebaceous cyst, "Grutzbalg"). Thus, the defining feature of the "atheroma" is the presence of a necrotic fatty mass contained by fibrous tissue (Fig. 3).

This characteristic is remarkably analogous to the capsule surrounding an abscess, and like an abscess, an atherosclerotic plaque can rupture. How inflammation effects the development of a fibroatheroma is complicated. Because the definition of fibroatheroma must include the presence of a lipid core, the origin and development of the core is key towards the understanding of disease progression. As a plaque enlarges, the lipid core becomes consolidated into a relatively avascular hypocellular mass containing cholesterol monohydrate, cholesterol esters, phospholipids, and cellular debris. Recent studies from a number of investigators have shown that necrotic core formation is mostly attributed to macrophage cell death either through necrosis or apoptosis [48].

Macrophages of atherosclerotic lesions from humans and animals are often co-localized to areas of SMC apoptosis. In culture, intimal SMCs are short-lived compared with those derived from the media as a result of increased propensity towards apoptosis [49]. Further, macrophages in co-culture have been shown to actually promote SMC apoptosis [49, 50]. It is postulated that although apoptosis is usually not associated with inflammation, under certain conditions where the rate of apoptosis exceeds the clearance capacity by macrophages, apoptotic cell death may proceed to secondary necrosis [51]. The activation of inflammatory responses by massive apop-

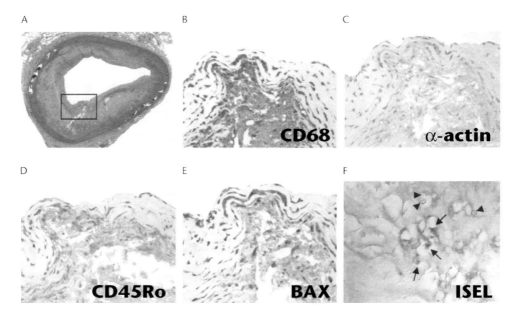

Figure 3
Identification of apoptosis in a coronary lesion classified as thin-cap fibroatheroma. The various cell types were detected using specific monoclonal antibodies for SMCs (α-actin, B), macrophages (KP-1/CD68, C), or T-lymphocytes (CD45Ro, D). Cells committed to apoptosis were identified using an antibody directed against BAX, a pro-apoptotic protein of the BCL-2 family (E). DNA fragmentation staining, an assay for apoptosis, was performed using in-situ-end labeling (ISEL, F). The positive nuclei were visualized with diaminobenzidine (dark brown reaction); the methyl green counterstain yields blue-green nuclei. (A) Movat pentachrome stained section showing an eccentric thin-cap fibroatheroma (x20). The area represented by the black box is shown in serial sections B–E (x100, the counterstain is hematoxylin). (B) Immunostaining for α-actin; note the absence of SMCs. (C) CD68 staining demonstrating infiltration of the fibrous cap by macrophages. (D) CD45RO staining showing a paucity of T-lymphocytes. (E) Staining for BAX; note the intense immunoreactivity colocalized to areas rich in macrophages. (F) Interference contrast-microscopy showing DNA fragmentation staining in an area of fibrous thinning represented by the black box in E. Note the nuclear fragments staining positive (arrows); non-apoptotic nuclei are stained bluish-green (arrowheads, x1,000).

tosis has been recently demonstrated *in vivo*. In an animal model of balloon arterial rat carotid injury, Schaub et al. showed that SMC apoptosis initiated by transient transfection with the Fas and/or the Fas-Associated Death Domain (FADD) actively promotes macrophage recruitment into vascular lesions through the release of chemokines MCP-1 and IL-8 [52].

Complications of lesion progression may further occur through the release of plaque destabilizing and thrombogenic molecules from the death of resident macrophages. Macrophages exert a tendency to become massively loaded with cholesteryl ester, a process known as foam cell formation. The pathway by which macrophages accumulate cholesteryl ester is complex and is closely facilitated by integral membrane enzyme ACAT-1, which catalyzes the esterification of the cholesterol to fatty acids [53]. It is suspected that excess free cholesterol may be among the inducers of macrophage death. Yao and Tabas recently explored the selective activation of apoptotic pathways in macrophages exposed to free cholesterol [54]. Within hours after free cholesterol loading there was detectable cytochrome c release into the cytosol, and activation of caspase-9 and BAX independent of Fas activation. Interestingly, only 15–25% of cells experienced caspase-dependent death, while virtually all cells developed mitochondrial dysfunction and death with prolonged exposure to cholesterol [54]. These data suggest that both caspase-dependent and independent pathways activated by free cholesterol may be involved in controlling macrophage populations by "physiologic" apoptosis in addition to perhaps providing a mechanism of lesion necrosis possibly contributing to plaque disruption and thrombosis.

The tumor-suppressor protein p53 exhibits both antiproliferative and pro-apoptotic actions and is another potential inducer of macrophage cell death [55]. *In vivo* studies have shown that p53 may contribute to advanced lesion formation. When APOE*3-Leiden transgenic mice were lethally radiated and reconstituted with bone marrow derived from p53$^{-/-}$ or control p53$^{+/+}$ donor mice, the p53 null mice showed significantly greater lesion area accompanied by increased necrosis and a tendency towards decreased apoptosis than mice receiving p53$^{+/+}$ bone marrow [56]. Similarly, von der Thusen et al. have shown that p53 over expression in apoE$^{-/-}$ mice leads to a decrease in the cellular and extracellular content of the fibrous cap, which induced the presence of vulnerable plaque that resulted in a higher frequency of plaque rupture [57]. Taken collectively, these studies suggest that the tumor suppressor protein p53 is an essential gene in cell proliferation and cell death, which may play an important role in lesion instability. Increased p53 expression has been documented in human atherosclerotic lesions, both in lipid-laden macrophages and vascular SMCs [58].

The thin-cap fibroatheroma – a type of vulnerable plaque

While Little, in 1990 [59], first coined the term "vulnerable plaque" to identify lesion sites that eventually form luminal thrombi Muller, in 1992 [60], proposed that plaque vulnerability requires a trigger mechanism for thrombus formation. As appropriately stated "recognition of the circadian variation – and the possibility of frequent triggering – of the onset of acute disease suggests the need for pharmacologic protection of patients during the vulnerable periods and provides clues to the mechanism of disease" [61]. The importance of mental or physical stress in provoking acute cardiac events was exemplified in a later report by Kloner demonstrating a higher incidence of sudden coronary death soon after the San Francisco earthquake than in weeks before or after this catastrophic event [62]. Peter Libby characterized the morphologic substrate of the vulnerable plaque as a "lesion composed of a lipid-rich core in the center and an overlying cap rich in macrophages" [63]. Our laboratory has further defined plaque vulnerability based on actual fibrous cap thickness at rupture sites. Accordingly, ruptured plaques were characterized as those with fibrous caps < 65 μm and heavily infiltrated by macrophages [64]. Although many investigators believe that macrophage infiltration is essential to lesions that rupture, the time-course of inflammation within the fibrous cap is unknown. Such knowledge would be invaluable for implementing treatment strategies for improving lesion stability. In addition to an inflamed cap, the unstable atheroma contains a substantial volume of necrotic, lipid-laden debris. The consistency of the lipid core is several magnitudes softer than the typical fibrous cap, with a semi-fluid consistency at body temperature. This mechanical property is likely to be a critical factor in determining plaque stability; the softer the lipid core, the more stress the overlying fibrous cap must withstand [65].

The origin of macrophages within the fibrous cap

Although the precise origin of macrophages within the fibrous cap is unknown specific signaling mechanisms including adhesion molecules, MCP-1, and MCS-F likely facilitate the recruitment and maturation of macrophages within the cap. In particular, those lesions involved in acute coronary syndromes have been shown to demonstrate various subsets of macrophages, some of which contain the catalytic enzyme myeloperoxidase [66]. It has been suggested that thin-cap fibroatheromas are those lesions in which the macrophage infiltration is predominantly from the luminal surface and not from the intraplaque vasa vasorum extending from the adventitia. Specific signals however, that selectively induce macrophage infiltration only from the luminal surface, have not yet been identified. It is conceivable that macrophages that localize towards the lumen actually never penetrate deep within the plaque and those macrophages that participate in necrosis and expansion of the necrotic core may be of an entirely different origin. Rather than migration alone however, a certain percentage of macrophages display characteristic patterns of cell turnover as plaque progress. In a study by Lutgen et al., double staining showed a high degree of DNA synthesis in macrophages of Type II fatty streak lesions while more advanced plaques showed a decline in cell proliferation; early plaques showed minimal evidence of apoptosis [67, 68]. Similar bursts of monocyte/macrophage proliferation in early fatty streaks have been described in murine models of atherosclerosis [68]. Interestingly, ruptured plaques demonstrated resurgence in DNA synthesis and increased cell apoptosis. These data emphasize the findings that ruptured lesions are very active plaques.

Fibrous cap thinning

Activation of matrix metalloproteinase

Despite many theories, the precise mechanism(s) responsible for fibrous cap thinning and plaque rupture are not known. The most comprehensive explanation of rupture is that put forward by Libby and colleagues [69], a logical extension of the inflammation hypothesis by Ross [70]. This hypothesis is predicated on the belief that inflammation and the production of cytokines are critical factors, driving the expression of proteases and inhibition of proteolytic inhibitors. One limitation of the inflammation hypothesis is the uncertainty when the inflammatory or immune process becomes critical to lesion instability. For example, proteolytic activity is elevated even in early lesion progression in experimental animals that do not rupture [71]. Further, the concept of net balance between matrix metalloproteinases (MMPs) and their inhibitors is becoming more complex. Recent data suggest that MMPs retained on the cell surface by extracellular matrix adhesion receptors are protected from their natural inhibitors [72], which may argue the balance theory between MMPs and their respective inhibitors. While the finding of proteolytic activity in the atherosclerotic plaque is clearly established, the time-course of net activity in relationship to rupture will probably remain unknown until a reproducible animal model of advanced atherosclerosis and rupture is established.

A recent study suggests that (MMPs) may influence lesion progression. In a transgenic model of selective expression of human MMP-1 in macrophages, crossed onto an apoE-null background, lesion size after 16–25 weeks of cholesterol feeding showed a paradoxical decrease compared with control littermates [73]. Rather than a promoter of plaque rupture, these data suggest a beneficial role of MMP-1 in plaque progression. Alternatively, the localized expression of MMP-1 specifically in the fibrous cap of an advanced lesion may promote plaque instability. The recent observation by Schonbeck et al. that stromelysin-3, a protease itself able to digest proteolytic inhibitors, is present only in advanced human lesions offers intriguing possibilities [74]. Stromelysin-3, a member of the serpin family has been shown to co-localize with CD40 expression on endothelial cells, SMCs, and monocytes in advanced human atheroma [75]. Activated T-lymphocytes express the CD40 ligand surface molecule, which, when activated, promotes the expression of adhesion molecules, cytokines, MMPs, and tissue factor [76]. The regulation of stromelysin-3 by CD40 ligand (CD40L) may be crucial to the progression of stable plaque to one prone to rupture and thrombosis. Interruption of CD40–CD40L signaling by an anti-CD40L antibody has been demonstrated to limit experimental autoimmune diseases, such as collagen-induced arthritis, lupus nephritis, acute or chronic graft-versus-host disease, multiple sclerosis and thyroiditis. Mach et al. showed reduction of atherosclerosis by inhibition of CD40 signaling (antibody directed against CD154 pathway) in mice [77]. Furthermore, atheroma of mice treated with anti-CD40L antibody contained significantly fewer macrophages and T lymphocytes, and exhibited decreased expression of VCAM-1 [77].

Apoptotic cell death and plaque instability

The significance of apoptotic cell death of macrophages and SMCs is becoming recognized as a major factor in perhaps causing plaque instability. The fibrous cap of ruptured plaques typically show little accumulated proteoglycans while the majority of matrix represents attenuated strands collagen Type I [78]. The absence of SMCs within the fibrous cap would greatly impair the accumulation of matrix proteins influential in maintaining its strength. Along this notion, plaque rupture sites of human aorta [79, 80] and coronary arteries [81] consistently show only a paucity of α-actin positive SMCs. These morphologic studies suggest that the overall loss of SMCs within the fibrous cap represent a chronic process before the actual rupture event. Under normal conditions, SMCs express Fas, but do not undergo apoptosis. Pretreatment of SMCs in culture however, with the cytokines TNF-α, IL-1, and IFN-γ results in Fas-induced SMC apoptosis [82]. Human atherosclerotic plaques show staining for both Fas and TUNEL in intimal SMCs cells in areas containing a high density of T-cells and macrophages, suggesting the induction of SMC apoptosis by activated T-cells [83]. The lack of survival factors such as insulin-like growth factor-1 and its receptor may also contribute to triggering SMC apoptosis potentially leading to plaque weakening and rupture [84].

There is a likely balance between inhibitors and inducers of apoptosis that occur in the many micro-environments with the advanced plaque. Potential inhibitors of apoptosis include shear stress, growth factors (PDGF, M-CSF, bFGF), and antioxidants. Interestingly, the phagocytosis of platelets has shown to highly enhance the lifespan of monocytes/macrophages by inhibition of apoptosis [85]. The initiators and executers of vascular cell death include a family of cysteine proteases known as caspases, which play a role in many forms of apoptosis. Caspases are multifunctional proteins, some of which act as pro-inflammatory mediators (pro-caspase-1, -4, -5, -m11 and -13), initiators (pro-caspase-2, -8, -9, -10 and -12), or functional effectors of apoptosis (pro-caspase-3, -6, and -7) [86]. In addition to their participation in cell death, a recent study suggests that activation of caspase-3 and -9 may play a role in the differentiation of human peripheral blood monocytes into macrophages in response to M-CSF [87].

Caspase-1, also known as IL-1-converting enzyme, is particularly intriguing since it is essential for the proteolytic maturation of IL-1 and IL-18, which further promotes the maturation and secretion of IFN-γ. Human atheroma express IL-18 and elevated levels of its receptor subunits IL-18Rα/β have been demonstrated in endothelial cells, SMCs, and macrophages (Fig. 4) [88, 89].

Further apoE-null mice administered an expression-plasmid DNA encoding for murine IL-18 binding protein (an endogenous inhibitor of IL-18) prevented fatty streak development of the thoracic aorta and slowed the progression of advanced lesions in the aortic sinus [90]. In another laboratory, exogenous IL-18 increased lesion size in both the ascending aorta and aortic arch compared with those mice injected with saline vehicle [91]. To determine the role of IFN-γ production in this response, exogenous IL-18 was administered to apoE-null mice that were IFN-γ-deficient. The lack of IFN-γ ablated the effects of IL-18 on atherosclerosis. These data further corroborate that IL-18 is a pro-atherogenic cytokine whose effect during atherosclerotic development is dependent on the presence of IFN-γ.

Two main pathways are described to trigger caspase activation in cell killing [92]. Caspases are present in the cytoplasm as inactive precursors that must be cleaved, after conserved aspartate residues to be activated. The intrinsic pathway of cell death involves a dysfunctional mitochondrial that permits the release of pro-apoptotic molecules into the cytosol. One of these molecules, cytochrome c, oligomerizes the adaptor molecule Apaf-1 to recruit and activate the initiator caspase-9. In turn, this molecule cleaves and activates downstream effector enzymes such as caspase-3. Alternatively the extrinsic pathway to cell death involves plasma membrane death receptors. The engagement of these receptors, trimerize and recruit the adaptor molecule FADD that, in turn, interacts with and activates an initiator enzyme, usually caspase-8. This enzyme, either directly or through the mitochondrial pathway, activates downstream effector enzymes including caspase-3. In both pathways, effector caspases trigger the limited proteolytic cleavage of intracellular structural and regulatory proteins; this leads to membrane blebbing, chromatin condensation and nuclear fragmentation that characterize apoptosis.

An initial event in atherosclerosis is the accumulation of low-density lipoproteins (LDLs) in the sub-endothelial space where they are susceptible to further modifications, especially oxidative changes. Mild oxidization of LDL induces apoptosis in endothelial and SMCs and is mediated principally by members of the TNF receptor family, including Fas and TNF receptors I and II. A mild oxidation of LDL causes up-regulation and expression of Fas ligand (FasL) since blocking antibodies to FasL reduce apoptosis in response to oxLDL by 50% [93, 94]. On the contrary, highly oxLDL is rapidly taken up by macrophages to form foam cells and is cytotoxic causing necrosis and apoptosis [95]. Therefore, it is speculated that highly oxLDL is involved in endothelial injury, lipid core formation, plaque rupture and subsequent thrombosis. Along these lines we have assessed apoptotic cell death in stable and ruptured plaques [81]. In a series of coronary arteries from sudden coronary death patients exhibiting plaque rupture as the culprit lesion, extensive macrophage apoptosis was found localized to the rupture site, whereas the frequency of apoptosis in

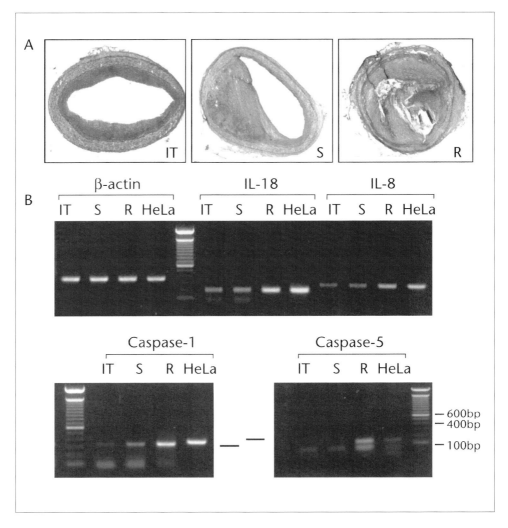

Figure 4

Comparison of RT-PCR of caspases-1 and -5 and interleukins IL-8 and IL-1 in stable and rup-tured plaques. A – Micrographs of cross-sections of different lesion types from a sudden coronary death; IT = intimal thickening, S = stable plaque, R = acute rupture (Movat pen-tachrome stain x 20). B – RT-PCR products (β-actin, interleukin-18 and -8, and caspase-1 and -5) from the lesions from panel A. RT-PCR products from HeLa cell lysates are shown as a positive control. Under the same PCR conditions (5 µl of RNA extract), similar band inten-sity for β-actin was noted for the various lesions types. In contrast, considerably more intense bands are obtained for all RT-PCR products in plaque rupture compared with intimal thickening and stable plaque.

remote areas of the fibrous cap was considerably less. Biochemical analysis showed the expression and selective activation of the pro-apoptotic enzyme, caspase-1 in ruptured arteries compared with stable plaque.

The role of myeloperoxidase in the development of coronary artery disease

Myeloperoxidase (MPO), alongside with its reactions products, have been identified in human atherosclerotic plaques [96]. MPO, a heme enzyme secreted by activated phagocytes, constitutes approximately 5% and 1% of total protein in human neutrophils and macrophages, respectively, and it is proposed that MPO modifies targets in the arterial wall through processes of oxidation. Catalytically active MPO is found to co-localized with foam cells [97] within plaques and recent studies suggest that macrophage MPO may be responsible for disruption of the fibrous cap [66]. Subsets of macrophages rich in myeloperoxidase become more frequent with lesion progression and are maximal in lesions with fibrous cap rupture. Preliminary data in our laboratory demonstrate that MPO expressing macrophages are more prevalent in ruptures than erosions (67 ± 28 *versus* 5 ± 4, p = 0.02), represented 13% and 1.4% of total macrophage content, respectively whereas MPO-positive macrophages are typically absent in stable plaques. Further, macrophages were shown to be more numerous in patients with hypercholesterolemia, and the macrophage/T-cell density is significantly increased in diabetics. Thus these findings suggest that acute plaque rupture is associated with an influx of macrophages including subsets of MPO-expressing macrophages, and that increased macrophage density in coronary plaques is associated with hypercholesterolemia and diabetes mellitus.

The pro-inflammatory properties of MPO are thought to contribute to plaque destabilization by promoting extracellular matrix degradation partly through activation of MMPs. MPO catalyzes the generation of hypochlorous acid (HOCl), a potent cytotoxic oxidant, which has been shown to convert latent collagenase-2 (MMP-8) and MMP-9 into active enzymes by proteolytic cleavage. Many MPO-positive cells have been shown to contain cathepsin G, leucocyte elastase, and MMP-9 enzymes, which alone or collectively can potentially destroy the fibrous cap. HOCl can inhibit the tissue inhibitor of matrix metalloproteinase-1 (TIMP-1) in a concentration dependent manner and can degrade collagen and elastin *in vitro*. Recently, HOCl production by MPO has been shown to activate thiol residues converting latent MMP-7 (matrilysin) to an active form [98]. The degradation of proteoglycans in advanced human atheroma (in particular, versican) has been attributed to the expression of matrilysin by resident macrophages [99]. MPO has also been implicated as an enzymatic catalyst of LDL oxidation *in vivo*, converting lipoproteins into a high-uptake form for macrophages resulting in cholesterol deposition and foam cell formation [100]. MPO has been observed to catalytically consume nitric oxide as a physiologic substrate, thereby regulating NO bioavailability during acute inflammation [101]. Impaired endothelium-dependent relaxation has been attributed to decreased NO from substrate radicals generated by MPO. Finally, HOCl may also cause SMCs death whereas taurine prevents the cytotoxic effect of HOCl [66]. Thus, there appears to be a redundancy of pathways by which the fibrous cap may rupture contingent of the co-ordinated activation of multiple cellular elements including MPO.

The clinical utility of MPO is also becoming recognized as a marker of individuals at risk for coronary artery disease (CAD). In a recent case controlled study of over 300 patients, Zhang et al. found leukocyte- and blood-MPO levels to be significantly greater in patients with CAD than in controls, even after adjusting for traditional cardiovascular risk factors, Framingham risk score, and white blood cell counts [102]. These findings support a potential role for MPO as an independent marker for increased coronary risk and may prove to be predictive of coronary events even in patients who might otherwise not be identified by routine screening methods. In another study, Buffon and colleagues sampled blood from the aorta and great cardiac vein and used neutrophil activation (i.e., the decrease in neutrophil MPO content in the blood) as an index of local coronary inflammation [103]. Since the right coronary artery does not drain into the great cardiac vein, the use of selective sampling allowed for discriminating inflammation in the left coronary artery. In unstable angina patients with a culprit lesion in the left coronary artery, evidence of inflammation was, as expected, found in the left coronary artery. Patients with unstable angina however, had evidence of inflammation in the left coronary artery even if it was free of substantial atherosclerosis and the culprit stenosis was in the right. Chronic stable angina patients failed to shown significant evidence of coronary inflammation, despite the fact that angiographic plaque burden was similar in extent to that in patients with unstable angina. There was also no evidence of inflammation in the coronary arteries of patients who had multiple episodes of variant angina and recurrent myocardial ischemia, which is believed to result from a different mechanism. Thus, ischemia alone is not likely to contribute to the measurable inflammatory state found in patients with unstable angina. Overall, the study argues the concept that the link between inflammation and active coronary disease does not arise a single vulnerable plaque in unstable coronary syndromes.

Fibrous cap atrophy – Is inflammation really necessary?

It is likely that plaque instability is the result of a number of factors that are collectively responsible for thinning and eventual rupture of the fibrous cap. Potential mechanism(s) of fibrous cap rupture, as already discussed, focus around apoptotic cell death and the liberation of specific MMPs by inflammatory cells. Another suggested mechanism is high shear stress, which may also influence the composition and configuration of the fibrous cap [104]. It is well established that lumen area is conserved in the early phases of plaque progression, through mechanisms involving compensatory enlargement of the vessel [105]. Continued plaque growth however, leads to an uncompensated reduction in lumen area and a resultant increase in surface shear forces. To answer some critical questions involving shear stress and intimal hyperplasia, Clowes laboratory developed a primate prosthetic graft models with or without placement of a distal fistula to examine the effects of varying conditions of shear. When bilateral aorto-iliac PTFE grafts were implanted simultaneously with the distal placement of a bilateral femoral arteriovenous fistula, they develop a thickened endothelialized intima over two months [106]. When one of the fistulae was ligated (reduced blood flow condition), neointimal SMCs begin to proliferate reaching a maximum at four days with cell quiescence by 14 days. The increased proliferative response corresponded with continued intimal growth over a period of 14–28 days. To determine if the increase in intimal thickness was reversible, the authors implanted bilateral aorto-iliac PTFE grafts without fistulas for two months at which time one graft was left alone for an additional two months (normal flow for four months) while the other was switched to two months of high flow by again creating an arteriovenous fistula [107]. Simulated high-flow conditions resulted in a dramatic reduction in intimal area and SMCs proliferation, without evidence of inflammation in response to increased wall shear stress. A significant loss in extracellular matrix and cell apoptosis was responsible for the increase in intimal thinning. Further, high flow was accompanied by a four-fold increase in endothelial cell nitric oxide synthase (eNOS). Endothelial-derived NO is an important regulator of the pathophysiology of arterial disease and has been shown to inhibit SMC proliferation, increase apoptotic cell death, as well as regulate PDGF synthesis. This model helps to promote the theory that fibrous caps can thin after they are formed and that flow characteristics may be all important.

Elevated inflammatory markers with adverse coronary prognosis

We have previously described clinical correlates of plaque rupture in comparison to erosion in patients dying sudden coronary death. The major clinical parameters that consistently show correlation with plaque rupture are high total cholesterol (TC), low high-density cholesterol (HDL-C), and high TC/HDL-C ratio [64]. Moreover, preliminary data from our laboratory suggests a correlation of plaque macrophages with serum TC and TC/HDL ratio at sites of maximum coronary artery narrowing. Smoking is also a strong predictor of coronary thrombosis [108]. In regards to blood pressure, the risk is counterintuitive since normotensives die more frequently from plaque rupture than hypertensives (75% *versus* 36%) [109]. In particular, diabetics have a higher frequency of healed myocardial infarction and a lower incidence of acute coronary thrombi compared to non-diabetics.

Beyond the traditional risk factors, there is a continuing search for other clinical markers that may predict future coronary events. Because of the multiple lines of evidence supporting the view of atherosclerosis as a chronic inflammatory disease, many have focused attention on plasma levels of inflammatory mediators that may potentially diagnose individuals at a higher risk for plaque rupture. Data from large-scale population-based studies have demonstrated that increased circulating levels of numerous markers of inflammation such as soluble ICAM-1, P-selectin, and IL-6, C-reactive protein (CRP) and TNF-α [110]. Of all the plasma markers thus far explored however, CRP is perhaps the most predictive of future coronary events [111]. CRP, a member of the pentraxin family of proteins is a hepatic acute phase reactant, increasing 1,000-fold in response to infection, ischemia, trauma, burns and inflammatory conditions [112]. In epidemiological studies, which have included elderly and middle-aged individuals, high CRP is a strong predictor of first-ever myocardial infarction [113], stroke [114] or the development of peripheral vascular disease [115]. Plasma CRP levels in the highest tertile with an average follow-up of eight years are associated with a two-fold increase in future vascular events even after adjusting for other cardiovascular risk factors. This is true for both men and women and algorithms that combine CRP and lipid testing may further improve risk assessment and clinical utility for outpatient use [116–118]. In a recent study from our laboratory, we assessed elevations in CRP by high-sensitivity assay (hs-CRP) in postmortem sera from 302 autopsy patients dying of CAD in the absence of overt inflammatory conditions [119]. Seventy-three patients had coronary thrombi involving both plaque rupture (n = 55) and erosion (n = 18), while 71 individuals had sudden coronary death with stable coronary plaque; there were 158 control cases (unnatural sudden death and non-cardiac natural death without conditions known to elevate CRP). The median sCRP (mg/ml) was 3.2 for rupture, 2.9 for erosion, 2.5 for stable plaques, control patients showed 1.4. The mean log hsCRP was significantly greater in individuals with culprit plaques compared with control patients. The mean staining intensity for CRP of macrophages and lipid cores in plaques was also significantly greater in cases with high versus low serum CRP as were mean number of thin-cap atheromas. These data suggest that hsCRP is a good marker for coronary atherosclerosis, especially in those lesions rich in lipid core and macrophages. Despite an increase in hs-CRP in individuals with culprit plaques however significant increases or spikes in serum hsCRP could not be discerned in patients with fatal acute coronary thrombosis compared with patients dying with stable plaque.

Plaque erosion

A second mechanism of coronary thrombosis, known as plaque erosion, does not involve disruption of the fibrous cap. The underlying lesion contains an abundance of SMCs, and proteoglycan matrix and the thrombus is confined to the luminal surface with no established communication with the deep underlying plaque. The plaque substrate mostly resembles pathologic intimal thickening such that there are mostly lipid-rich pools in the absence of a prominent necrotic core; calcification is rare. Most eroded plaques are eccentric with less severe luminal narrowing than in ruptures [120]. Unlike the prominent fibrous cap inflammation described in ruptures, eroded surfaces contain few or no macrophages and a decreased numbers of T-cells [6, 78, 120]. The lack of an obvious inflammatory response in plaque erosion is perplexing and cast doubt on whether this lesion truly represents an atherosclerotic process. In our experience, erosions account for approximately 35–40% of all cases of thrombotic sudden coronary death, and are especially common in young women and men [6]. Besides the thrombus, the most striking aspects of this lesion are the absence of luminal endothelium and that SMCs near the erosion site appear "activated" often displaying bizarre shapes with hyperchromatic nuclei and prominent nucleoli.

The extensive nature of proteoglycan matrix in plaque erosion is remarkable and a recent study from our laboratory explored the possibility of whether the accumulation of specific types of proteoglycans discriminate among lesions types associated with sudden coronary events. Plaque erosions demonstrated a selective increase in hyaluronan content at the plaque/thrombus interface compared with the fibrous caps of ruptures or stable plaques [78]. In fact, plaque rupture sites contain very little proteoglycan content relative to stable or eroded lesions. On this basis, we postulate that hyaluronan may provide a high-risk substrate for the development of thrombosis in erosion. Indirect support for this hypothesis comes from culture models demonstrating a decreased potential for endothelial cell adherence, growth and survival on hyaluronan substrates [121]. Further, the major cell surface receptor for hyaluronan CD44 was found highly localized to a subset of SMCs at the plaque/ thrombus interface as well as in some platelets and inflammatory cells within the thrombus. The de-endothelialized surface of erosion may expose hyaluronan, thereby promoting platelet attachment *via* a CD44-dependent mechanism [122]. Moreover, the expression of CD44 in erosion may also promote vascular cell activation and migration of SMCs to the wounded edge represented by the loss of endothelium. Consistent with a wounding hypothesis, acute erosions are often superimposed on what appears to be repeated episodes of thrombosis and healing such that layers of platelets and fibrin are commonly found deep within the plaque.

Vascular remodeling

In the late 1980s Glagov introduced the concept of compensatory enlargement to explain vessel expansion in response to increasing plaque burden. This mechanism would allow the maintenance of the vessel lumen until a critical narrowing of 40% occurs [105]. In atherosclerotic left anterior coronary arteries obtained at autopsy, lumen size has been shown to be independent of cross-sectional area luminal-narrowing, which is a common angiographic measure of the degree of atherosclerotic plaque [123]. Positive remodeling has also been demonstrated in patients with unstable coronary syndromes by IVUS [124]. Negative remodeling occurs in 15% of human epicardial segments. IVUS measurements show that the necrotic core cavity in ruptured plaques is larger in lesions with adaptive vascular remodeling and there is a linear relationship between overall plaque and vessel size but not the degree of lumen narrowing [125]. Further, plaques that rupture have a larger vessel area, which correlates positive with macrophages and T-cells and negative with SMCs and collagen [126]. Pasterkamp et al. have showed that lipid-rich femoral plaques are positively remodeled, which is influenced by systemic factors although macrophage infiltration appears to be under local influences and not systemic. In apoE$^{-/-}$ and apoE*3-Leiden mouse models, Lutgens et al. have also shown compensatory enlargement of the carotid artery (55% and 38%, respectively), with a correlation between plaque and lumen area; medial thinning and elastolysis was also observed [127].

In a study of morphologic predictors of arterial remodeling in coronary atherosclerosis, we found marked expansion of the internal elastic lamina (IEL) in plaque ruptures, or lesions with intraplaque hemorrhage (including thin-cap fibroatheromas) while in erosion and total occlusions, there was shrinkage of the IEL [128]. Macrophage burden, lipid core size, calcium, and medial atrophy were all associated with positive remodeling. The fibrous area however, showed a negative relationship with remodeling. It has been suggested in abdominal aortic aneurysms that MMPs play an important role and that in animals aneurysms can be created by target gene disruption of MMP-9, a secretary product of macrophages in mice [129]. Macrophage infiltration had been shown to correlate with increasing aneurysm diameter and MMP-9 is elevated in circulating plasma of patients with abdominal aneurysms [130]. MMP-12 plays a similar role because it is selectively expressed by macrophages within the aneurismal tissue [131].

Conclusion

Inflammation is an important component of coronary plaques having an influence on both lesion progression and plaque stability. Great strides in our understanding of the relationship between inflammation and atherosclerosis have been achieved through the examination of human disease in surgical specimens and in sudden coronary death patients at autopsy. The targeted expression or deletion of critical genes in mouse models of hyperlipidemia has also furthered our knowledge of inflammation in plaques. Suppression of the inflammatory response within plaques may be an important therapeutic strategy towards lesion stability. For example, lipid lowering by HMG-CoA reductase inhibitors in experimental atherosclerosis has been shown to cause an accumulation of SMCs and collagen matrix with a corresponding reduction in tissue factor, MMP activity, macrophage content, extracellular lipid, calcification, and decreased rate of apoptosis [132–135]. These results however, cannot be easily applied to human disease since unlike animal models we cannot appreciate the nature of the lesions being treated. Furthermore, patients most likely manifest the their disease episodically [136]. As a practical application only modest lipid lowering is achievable in man, and long-term treatment is required for a clinical benefit. The development of more sensitive imaging techniques is required to monitor symptomatic disease prior to and following treatment. Other avenues that may be useful will be detailed morphologic studies of arteries following long-term lipid lowering treatment in symptomatic patients such as those already performed in carotid plaques [137]. Perhaps systemic treatment with potent new anti-inflammatory drugs in combination with lipid lowering may be another area where dramatic benefits can be achieved especially in asymptomatic patients in whom vulnerable plaques can be identified.

Acknowledgements
This work was supported in part by research grants from the National Institute of Health (RO1 HL-71148-01 to RV).

References

1   *2002 Heart and Stroke Statistical Update*. American Heart Association, Dallas, Texas: American Heart Association, 2001

2   Stary HC, Chandler AB, Glagov S, Guyton JR, Insull W Jr, Rosenfeld ME, Schaffer SA, Schwartz CJ, Wagner WD, Wissler RW (1994) A definition of initial, fatty streak, and intermediate lesions of atherosclerosis. A report from the committee on vascular lesions of the council on arteriosclerosis, American Heart Association. *Arterioscler Thromb* 14: 840–856

3   Schwartz SM, deBlois D, O'Brien ER (1995) The intima. Soil for atherosclerosis and restenosis. *Circ Res* 77: 445–465

4   McCaffrey TA, Du B, Consigli S, Szabo P, Bray PJ, Hartner L, Weksler BB, Sanborn TA, Bergman G, Bush HL Jr (1997) Genomic instability in the Type II TGF-beta1 receptor gene in atherosclerotic and restenotic vascular cells. *J Clin Invest* 100: 2182–2188

5   Chatterjee SB, Dey S, Shi WY, Thomas K, Hutchins GM (1997) Accumulation of glycosphingolipids in human atherosclerotic plaque and unaffected aorta tissues. *Glycobiology* 7: 57–65

6   Virmani R, Kolodgie FD, Burke AP, Farb A, Schwartz SM (2000) Lessons from sudden

coronary death: A comprehensive morphological classification scheme for atherosclerotic lesions. *Arterioscler Thromb Vasc Biol* 20: 1262–1275

7   Velican D, Velican C (1980) Atherosclerotic involvement of the coronary arteries of adolescents and young adults. *Atherosclerosis* 36: 449–460

8   Strong JP, Malcom GT, McMahan CA, Tracy RE, Newman WP 3rd, Herderick EE, Cornhill JF (1999) Prevalence and extent of atherosclerosis in adolescents and young adults: Implications for prevention from the pathobiological determinants of atherosclerosis in youth study. *Jama* 281: 727–735

9   De Caterina R, Liao JK, Libby P (2000) Fatty acid modulation of endothelial activation. *Am J Clin Nutr* 71: 213S–223S

10   Collins RG, Velji R, Guevara NV, Hicks MJ, Chan L, Beaudet AL (2000) P-Selectin or intercellular adhesion molecule (ICAM)-1 deficiency substantially protects against atherosclerosis in apolipoprotein E-deficient mice. *J Exp Med* 191: 189–194

11   Methia N, Andre P, Denis CV, Economopoulos M, Wagner DD (2001) Localized reduction of atherosclerosis in von Willebrand factor-deficient mice. *Blood* 98: 1424–1428

12   Li H, Cybulsky MI, Gimbrone MA Jr, Libby P (1993) Inducible expression of vascular cell adhesion molecule-1 by vascular smooth muscle cells *in vitro* and within rabbit atheroma. *Am J Pathol* 143: 1551–1559

13   Richardson M, Hadcock SJ, DeReske M, Cybulsky MI (1994) Increased expression *in vivo* of VCAM-1 and E-selectin by the aortic endothelium of normolipemic and hyperlipemic diabetic rabbits. *Arterioscler Thromb* 14: 760–769

14   Cybulsky MI, Iiyama K, Li H, Zhu S, Chen M, Iiyama M, Davis V, Gutierrez-Ramos JC, Connelly PW, Milstone DS (2001) A major role for VCAM-1, but not ICAM-1, in early atherosclerosis. *J Clin Invest* 107: 1255–1262

15   Chan BM, Elices MJ, Murphy E, Hemler ME (1992) Adhesion to vascular cell adhesion molecule 1 and fibronectin. Comparison of alpha 4 beta 1 (VLA-4) and alpha 4 beta 7 on the human B cell line JY. *J Biol Chem* 267: 8366–8370

16   Patel SS, Thiagarajan R, Willerson JT, Yeh ET (1998) Inhibition of alpha4 integrin and ICAM-1 markedly attenuate macrophage homing to atherosclerotic plaques in ApoE-deficient mice. *Circulation* 97: 75–81

17   Collins T, Read MA, Neish AS, Whitley MZ, Thanos D, Maniatis T (1995) Transcriptional regulation of endothelial cell adhesion molecules: NF-kappa-B and cytokine-inducible enhancers. *Faseb J* 9: 899–909

18   Barnes PJ, Karin M (1997) Nuclear factor-kappa-B: A pivotal transcription factor in chronic inflammatory diseases. *N Engl J Med* 336: 1066–1071

19   Wilson SH, Best PJ, Edwards WD, Holmes DR Jr, Carlson PJ, Celermajer DS, Lerman A (2002) Nuclear factor-kappa-B immunoreactivity is present in human coronary plaque and enhanced in patients with unstable angina pectoris. *Atherosclerosis* 160: 147–153

20   Bourcier T, Sukhova G, Libby P (1997) The nuclear factor kappa-B signaling pathway participates in dysregulation of vascular smooth muscle cells *in vitro* and in human atherosclerosis. *J Biol Chem* 272: 15817–15824

21 Li D, Chen H, Romeo F, Sawamura T, Saldeen T, Mehta JL (2002) Statins modulate oxidized low-density lipoprotein-mediated adhesion molecule expression in human coronary artery endothelial cells: Role of LOX-1. *J Pharmacol Exp Ther* 302: 601–605

22 Cyrus T, Sung S, Zhao L, Funk CD, Tang S, Pratico D (2002) Effect of low-dose aspirin on vascular inflammation, plaque stability, and atherogenesis in low-density lipoprotein receptor-deficient mice. *Circulation* 106: 1282–1287

23 Baeuerle PA, Baltimore D (1989) A 65-kappa-D subunit of active NF-kappa-B is required for inhibition of NF-kappa-B by I kappa-B. *Genes Dev* 3: 1689–1698

24 Oitzinger W, Hofer-Warbinek R, Schmid JA, Koshelnick Y, Binder BR, de Martin R (2001) Adenovirus-mediated expression of a mutant I kappa-B kinase 2 inhibits the response of endothelial cells to inflammatory stimuli. *Blood* 97: 1611–1617

25 Lee R, Collins T (2001) Nuclear factor-kappa-B and cell survival: IAPs call for support. *Circ Res* 88: 262–264

26 Wang J, Wang S, Lu Y, Weng Y, Gown AM (1994) GM-CSF and M-CSF expression is associated with macrophage proliferation in progressing and regressing rabbit atheromatous lesions. *Exp Mol Pathol* 61: 109–118

27 Qiao JH, Tripathi J, Mishra NK, Cai Y, Tripathi S, Wang XP, Imes S, Fishbein MC, Clinton SK, Libby P et al (1997) Role of macrophage colony-stimulating factor in atherosclerosis: Studies of osteopetrotic mice. *Am J Pathol* 150: 1687–1699

28 Rajavashisth T, Qiao JH, Tripathi S, Tripathi J, Mishra N, Hua M, Wang XP, Loussararian A, Clinton S, Libby P et al (1998) Heterozygous osteopetrotic (op) mutation reduces atherosclerosis in LDL receptor-deficient mice. *J Clin Invest* 101: 2702–2710

29 Smith JD, Trogan E, Ginsberg M, Grigaux C, Tian J, Miyata M (1995) Decreased atherosclerosis in mice deficient in both macrophage colony-stimulating factor (op) and apolipoprotein E. *Proc Natl Acad Sci USA* 92: 8264–8268

30 Evanko SP, Raines EW, Ross R, Gold LI, Wight TN (1998) Proteoglycan distribution in lesions of atherosclerosis depends on lesion severity, structural characteristics, and the proximity of platelet-derived growth factor and transforming growth factor-beta. *Am J Pathol* 152: 533–546

31 Chang MY, Olin KL, Tsoi C, Wight TN, Chait A (1998) Human monocyte-derived macrophages secrete two forms of proteoglycan-macrophage colony-stimulating factor that differ in their ability to bind low density lipoproteins. *J Biol Chem* 273: 15985–15992

32 Skalen K, Gustafsson M, Rydberg EK, Hulten LM, Wiklund O, Innerarity TL, Boren J (2002) Sub-endothelial retention of atherogenic lipoproteins in early atherosclerosis. *Nature* 417: 750–754

33 Fukuchi M, Watanabe J, Kumagai K, Baba S, Shinozaki T, Miura M, Kagaya Y, Shirato K (2002) Normal and oxidized low density lipoproteins accumulate deep in physiologically thickened intima of human coronary arteries. *Lab Invest* 82: 1437–1447

34 Kockx MM, De Meyer GR, Muhring J, Jacob W, Bult H, Herman AG (1998) Apoptosis and related proteins in different stages of human atherosclerotic plaques. *Circulation* 97: 2307–2315

35   Buono C, Come CE, Witztum JL, Maguire GF, Connelly PW, Carroll M, Lichtman AH (2002) Influence of C3 deficiency on atherosclerosis. *Circulation* 105: 3025–3031

36   Borkowski P, Robinson MJ, Kusiak JW, Borkowski A, Brathwaite C, Mergner WJ (1995) Studies on TGF-beta 1 gene expression in the intima of the human aorta in regions with high and low probability of developing atherosclerotic lesions. *Mod Pathol* 8: 478–482

37   Mallat Z, Gojova A, Marchiol-Fournigault C, Esposito B, Kamate C, Merval R, Fradelizi D, Tedgui A (2001) Inhibition of transforming growth factor-beta signaling accelerates atherosclerosis and induces an unstable plaque phenotype in mice. *Circ Res* 89: 930–934

38   Lutgens E, Gijbels M, Smook M, Heeringa P, Gotwals P, Koteliansky VE, Daemen MJ (2002) Transforming growth factor-beta mediates balance between inflammation and fibrosis during plaque progression. *Arterioscler Thromb Vasc Biol* 22: 975–982

39   Tedgui A, Mallat Z (2001) Anti-inflammatory mechanisms in the vascular wall. *Circ Res* 88: 877–887

40   Wang P, Wu P, Siegel MI, Egan RW, Billah MM (1995) Interleukin (IL)-10 inhibits nuclear factor kappa B (NF kappa-B) activation in human monocytes. IL-10 and IL-4 suppress cytokine synthesis by different mechanisms. *J Biol Chem* 270: 9558–9563

41   O'Sullivan BJ, Thomas R (2002) CD40 ligation conditions dendritic cell antigen-presenting function through sustained activation of NF-kappa-B. *J Immunol* 168: 5491–5498

42   Mallat Z, Heymes C, Ohan J, Faggin E, Leseche G, Tedgui A (1999) Expression of interleukin-10 in advanced human atherosclerotic plaques: relation to inducible nitric oxide synthase expression and cell death. *Arterioscler Thromb Vasc Biol* 19: 611–616

43   Smith DA, Irving SD, Sheldon J, Cole D, Kaski JC (2001) Serum levels of the antiinflammatory cytokine interleukin-10 are decreased in patients with unstable angina. *Circulation* 104: 746–749

44   Mallat Z, Besnard S, Duriez M, Deleuze V, Emmanuel F, Bureau MF, Soubrier F, Esposito B, Duez H, Fievet C et al (1999) Protective role of interleukin-10 in atherosclerosis. *Circ Res* 85: e17–24

45   Pinderski Oslund LJ, Hedrick CC, Olvera T, Hagenbaugh A, Territo M, Berliner JA, Fyfe AI (1999) Interleukin-10 blocks atherosclerotic events *in vitro* and *in vivo*. *Arterioscler Thromb Vasc Biol* 19: 2847–2853

46   Pinderski LJ, Fischbein MP, Subbanagounder G, Fishbein MC, Kubo N, Cheroutre H, Curtiss LK, Berliner JA, Boisvert WA (2002) Over-expression of interleukin-10 by activated T lymphocytes inhibits atherosclerosis in LDL receptor-deficient mice by altering lymphocyte and macrophage phenotypes. *Circ Res* 90: 1064–1071

47   Stary HC, Chandler AB, Dinsmore RE, Fuster V, Glagov S, Insull W Jr, Rosenfeld ME, Schwartz CJ, Wagner WD, Wissler RW (1995) A definition of advanced types of atherosclerotic lesions and a histological classification of atherosclerosis. A report from the Committee on Vascular Lesions of the Council on Arteriosclerosis, American Heart Association. *Arterioscler Thromb Vasc Biol* 15: 1512–1531

48 Colles SM, Maxson JM, Carlson SG, Chisolm GM (2001) Oxidized LDL-induced injury and apoptosis in atherosclerosis. Potential roles for oxysterols. *Trends Cardiovasc Med* 11: 131–138

49 Bennett MR, Evan GI, Schwartz SM (1995) Apoptosis of human vascular smooth muscle cells derived from normal vessels and coronary atherosclerotic plaques. *J Clin Invest* 95: 2266–2274

50 Seshiah PN, Kereiakes DJ, Vasudevan SS, Lopes N, Su BY, Flavahan NA, Goldschmidt-Clermont PJ (2002) Activated monocytes induce smooth muscle cell death: Role of macrophage colony-stimulating factor and cell contact. *Circulation* 105: 174–180

51 Vivers S, Dransfield I, Hart SP (2002) Role of macrophage CD44 in the disposal of inflammatory cell corpses. *Clin Sci (Lond)* 103: 441–449

52 Schaub FJ, Han DK, Liles WC, Adams LD, Coats SA, Ramachandran RK, Seifert RA, Schwartz SM, Bowen-Pope DF (2000) Fas/FADD-mediated activation of a specific program of inflammatory gene expression in vascular smooth muscle cells. *Nat Med* 6: 790–796

53 Khelef N, Buton X, Beatini N, Wang H, Meiner V, Chang TY, Farese RV Jr., Maxfield FR, Tabas I (1998) Immunolocalization of acyl-coenzyme A:cholesterol O-acyltransferase in macrophages. *J Biol Chem* 273: 11218–11224

54 Yao PM, Tabas I (2001) Free cholesterol loading of macrophages is associated with widespread mitochondrial dysfunction and activation of the mitochondrial apoptosis pathway. *J Biol Chem* 276: 42468–42476

55 Tabas I (2001) p53 and atherosclerosis. *Circ Res* 88: 747–749

56 van Vlijmen BJ, Gerritsen G, Franken AL, Boesten LS, Kockx MM, Gijbels MJ, Vierboom MP, van Eck M, van De Water B, van Berkel TJ et al (2001) Macrophage p53 deficiency leads to enhanced atherosclerosis in APOE*3-Leiden transgenic mice. *Circ Res* 88: 780–786

57 von der Thusen JH, van Vlijmen BJ, Hoeben RC, Kockx MM, Havekes LM, van Berkel TJ, Biessen EA (2002) Induction of atherosclerotic plaque rupture in apolipoprotein E–/– mice after adenovirus-mediated transfer of p53I. *Circulation* 105: 2064–2070

58 Ihling C, Menzel G, Wellens E, Monting JS, Schaefer HE, Zeiher AM (1997) Topographical association between the cyclin-dependent kinases inhibitor P21, p53 accumulation, and cellular proliferation in human atherosclerotic tissue. *Arterioscler Thromb Vasc Biol* 17: 2218–2224

59 Little WC (1990) Angiographic assessment of the culprit coronary artery lesion before acute myocardial infarction. *Am J Cardiol* 66: 44G–47G

60 Muller JE, Stone PH, Turi ZG, Rutherford JD, Czeisler CA, Parker C, Poole WK, Passamani E, Roberts R, Robertson T et al (1985) Circadian variation in the frequency of onset of acute myocardial infarction. *N Engl J Med* 313: 1315–1322

61 Muller JE, Tofler GH, Stone PH (1989) Circadian variation and triggers of onset of acute cardiovascular disease. *Circulation* 79: 733–743

62 Leor J, Poole WK, Kloner RA (1996) Sudden cardiac death triggered by an earthquake. *N Engl J Med* 334: 413–419

63 Libby P, Geng YJ, Aikawa M, Schoenbeck U, Mach F, Clinton SK, Sukhova GK, Lee RT (1996) Macrophages and atherosclerotic plaque stability. *Curr Opin Lipidol* 7: 330–335

64 Burke AP, Farb A, Malcom GT, Liang YH, Smialek J, Virmani R (1997) Coronary risk factors and plaque morphology in men with coronary disease who died suddenly. *N Engl J Med* 336: 1276–1282

65 Loree HM, Tobias BJ, Gibson LJ, Kamm RD, Small DM, Lee RT (1994) Mechanical properties of model atherosclerotic lesion lipid pools. *Arterioscler Thromb* 14: 230–234

66 Sugiyama S, Okada Y, Sukhova GK, Virmani R, Heinecke JW, Libby P (2001) Macrophage myeloperoxidase regulation by granulocyte macrophage colony-stimulating factor in human atherosclerosis and implications in acute coronary syndromes. *Am J Pathol* 158: 879–891

67 Lutgens E, de Muinck ED, Kitslaar PJ, Tordoir JH, Wellens HJ, Daemen MJ (1999) Biphasic pattern of cell turnover characterizes the progression from fatty streaks to ruptured human atherosclerotic plaques. *Cardiovasc Res* 41: 473–479

68 Lessner SM, Prado HL, Waller EK, Galis ZS (2002) Atherosclerotic lesions grow through recruitment and proliferation of circulating monocytes in a murine model. *Am J Pathol* 160: 2145–2155

69 Libby P, Aikawa M (2002) Stabilization of atherosclerotic plaques: New mechanisms and clinical targets. *Nat Med* 8: 1257–1262

70 Ross R (1999) Atherosclerosis: An inflammatory disease. *N Engl J Med* 340: 115–126

71 Galis ZS, Sukhova GK, Libby P (1995) Microscopic localization of active proteases by in situ zymography: Detection of matrix metalloproteinase activity in vascular tissue. *Faseb J* 9: 974–980

72 Yu Q, Stamenkovic I (1999) Localization of matrix metalloproteinase 9 to the cell surface provides a mechanism for CD44-mediated tumor invasion. *Genes Dev* 13: 35–48

73 Lemaitre V, O'Byrne TK, Borczuk AC, Okada Y, Tall AR, D'Armiento J (2001) ApoE knockout mice expressing human matrix metalloproteinase-1 in macrophages have less advanced atherosclerosis. *J Clin Invest* 107: 1227–1234

74 Schonbeck U, Mach F, Sukhova GK, Atkinson E, Levesque E, Herman M, Graber P, Basset P, Libby P (1999) Expression of stromelysin-3 in atherosclerotic lesions: Regulation *via* CD40-CD40 ligand signaling *in vitro* and *in vivo*. *J Exp Med* 189: 843–853

75 Mach F, Schonbeck U, Sukhova GK, Bourcier T, Bonnefoy JY, Pober JS, Libby P (1997) Functional CD40 ligand is expressed on human vascular endothelial cells, smooth muscle cells, and macrophages: Implications for CD40–CD40 ligand signaling in atherosclerosis. *Proc Natl Acad Sci USA* 94: 1931–1936

76 Mach F, Schonbeck U, Bonnefoy JY, Pober JS, Libby P (1997) Activation of monocyte/macrophage functions related to acute atheroma complication by ligation of CD40: Induction of collagenase, stromelysin, and tissue factor. *Circulation* 96: 396–399

77 Mach F, Schonbeck U, Sukhova GK, Atkinson E, Libby P (1998) Reduction of atherosclerosis in mice by inhibition of CD40 signalling. *Nature* 394: 200–203

78 Kolodgie FD, Burke AP, Farb A, Weber DK, Kutys R, Wight TN, Virmani R (2002) Dif-

ferential accumulation of proteoglycans and hyaluronan in culprit lesions: Insights into plaque erosion. *Arterioscler Thromb Vasc Biol* 22: 1642–1648

79   Davies MJ, Richardson PD, Woolf N, Katz DR, Mann J (1993) Risk of thrombosis in human atherosclerotic plaques: Role of extracellular lipid, macrophage, and smooth muscle cell content. *Br Heart J* 69: 377–381

80   Lendon CL, Davies MJ, Born GV, Richardson PD (1991) Atherosclerotic plaque caps are locally weakened when macrophages density is increased. *Atherosclerosis* 87: 87–90

81   Kolodgie FD, Narula J, Burke AP, Haider N, Farb A, Hui-Liang Y, Smialek J, Virmani R (2000) Localization of apoptotic macrophages at the site of plaque rupture in sudden coronary death. *Am J Pathol* 157: 1259–1268

82   Geng YJ, Wu Q, Muszynski M, Hansson GK, Libby P (1996) Apoptosis of vascular smooth muscle cells induced by *in vitro* stimulation with interferon-gamma, tumor necrosis factor-alpha, and interleukin-1 beta. *Arterioscler Thromb Vasc Biol* 16: 19–27

83   Geng YJ, Henderson LE, Levesque EB, Muszynski M, Libby P (1997) Fas is expressed in human atherosclerotic intima and promotes apoptosis of cytokine-primed human vascular smooth muscle cells. *Arterioscler Thromb Vasc Biol* 17: 2200–2208

84   Okura Y, Brink M, Zahid AA, Anwar A, Delafontaine P (2001) Decreased expression of insulin-like growth factor-1 and apoptosis of vascular smooth muscle cells in human atherosclerotic plaque. *J Mol Cell Cardiol* 33: 1777–1789

85   Geng YJ, Libby P (2002) Progression of atheroma: A struggle between death and pro-creation. *Arterioscler Thromb Vasc Biol* 22: 1370–1380

86   Earnshaw WC, Martins LM, Kaufmann SH (1999) Mammalian caspases: Structure, activation, substrates, and functions during apoptosis. *Annu Rev Biochem* 68: 383–424

87   Sordet O, Rebe C, Plenchette S, Zermati Y, Hermine O, Vainchenker W, Garrido C, Solary E, Dubrez-Daloz L (2002) Specific involvement of caspases in the differentiation of monocytes into macrophages. *Blood* 100: 4446–4453

88   Gerdes N, Sukhova GK, Libby P, Reynolds RS, Young JL, Schonbeck U (2002) Expression of interleukin (IL)-18 and functional IL-18 receptor on human vascular endothelial cells, smooth muscle cells, and macrophages: implications for atherogenesis. *J Exp Med* 195: 245–257

89   Mallat Z, Corbaz A, Scoazec A, Besnard S, Leseche G, Chvatchko Y, Tedgui A (2001) Expression of interleukin-18 in human atherosclerotic plaques and relation to plaque instability. *Circulation* 104: 1598–1603

90   Mallat Z, Corbaz A, Scoazec A, Graber P, Alouani S, Esposito B, Humbert Y, Chvatchko Y, Tedgui A (2001) Interleukin-18/interleukin-18 binding protein signaling modulates atherosclerotic lesion development and stability. *Circ Res* 89: E41–45

91   Whitman SC, Ravisankar P, Daugherty A (2002) Interleukin-18 enhances atherosclerosis in apolipoprotein E (–/–) mice through release of interferon-gamma. *Circ Res* 90: E34–38

92   Hengartner MO (2000) The biochemistry of apoptosis. *Nature* 407: 770–776

93   Napoli C, Quehenberger O, De Nigris F, Abete P, Glass CK, Palinski W (2000) Mildly

oxidized low density lipoprotein activates multiple apoptotic signaling pathways in human coronary cells. *Faseb J* 14: 1996–2007

94 Lee T, Chau L (2001) Fas/Fas ligand-mediated death pathway is involved in oxLDL-induced apoptosis in vascular smooth muscle cells. *Am J Physiol Cell Physiol* 280: C709–718

95 Martinet W, Knaapen MW, De Meyer GR, Herman AG, Kockx MM (2002) Elevated levels of oxidative DNA damage and DNA repair enzymes in human atherosclerotic plaques. *Circulation* 106: 927–932

96 Heinecke JW (1999) Mechanisms of oxidative damage by myeloperoxidase in atherosclerosis and other inflammatory disorders. *J Lab Clin Med* 133: 321–325

97 Daugherty A, Dunn JL, Rateri DL, Heinecke JW (1994) Myeloperoxidase, a catalyst for lipoprotein oxidation, is expressed in human atherosclerotic lesions. *J Clin Invest* 94: 437–444

98 Fu X, Kassim SY, Parks WC, Heinecke JW (2001) Hypochlorous acid oxygenates the cysteine switch domain of pro-matrilysin (MMP-7). A mechanism for matrix metalloproteinase activation and atherosclerotic plaque rupture by myeloperoxidase. *J Biol Chem* 276: 41279–41287

99 Halpert I, Sires UI, Roby JD, Potter-Perigo S, Wight TN, Shapiro SD, Welgus HG, Wickline SA, Parks WC (1996) Matrilysin is expressed by lipid-laden macrophages at sites of potential rupture in atherosclerotic lesions and localizes to areas of versican deposition, a proteoglycan substrate for the enzyme. *Proc Natl Acad Sci USA* 93: 9748–9753

100 Podrez EA, Schmitt D, Hoff HF, Hazen SL (1999) Myeloperoxidase-generated reactive nitrogen species convert LDL into an atherogenic form *in vitro*. *J Clin Invest* 103: 1547–1560

101 Eiserich JP, Baldus S, Brennan ML, Ma W, Zhang C, Tousson A, Castro L, Lusis AJ, Nauseef WM, White CR et al (2002) Myeloperoxidase, a leukocyte-derived vascular NO oxidase. *Science* 296: 2391–2394

102 Zhang R, Brennan ML, Fu X, Aviles RJ, Pearce GL, Penn MS, Topol EJ, Sprecher DL, Hazen SL (2001) Association between myeloperoxidase levels and risk of coronary artery disease. *Jama* 286: 2136–2142

103 Buffon A, Biasucci LM, Liuzzo G, D'Onofrio G, Crea F, Maseri A (2002) Widespread coronary inflammation in unstable angina. *N Engl J Med* 347: 5–12

104 Clowes AW, Berceli SA (2000) Mechanisms of vascular atrophy and fibrous cap disruption. *Ann NY Acad Sci* 902: 153–161; discussion 161–152

105 Glagov S, Weisenberg E, Zarins CK, Stankunavicius R, Kolettis GJ (1987) Compensatory enlargement of human atherosclerotic coronary arteries. *N Engl J Med* 316: 1371–1375

106 Geary RL, Kohler TR, Vergel S, Kirkman TR, Clowes AW (1994) Time course of flow-induced smooth muscle cell proliferation and intimal thickening in endothelialized baboon vascular grafts. *Circ Res* 74: 14–23

107 Mattsson EJ, Kohler TR, Vergel SM, Clowes AW (1997) Increased blood flow induces regression of intimal hyperplasia. *Arterioscler Thromb Vasc Biol* 17: 2245–2249

108 Burke AP, Farb A, Malcom GT, Liang Y, Smialek J, Virmani R (1998) Effect of risk factors on the mechanism of acute thrombosis and sudden coronary death in women. *Circulation* 97: 2110–2116

109 Burke AP, Farb A, Liang YH, Smialek J, Virmani R (1996) Effect of hypertension and cardiac hypertrophy on coronary artery morphology in sudden cardiac death. *Circulation* 94: 3138–3145

110 Blake GJ, Ridker PM (2002) Inflammatory bio-markers and cardiovascular risk prediction. *J Intern Med* 252: 283–294

111 Blake GJ, Ridker PM (2002) C-reactive protein, subclinical atherosclerosis, and risk of cardiovascular events. *Arterioscler Thromb Vasc Biol* 22: 1512–1513

112 Westhuyzen J, Healy H (2000) Review: Biology and relevance of C-reactive protein in cardiovascular and renal disease. *Ann Clin Lab Sci* 30: 133–143

113 Sakkinen P, Abbott RD, Curb JD, Rodriguez BL, Yano K, Tracy RP (2002) C-reactive protein and myocardial infarction. *J Clin Epidemiol* 55: 445–451

114 Winbeck K, Poppert H, Etgen T, Conrad B, Sander D (2002) Prognostic relevance of early serial C-reactive protein measurements after first ischemic stroke. *Stroke* 33: 2459–2464

115 Schillinger M, Exner M, Mlekusch W, Rumpold H, Ahmadi R, Sabeti S, Haumer M, Wagner O, Minar E (2002) Vascular inflammation and percutaneous transluminal angioplasty of the femoropopliteal artery: Association with restenosis. *Radiology* 225: 21–26

116 Ridker PM (2001) High-sensitivity C-reactive protein: Potential adjunct for global risk assessment in the primary prevention of cardiovascular disease. *Circulation* 103: 1813–1818

117 Ridker PM, Stampfer MJ, Rifai N (2001) Novel risk factors for systemic atherosclerosis: A comparison of C-reactive protein, fibrinogen, homocysteine, lipoprotein(a), and standard cholesterol screening as predictors of peripheral arterial disease. *Jama* 285: 2481–2485

118 Libby P, Ridker PM, Maseri A (2002) Inflammation and atherosclerosis. *Circulation* 105: 1135–1143

119 Burke AP, Tracy RP, Kolodgie F, Malcom GT, Zieske A, Kutys R, Pestaner J, Smialek J, Virmani R (2002) Elevated C-reactive protein values and atherosclerosis in sudden coronary death: Association with different pathologies. *Circulation* 105: 2019–2023

120 Farb A, Burke AP, Tang AL, Liang TY, Mannan P, Smialek J, Virmani R (1996) Coronary plaque erosion without rupture into a lipid core. A frequent cause of coronary thrombosis in sudden coronary death. *Circulation* 93: 1354–1363

121 Relou IA, Damen CA, van der Schaft DW, Groenewegen G, Griffioen AW (1998) Effect of culture conditions on endothelial cell growth and responsiveness. *Tissue Cell* 30: 525–530

122 Koshiishi I, Shizari M, Underhill CB (1994) CD44 can mediate the adhesion of platelets to hyaluronan. *Blood* 84: 390–396

123 Clarkson TB, Prichard RW, Morgan TM, Petrick GS, Klein KP (1994) Remodeling of coronary arteries in human and nonhuman primates. *Jama* 271: 289–294

124 Schoenhagen P, Ziada KM, Kapadia SR, Crowe TD, Nissen SE, Tuzcu EM (2000) Extent and direction of arterial remodeling in stable versus unstable coronary syndromes: An intravascular ultrasound study. *Circulation* 101: 598–603

125 von Birgelen C, Klinkhart W, Mintz GS, Papatheodorou A, Herrmann J, Baumgart D, Haude M, Wieneke H, Ge J, Erbel R (2001) Plaque distribution and vascular remodeling of ruptured and nonruptured coronary plaques in the same vessel: An intravascular ultrasound study *in vivo. J Am Coll Cardiol* 37: 1864–1870

126 Pasterkamp G, Schoneveld AH, van der Wal AC, Haudenschild CC, Clarijs RJ, Becker AE, Hillen B, Borst C (1998) Relation of arterial geometry to luminal narrowing and histologic markers for plaque vulnerability: The remodeling paradox. *J Am Coll Cardiol* 32: 655–662

127 Lutgens E, de Muinck ED, Heeneman S, Daemen MJ (2001) Compensatory enlargement and stenosis develop in apoE(–/–) and apoE*3-Leiden transgenic mice. *Arterioscler Thromb Vasc Biol* 21: 1359–1365

128 Burke AP, Kolodgie FD, Farb A, Weber D, Virmani R (2002) Morphological predictors of arterial remodeling in coronary atherosclerosis. *Circulation* 105: 297–303

129 Pyo R, Lee JK, Shipley JM, Curci JA, Mao D, Ziporin SJ, Ennis TL, Shapiro SD, Senior RM, Thompson RW (2000) Targeted gene disruption of matrix metalloproteinase-9 (gelatinase B) suppresses development of experimental abdominal aortic aneurysms. *J Clin Invest* 105: 1641–1649

130 Annabi B, Shedid D, Ghosn P, Kenigsberg RL, Desrosiers RR, Bojanowski MW, Beaulieu E, Nassif E, Moumdjian R, Beliveau R (2002) Differential regulation of matrix metalloproteinase activities in abdominal aortic aneurysms. *J Vasc Surg* 35: 539–546

131 Curci JA, Liao S, Huffman MD, Shapiro SD, Thompson RW (1998) Expression and localization of macrophage elastase (matrix metalloproteinase-12) in abdominal aortic aneurysms. *J Clin Invest* 102: 1900–1910

132 Verhamme P, Quarck R, Hao H, Knaapen M, Dymarkowski S, Bernar H, Van Cleemput J, Janssens S, Vermylen J, Gabbiani G et al (2002) Dietary cholesterol withdrawal reduces vascular inflammation and induces coronary plaque stabilization in miniature pigs. *Cardiovasc Res* 56: 135

133 Aikawa M, Rabkin E, Sugiyama S, Voglic SJ, Fukumoto Y, Furukawa Y, Shiomi M, Schoen FJ, Libby P (2001) An HMG-CoA reductase inhibitor, cerivastatin, suppresses growth of macrophages expressing matrix metalloproteinases and tissue factor *in vivo* and *in vitro. Circulation* 103: 276–283

134 Martinet W, Knaapen MW, De Meyer GR, Herman AG, Kockx MM (2001) Oxidative DNA damage and repair in experimental atherosclerosis are reversed by dietary lipid lowering. *Circ Res* 88: 733–739

135 Kockx MM, Seye C, De Meyer GR, Knaapen MW (2000) Decreased apoptosis and tissue factor expression after lipid lowering. *Circulation* 102: E99

136 Burke AP, Kolodgie FD, Farb A, Weber DK, Malcom GT, Smialek J, Virmani R (2001)

Healed plaque ruptures and sudden coronary death: Evidence that subclinical rupture has a role in plaque progression. *Circulation* 103: 934–940

137 Crisby M, Nordin-Fredriksson G, Shah PK, Yano J, Zhu J, Nilsson J (2001) Pravastatin treatment increases collagen content and decreases lipid content, inflammation, metalloproteinases, and cell death in human carotid plaques: Implications for plaque stabilization. *Circulation* 103: 926–933

138 Tedgui A, Mallat Z (2001) Anti-inflammatory mechanisms in the vascular wall. *Circ Res* 88: 877–887

Inflammatory cells and their metalloproteinases in cardiac disease

The role of matrix metalloproteinases in LV remodeling following myocardial infarction

Esther E.J.M. Creemers[1], Jack P.M. Cleutjens[1], Jos F.M. Smits[2] and Mat J.A.P. Daemen[1]

Department of [1]Pathology and [2]Pharmacology, Cardiovascular Research Institute Maastricht (CARIM), University of Maastricht, 6200 MD Maastricht, The Netherlands

Introduction

The major function of the extracellular matrix (ECM) is to provide a mechanical framework to hold cells together in tissue and organs. Besides this function, it is becoming widely accepted that the ECM is a dynamic entity that interacts with cells and regulates cell phenotype. In this regard, the matrix profoundly affects cell behavior through signaling by integrins, which form direct contacts between cells and the ECM [1]. Second, proteoglycans in the ECM sequester growth factors like TGF-β, FGF, VEGF and various cytokines that regulate some of the most fundamental cellular processes, such as proliferation, differentiation and survival [2]. Third, in order for cells to migrate, they have to disconnect from the ECM and degrade the matrix molecules that lie along the path they want to traverse. To control their ECM turnover, to release growth factors from the ECM and to migrate through the ECM, cells produce a wide range of proteolytic enzymes, in particular the matrix metalloproteinases (MMPs). MMPs are involved in many physiological processes, such as embryonic development, ovulation, bone remodeling and wound healing and their enhanced activity has been implicated in numerous disease processes associated with inflammatory destruction or invasion of metastatic cancer [3–7]. MMPs, which are present in the myocardium are the driving force behind myocardial matrix remodeling. Recent studies have demonstrated that preventing the breakdown of the myocardial extracellular matrix with pharmacological broad spectrum MMP inhibitors in animal models of cardiomyopathy and myocardial infarction has favorable effects on the left ventricular (LV) remodeling process. This led to the proposal that MMP inhibitors could potentially be used as therapy for patients at risk for the development of heart failure. In the present chapter, we describe the biology of MMPs and discuss new insights into the role of MMPs in the LV remodeling process after myocardial infarction (MI). Attention will be paid to the central role of the plasminogen system, as an important activator of MMPs and we will speculate on the use of MMP inhibitors as potential therapy for heart failure.

Inflammation and Cardiac Diseases, edited by Giora Z. Feuerstein, Peter Libby and Douglas L. Mann
© 2003 Birkhäuser Verlag Basel/Switzerland

Table 1 - MMPs and their substrates

Enzyme	MMP classification	Substrate
Collagenases		
Interstitial collagenase	MMP-1	Collagens I-III, VII, X, gelatin, entactin, aggrecan, L-selectin, proTNF, IL-1β, MMP-2 and -9
Neutrophil collagenase	MMP-8	Collagens I-III, V, VII, VIII and X, gelatin, fibronectin, aggrecan
Collagenase-3	MMP-13	Collagens I-III, IV, IX, X, gelatin, fibronectin, laminin, tenascin, osteonectin, MMP-9
Gelatinases		
Gelatinase A	MMP-2	Collagens I, IV, V, VII, X, gelatin, fibronectin, laminin, aggrecan, tenascin-C, vitronectin, elastin, osteonectin, proTNF, IL-1β, MMP-1, -9, -13
Gelatinase B	MMP-9	Collagens IV, V, VII, XIV, gelatin, aggrecan, elastin, entactin, vitronectin, proTNF, IL-1β
Stromelysins		
Stromelysin 1	MMP-3	Collagens III, IV, IX, X, gelatin, fibronectin, laminin, tenascin-C, vitronectin, elastin, casein, proTNF, IL-1β, MMP-1, -7, -8, -9 and -13
Stromelysin 2	MMP-10	Collagen III, IV, V, gelatin, elastin, fibronectin, aggrecan, MMP-1, MMP-8
Stromelysin 3	MMP-11	Collagen IV, fibronectin, gelatin, laminin, aggrecan

The family members of matrix metalloproteinases (MMPs)

Matrix metalloproteinases (MMPs) are a family of zinc-containing endoproteinases that share structural domains, but differ in substrate specificity, cellular sources, and inducibility. The list of MMPs has grown rapidly in the past several years and by now, over 20 mammalian members have been cloned and identified (Tab. 1).

MMPs share the following functional features:

1. They degrade ECM components;
2. They are secreted in a latent proform and require activation for proteolytic activity;
3. They contain Zn^{2+} at their active site;

Table 1 - continued

Enzyme	MMP classification	Substrate
Membrane-type MMPs		
MT1-MMP	MMP-14	Collagens I–IV, fibronectin, laminin, vitronectin, elastin proteoglycans, proTNF, MMP-2 and -13
MT2-MMP	MMP-15	Collagens I–IV, gelatin, laminin, fibronectin, fibrin, aggrecan, proTNF, MMP-2
MT3-MMP	MMP-16	Collagens I–IV, gelatin, laminin, fibronectin, fibrin, MMP-2
MT4-MMP	MMP-17	Fibrin, proTNF
MT5-MMP	MMP-24	Collagens I–IV, gelatin, laminin, fibronectin, fibrin, MMP-2
MT6-MMP (leukolysin)	MMP-25	Collagen IV, gelatin, fibronectin, fibrin
Others		
Matrilysin	MMP-7	Gelatin, fibronectin, laminin, collagen IV, vitronectin, tenascin-C, elastin, aggrecan, proTNF, MMP-1, -2, -9
Matrilysin-2 (endometase)	MMP-26	Gelatin, fibronectin, vitronectin, fibrinogen
Metalloelastase	MMP-12	Elastin
	MMP-19	Gelatin, fibronectin, laminin, collagen IV, tenascin-C, nidogen, aggrecan
Enamelysin	MMP-20	Aggrecan
CA-MMP	MMP-23	
Epilysin	MMP-28	

4. They need calcium for stability;
5. They function at neutral pH; and
6. They are inhibited by specific tissue inhibitors of metalloproteinases (TIMPs).

Based on their substrate specificity and primary structure, the MMP family can be subdivided into the four groups shown in Table 1. The first group, the collagenases, can all cleave fibrillar collagens (Type I, II and III collagen). These collagens are known to be extremely resistant to cleavage by most proteinases because they are tightly apposed and consist of highly cross-linked fibrils. Group 2, the gelatinases is well-known for its ability to degrade gelatins and Type IV collagen in basement membranes. Group 3 constitutes the stromelysins, so-named because they are active against a broad spectrum of ECM components, including proteoglycans, laminins, fibronectin, vitronectin and some types of collagens. Although most MMPs are secreted proteins, the recently described membrane-type MMPs are anchored to the cell membrane by a transmembrane domain. These MT-MMPs concentrate proteolytic activity to the cell surface and are also able to activate other MMPs.

This substrate-based subdivision of MMPs turned out to be useful in the past, however as more is known about the enzymatic activities and substrates, its usefulness becomes less clear because the substrate profile of the enzymes is often more gradual than absolute. It is also becoming increasingly clear that matrix degradation is not the only function of MMPs, but that they can act on a variety of non-matrix proteins as well. For example, several MMPs directly activate growth factors and chemokines, such as TGF-β, TNF-α, insulin-like growth factor-1, epidermal growth factor, fibroblast growth factor (FGFs), and monocyte chemoattractant protein (MCP)-3 [8–13]. In addition, fragments of matrix proteins released by MMPs can act as chemoattractants for distant cells. Therefore MMPs should not be viewed solely as proteinases of matrix degradation, but as extracellular processing enzymes critically involved in cell-cell and cell-matrix signalling [14].

Regulation of MMP activity

Since MMPs, once activated, are collectively capable of degrading the complete ECM, it is important that the activity of these enzymes is kept under tight control. The activity of MMPs is controlled at the following three levels: transcription, activation of the latent pro-enzymes and inhibition by their endogenous inhibitors, the TIMPs.

Regulation of MMP expression

The expression of most MMPs is generally found at low levels in normal adult tissue, but is upregulated during certain physiological and pathological remodeling processes. Induction or stimulation at the transcriptional level is mediated by a variety of inflammatory cytokines, hormones and growth factors, such as IL-1, IL-6, TNF-α, epidermal growth factor (EGF), platelet derived growth factor (PDGF), basic fibroblast growth factor (bFGF) and CD40 [15, 16]. In addition, a cell-surface protein that induces MMP expression, termed extracellular matrix metalloproteinase inducer (EMMPRIN) has been identified in both normal and diseased human tissue [17]. Other factors, like corticosteroids, retinoic acid, heparin and IL-4 have been demonstrated to inhibit MMP gene expression [18]. Not all MMPs react similarly to the same stimulus. For example TGF-β stimulates MMP-2 and

MMP-9, but inhibits MMP-1 and MMP-3 synthesis [19]. In case of interferon-γ (IFN-γ), the impact on MMP expression is cell-type specific. Whereas IFN-γ increases MMP-1 expression in keratinocytes, it decreases MMP-1 expression in macrophages and fibroblasts [20].

Activation mechanisms of latent MMPs

Although transcriptional regulation is essential for MMP production, matrix degradation requires the latent enzymes to be activated by proteolytic cleavage. Three different activation mechanisms have been described: (1) stepwise activation, (2) activation at the cell surface by MT-MMPs and (3) intracellular activation [21].

The first step during stepwise activation of MMPs often involves proteinases such as plasmin, trypsin, chymase, elastase or kallikrein. Of these proteinases, plasmin is thought to be the most potent physiological activator in vivo [22]. Plasmin attacks the proteinase susceptible region in the "propeptide domain" of the MMP, which induces conformational changes in the propeptide and renders the activation site to be cleaved by a second proteinase, usually another MMP [21].

Cell surface activation of MMPs is considered to be important for pericellular degradation of the ECM during cell migration. Besides the plasminogen system, also other enzymes are capable of activating MMPs at the plasma membrane. In 1994, Sato et al. cloned a membrane-type MMP (MT1-MMP) and identified it as an activator of proMMP-2 on the plasma membrane [23, 24]. Currently six MT-MMPs have been cloned and it has been demonstrated that MT-MMPs also activate other MMPs [21, 25].

The first evidence that members of the MMP family are activated intracellularly came from Pei and Weiss in 1995 [26]. They demonstrated that stromelysin-3 (MMP-11) could be activated by the Golgi-associated subtilisin-like proteinase, furin, and could be secreted as an active enzyme. Subsequently, Sato et al. reported that MT1-MMP, expressed in *E. coli* was also activated by furin, indicating that MT-MMPs are also likely to be activated intracellularly [27]. The precise molecular mechanism of intracellular activation and the contribution to extracellular MMP activity has, however, not been clarified.

Endogenous MMP inhibitors

Fully activated MMPs can be inhibited by interaction with naturally occurring, specific inhibitors, the TIMPs. TIMPs are expressed by a variety of cell types and are present in most tissues and body fluids. At present, the TIMP family consists of four structurally-related members, TIMP-1, -2, -3 and -4. TIMPs bind non-covalently to active MMPs in a 1:1 molar ratio. Inhibition is accomplished by their ability to interact with the zinc-binding site within the catalytic domain of active MMPs. There is a certain degree of specificity in the activity of different TIMPs towards distinct members of the MMP family. Whereas TIMP-1 potently inhibits the activity of most MMPs, with the exception of MMP-2 and MT1-MMP, TIMP-2 is a potent inhibitor of most MMPs, except MMP-9. Although the role of TIMPs is clearly important in the prevention of excessive matrix degradation by MMPs, recent studies suggest that TIMPs are multifunctional proteins with more diverse biological actions. In this regard, it has been reported that TIMP-1 and TIMP-2 exhibit growth factor-like activity and can inhibit angiogenesis [28–30], whereas TIMP-3 has been implicated in apoptosis [31]. TIMP-4 might be of particular interest in cardiac research since it shows a high level of expression in adult human cardiac tissue [32, 33].

In addition to the TIMPs family, there are also several other naturally occurring inhibitors of MMPs, of which α-macroglobulin is the most prominent. This macroglobulin is a large (750 kDa) protein produced by the liver. It can inhibit all four classes of proteinases (i.e., cysteine-, aspartic-, serine- and metalloproteinases) and not just MMPs. However, the large size of α-macroglobulin may exclude it from many sites of connective tissue turnover, which may limit its effectiveness as an inhibitor.

MMPs in cardiac diseases

Recent evidence implicates the MMP family as potential mediators of cardiac diseases, in particular in LV dilatation and the development of heart failure. This evidence is based on four lines of investigation, elaborated in the following four paragraphs. The first line of evidence proves that MMPs are extensively overexpressed in the diseased myocardium. Second, several laboratories have shown that pharmacological inhibition of MMPs attenuates LV remodeling after myocardial infarction. Third, gene targeting studies in mice indicate a specific role for MMP-9 in LV dilatation and cardiac rupture after infarction, and fourth, increased MMP activity (by overexpression of MMP-1 or TIMP-1 deficiency) was demonstrated to induce LV dilatation.

Increased MMP activity in cardiac diseases

In 1975, Montfort and Perez-Tamayo demonstrated that collagenase is present in the normal myocardium. It was located in the interstitium, in the neighborhood of its substrate, fibrillar collagen [34]. It is now known that myocardial MMPs are produced by fibroblast-like cells, inflammatory cells as well as by cardiomyocytes, that they are predominantly present in their latent form and that they are increas-

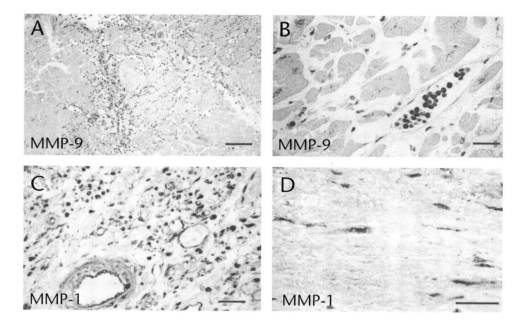

Figure 1

MMP-1 and -9 immunoreactivity in human myocardium.

A. Photomicrograph of human myocardium, three days after infarction demonstrating that MMP-9 is present in inflammatory cells that invade the infarcted ventricle; B. In relative normal areas of the myocardium, at 4–5 days post-MI, MMP-9 containing inflammatory cells are detected inside vessels; C. MMP-1 is expressed by a wider range of cell types than MMP-9. Note the MMP-1 containing endothelial cells, smooth muscle cells and interstitial cells in the granulation tissue at seven days post-MI; D. In scar tissue of a few months post-MI, MMP-1 is confined to fibroblast-like cells, suggesting that this enzyme is involved in the remodeling of the scar. (Scale bar represents 100 µm in panel A, and 20 µm in panels B–D.)

ingly expressed and activated in several pathological conditions of the heart [35–41]. Figure 1 illustrates that MMPs are abundantly present in the human infarcted myocardium, where MMP-9 immunoreactivity is largely confined to invading inflammatory cells and MMP-1 is located in a wider range of cell types in granulation and scar tissue. Others have demonstrated increased expression and activity of MMP-1, -2, -3 and -9 as well in infarcted rat and porcine hearts [42–47]. Although the data on the exact time-course of post-infarction myocardial MMP activity is diverse, it becomes more and more clear that MMP activation starts early (< 1 day post MI) [44]. TIMPs are normally in delicate balance with the MMPs, but a loss of TIMP-mediated inhibitory control has also been reported to occur in several cardiac pathologies [39, 40, 48, 49].

Pharmacological inhibition of MMPs attenuates LV remodeling

The role of MMPs during the healing and remodeling process of the left ventricle after myocardial infarction is being clarified in studies using broad range MMP inhibitors and genetically modified mice. In 1999, it was first demonstrated by Rohde et al. that *in vivo* MMP inhibition attenuates early LV dilatation, four days after experimental MI in mice [50]. Our laboratory has studied the effects of a broad range MMP inhibitor on LV remodeling as well, and we also found a significant reduction in LV dilatation, at one and two weeks post-MI in mice [51]. In another study, Lindsey et al. demonstrated that MMP inhibitor treatment attenuated LV dilatation four weeks post-MI in rabbits [52]. However, the latter study did not observe a reduction in LV dilatation in the early phase post-MI as was seen in the study of Rohde et al., but exclusively at the four weeks timepoint. The use of a selective MMP inhibitor (a broad range MMP inhibitor that did not inhibit MMP-1), the fact that treatment was started at different timepoints after MI, or the species differences might have accounted for the discrepancy in results between these two studies. Together, these studies have implicated the MMP family as potential mediators of cardiac dilatation and progression to heart failure, and have emerged MMP inhibitors as a therapeutic strategy to improve LV remodeling following MI. That MMP inhibition may not only be beneficial in the setting of MI has been demonstrated by the group of Spinale et al., who reported that MMP inhibitor treatment also attenuates the development of congestive heart failure in an experimental model of rapid cardiac pacing in pigs and in hypertensive rats [53, 54].

Besides this reduction in LV dilatation, MMP inhibitor treatment also resulted in a delay in infarct healing, clearly evidenced by larger necrotic areas (56%), thicker infarcted walls (32%), lower cell densities (37%) and a reduction in the deposition of collagen (68%) in the mouse heart, at one and two weeks post-MI [51]. Delayed wound healing by MMP inhibition has also been demonstrated in vascular and dermal wounds, where MMP activity facilitated the migration of inflammatory cells and smooth muscle cells into the wound [5, 55, 56]. The inhibitory effects of MMP inhibition on collagen deposition may seem paradoxical, since it may be expected that MMP inhibition reduces collagen degradation and thus promotes collagen accumulation. An inhibitory effect of MMP inhibition on collagen deposition is however not new, since MMP inhibitor treatment has comparable effects during neointima formation [56]. There are several possible explanations for these effects of MMP inhibition. First, the delay in healing reduced the migration of myofibroblast-like cells into the infarct. Since myofibroblasts are the main cell type responsible for collagen synthesis, a lower number of myofibroblasts may result in a reduction of collagen deposition. Second, MMPs may interfere in other pathways than ECM degradation, that are active during the repair process of the heart. In this view, MMPs regulate the activity of certain growth factors, like TNF-α, TGF-β and IL-1 [8, 57]. Decreased activity of TGF-β might reduce the synthesis of new collagen fibers [58].

An important role for MMP-9 in post-infarction remodeling

The particular importance of MMP-9 activity during infarct healing and LV remodeling has recently been demonstrated in two studies. In the first study, Heymans et al. reported that MMP-9 deficiency in mice retarded the wound healing process after myocardial infarction, which was demonstrated by a reduced leukocyte influx into the infarct and by larger residual necrotic areas [59]. In addition, that study demonstrated that lack of proteolytic activity of MMP-9 almost completely protected against infarct rupture, an acute and usually fatal event after MI. The significance of MMP-9 activity in early infarct healing and rupture was emphasized by the observation that MMP-9 was predominantly found in leukocytes and macrophages and that its activity peaked around day two, the period in which most of the ruptures occur. This indicates that by degrading matrix molecules, MMP-9 allows inflammatory cells to infiltrate the infarct and to disrupt the collagen network, a prerequisite for cardiac rupture [60]. In the second study, Ducharme et al. demonstrated that targeted deletion of MMP-9 attenuated LV dilatation as well, at 15 days post-MI [61]. Limited LV dilatation was accompanied with a reduced inflammatory response and a decrease in collagen deposition in the infarct of MMP-9 deficient mice. Interestingly, these MMP-9 null mice had increased expression of MMP-3 and MMP-13 in ventricular tissue compared to the wild-types. This indicates that compensatory up-regulation of other MMPs with possible overlapping MMP substrates should be taken into consideration when interpreting MMP deletion experiments [62].

Increased MMP activity induces LV dilatation

A causal relationship between proteolytic activity, architectural remodeling of the heart and cardiac performance has also been demonstrated by studying the consequences of increased MMP activity, especially in transgenic mice overexpressing myocardial MMP-1 (an interstitial collagenase that is normally absent in the mouse genome) and in TIMP-1$^{-/-}$ deficient mice. At an age of six months, the MMP-1 transgenic mice exhibited left ventricular hypertrophy and hypercontractility, while at an age of 12 months these mice displayed a loss of cardiac interstitial collagen, coincident with marked LV dilatation and systolic dysfunction [63]. TIMP-1 deficient mice developed an increase in LV end-diastolic volume and mass by four months of age, indicating that TIMP-1-mediated inhibitory control of MMP activity is necessary for the maintenance of LV myocardial geometry [64].

Polymorphisms in MMP genes

Interestingly, in the promoters of MMP-1, MMP-3, MMP-7, MMP-9 and MMP-12 polymorphisms have been identified that influence MMP gene expression [65]. These observations also indicate that variations in the levels of MMP transcription in patients suffering from myocardial infarction might contribute to differences in infarct healing, LV remodeling and the transition to end-stage heart failure or cardiac rupture. Polymorphisms in MMP-3, MMP-7, MMP-9 and MMP-12 have already been associated with susceptibility to cardiovascular diseases such as coronary artery disease and abdominal aortic aneurysms [65–67]. Further research is needed to identify a possible correlation between the progression to heart failure and MMP polymorphisms. The observation that levels of MMPs and TIMPs are altered in the serum of patients after myocardial infarction has raised the possibility that MMP/TIMP levels could predict clinical outcome [68, 69]. Correlations of serum TIMP-1 levels with LV end systolic volumes and with LV ejection fractions have already been found [68].

The plasminogen system as a regulatory system for MMP activity in the heart

Plasmin, one of the serine proteases, is the active enzyme of the plasminogen system and degrades a variety of ECM components. A relevant feature of plasmin is the proteolytic amplification that can be achieved by activating several MMPs [70]. The generation of plasmin is primarily controlled by the balance between the plasminogen activators (tPA and uPA) and their physiological inhibitors, the plasminogen activator inhibitors (PAIs). Two recent studies identified the plasminogen system as an important regulatory system in the onset of cardiac wound healing after myocardial infarction. In a study from our laboratory it was demonstrated that infarct healing was virtually abolished in plasminogen deficient (Plg$^{-/-}$) mice, until at least five weeks after MI [71]. In the second study, Heymans et al. demonstrated that uPA deficiency or adenoviral PAI-1 overexpression, but not tPA or uPAR deficiency resulted in impaired cardiac healing. In addition, this delay in infarct healing in uPA deficient mice or after adenoviral PAI-1 overexpression, protected against cardiac rupture [59]. Three distinct observations strongly suggest that the effects of plasminogen and uPA deficiency are mediated by reduced activation of MMPs. First, uPA was co-expressed with MMP-9 in infiltrating leukocytes [59]. Second, MMP activity was reduced in both uPA$^{-/-}$ and Plg$^{-/-}$ infarcts. And third, MMP inhibition by pharmacological tools has comparable, although less pronounced effects on infarct healing and cardiac rupture as uPA/plasminogen deficiency. It is however surprising that LV dilatation was not attenuated in these scarless Plg$^{-/-}$ or uPA$^{-/-}$ infarcted hearts, since this was a prominent effect seen after MMP inhibitor treatment. Besides degrading ECM components and activating MMPs, which are essential conditions for cell migration, the plasminogen system may act through other mechanisms. In this regard, plasmin can activate or liberate growth factors from the ECM. For example, TGF-β1, a potent inhibitor of cell proliferation and a mediator of collagen deposition, is activated by plasmin [72]. Reduced activation of latent TGF-β1 was indeed found in four day old infarcts of uPA deficient mice, indicating that the downstream pathway of the plasminogen system in infarct healing also includes the activation of TGF-β1.

These findings with respect to components of the plasminogen system may indicate that increased expression of plasminogen or uPA may predispose to cardiac rupture, whereas increased levels of PAI-1 may be protective [59]. On the other hand, as the principle inhibitor of fibrinolysis, it has been reported that high PAI-1 levels may accelerate the atherosclerotic process by allowing fibrin deposition and thrombosis within developing lesions. So far, epidemiological studies have related increased levels of PAI-1, due to genetic or metabolic determinants, to atherothrombosis [73].

MMP inhibitors as a new therapy for heart failure

The positive effects of MMP inhibition on LV dilatation in animal models led to the proposal to use MMP inhibitors as a potential therapy for patients at risk for the development of heart failure after MI. Although the promising results in animal studies encourage the design of clinical trails with MMP inhibitors, several issues have to be studied more extensively. First, the precise effect of MMP inhibitor treatment on cardiac function has to be studied more exensively. Second, the timing of MMP inhibitor administration after infarction has to be resolved and third, the choice between narrow *versus* broad range MMP inhibitiors has to be made.

With respect to evaluation of cardiac function after MMP inhibitor treatment, most studies used short-axis echocardiography to study cardiac function in infarcted mice. Recent advances in conductance technology allows us to measure left ventricular pressure-volume loops in the mouse heart. This technique, which can be used in closed thorax preparations will probably be critical for the assesment of cardiac function in MMP inhibitor treated or MMP knock-out mice [74]. Although the mouse-infarct model is an excellent model to initially study the effects of pharmacological agents on cardiac function and LV remodeling, it will be nessecary to evaluate the effects in other species before extrapolation to humans.

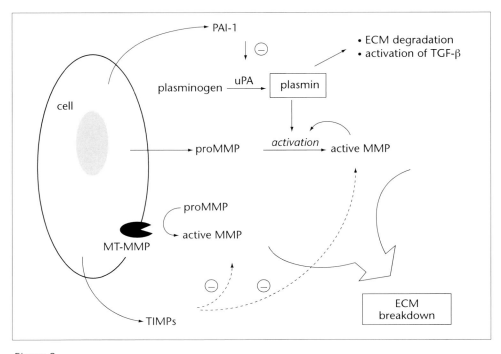

Figure 2
Regulation of extracellular matrix degradation in the infarcted heart.
Circulating plasminogen is cleaved by urokinase plasminogen activator (uPA), to form pro-
teolytic active plasmin. Besides degrading several ECM components directly, plasmin is
involved in the activation of latent MMPs and regulates the activation and/or liberation of
growth factors (such as TGF-β) from the ECM. The activity of uPA and MMPs is tightly con-
trolled by their endogenous inhibitors: PAIs and TIMPs.

With respect to the timing of the MMP inhibitor administration, one should keep in mind that some of the animal studies described above started drug delivery before induction of the infarct. In patients, in which MMP inhibitors are to be given after infarction by definition, the positive effect on LV dilatation might be smaller, since early infarct expansion might not be prevented.

Selective *versus* broad range MMP inhibition is another important, yet unresolved issue with respect to the possible treatment of heart failure. Broad-range MMP inhibition might be favorable to achieve maximal effects on ECM degradation. However, possible disadvantages of broad-range MMP inhibition include negative side-effects such as musculoskeletal toxicity, as seen after treatment with marimastat [75]. With respect to the important role of MMPs in physiological processes, broad range MMP inhibition might affect normal tissue as well. Selective inhibition of one or a few carefully chosen MMPs might be better in this regard. Inhibition of a single MMP will probably be of little therapeutic value because it is known that heart failure is associated with an elevation of multiple MMPs. The issue of selective *versus* broad range MMP inhibition has been addressed in other fields of research as well. In dermal wound healing, selective inhibition of MMPs seems desirable, because non-specific MMP inhibition would most likely impair re-epithelialization, due to inhibition of MMP-1. Inhibition of MMP-13 would be more favorable in dermal wound healing, since MMP-13 has been held responsible for the degradation of Type I and III collagen and may play a role in the pathogenesis of chronic cutaneous wounds [76]. In cancer research, selective inhibition of the gelatinases (MMP-2 and MMP-9) has been demonstrated to prevent tumor growth and invasion [77]. Extrapolated from gene-targeting studies in mice, MMP-9 might be one of the candidates for selective inhibition after myocardial infarction, since the deficiency in MMP-9 alone reduced LV chamber enlargement after infarction [61]. Furthermore, MMP-9 gene disruption also prevented fatal cardiac rupture to occur [59]. Although the synthesis of selective MMP inhibitors for all individual MMPs is currently a focus for many pharmaceutical companies, there is still a long way to go to meet this goal [78]. Tetracyclines are frequently as effective as other MMP inhibitors *in vivo* and their beneficial influence on ECM degradation can usually be achieved at remarkably low (nanomolar) concentrations. Although the mechanism of MMP inhibition seems to be different using tetracycline when compared to broad range MMP inhibitors, the clinical effect, i.e., decreased ECM degradation might be the same. In combination with their clinical availability, low cost and well-recognized safety profile, the use of tetracyclines appears to represent an ideal starting point for clinical studies on MMP-inhibition after myocardial infarction [79].

Conclusion

Some of the current therapies after myocardial infarction retard the development of heart failure. However, none of these therapies are able to prevent the LV expansion process completely. For this reason, additional therapy for these patients is desirable. Animal studies suggest that inhibition of myocardial MMP activity may be a promising therapeutic approach to slow down the time-course of the development of heart failure and dysfunction. Further research is needed to evaluate long-term effects of MMP inhibitor treatment after infarction, to resolve the issue of selective *versus* broad-range MMP inhibition and to evaluate the best time window for treatment.

Acknowledgements
This work has been supported by a grant from the Netherlands Heart Foundation (NHS 99.054).

References

1   Ross RS, Borg TK (2001) Integrins and the myocardium. *Circ Res* 88: 1112–1119
2   Park PW, Reizes O, Bernfield M (2000) Cell surface heparan sulfate proteoglycans: Selective regulators of ligand-receptor encounters. *J Biol Chem* 275: 29923–29926
3   Shalinsky DR, Brekken J, Zou H, McDermott CD, Forsyth P, Edwards D, Margosiak S, Bender S, Truitt G, Wood A et al (1999) Broad antitumor and antiangiogenic activities of AG3340, a potent and selective MMP inhibitor undergoing advanced oncology clinical trials. *Ann NY Acad Sci* 878: 236–270
4   Lewis EJ, Bishop J, Bottomley KMK, Bradshaw D, Brewster M, Broadhurst MJ, Brown PA, Budd JM, Elliott L, Greenham AK et al (1997) Ro 32-3555, and orally active collagenase inhibitor, prevents cartilage breakdown *in vitro* and *in vivo*. *Br J Pharmacol* 121: 540–546
5   Witte MB, Thornton FJ, Kiyama T, Efron DT, Schultz GS, Moldawer LL, Barbul A (1998) Metalloproteinase inhibitors and wound healing: A novel enhancer of wound strength. *Surgery* 124: 464–470
6   Galardy RE, Cassabonne ME, Giese C, Gilbert JH, Lapierre F, Lopez H, Schaefer ME, Stack R, Sullivan M, Summers B et al (1994) Low molecular weight inhibitors in corneal ulceration. *Ann NY Acad Sci* 732: 315–323
7   Sierevolgel MJ, Pasterkamp G, Velema E, de Jaegere PPT, de Smet BJGL, Verheijen JH, de Kleijn DPV, Borst C (2001) Oral matrix metalloproteinase inhibition and arterial remodeling after balloon dilation. *Circulation* 103: 302–306
8   Gearing AJH, Beckett P, Christodoulou M, Churchill M, Clements J, Davidson AH, Drummond AH, Galloway WA, Gilbert R, Gordon JL et al (1994) Processing of tumour necrosis factor-alpha precursor by metalloproteinases. *Nature* 370: 555–557
9   Levi E, Fridman R, Miao HQ, Ma YS, Yayon A, Vlodavsky I (1996) Matrix metalloproteinase 2 releases active soluble ectodomain of fibroblast growth factor receptor 1. *Proc Natl Acad Sci USA* 93: 7069–7074
10   Suzuki M, Raab G, Moses MA, Fernandez CA, Klagsbrun M (1997) Matrix metalloproteinase-3 releases active heparin-binding EGF-like growth factor by cleavage at a specific juxtamembrane site. *J Biol Chem* 272: 31730–31737
11   McGeehan GM, Becherer JD, Bast RC, Boyer CM, Champion B, Connolly KM, Conway JG, Furdon P, Karp S, Kidao S et al (1994) Regulation of tumour necrosis factor-alpha by a metalloproteinase inhibitor. *Nature* 370: 558–561
12   Yu Q, Stamenkovic I (2000) Cell surface-localized matrix metalloproteinase-9 proteolytically activates TGF-beta and promotes tumor invasion and angiogenesis. *Genes Dev* 14: 163–176
13   McQuibban GA, Gong JH, Tam EM, McCulloch CA, Clark-Lewis I, Overall CM (2000) Inflammation dampened by gelatinase A cleavage of monocyte chemoattractant protein-3. *Science* 289: 1202–1206
14   Parks WC, Shapiro SD (2001) Matrix metalloproteinases in lung biology. *Respir Res* 2: 10–19

15 Malik N, Greenfield BW, Wahl AF, Kiener PA (1996) Activation of human monocytes through CD40 induces matrix metalloproteinases. *J Immunol* 156: 3952–3960

16 Schonbeck U, Mach F, Sukhova GK, Murphy C, Bonnefoy JY, Fabunmi RP, Libby P (1997) Regulation of matrix metalloproteinase expression in human vascular smooth muscle cells by T lymphocytes. *Circ Res* 81: 448–454

17 Spinale FG, Coker ML, Heung LJ, Bond BR, Gunasinghe HR, Etoh T, Goldberg AT, Zellner JL, Crumbley J (2000) A matrix metalloproteinase induction/activation system exists in the human left ventricular myocardium and is upregulated in heart failure. *Circulation* 102: 1944–1949

18 Wassenaar A, Verschoor T, Kievits F, Den Hartog MT, Kapsenberg ML (1999) CD40 engagement modulates the production of matrix metalloproteinases by gingival fibroblasts. *Clin Exp Immunol* 115: 161–167

19 Mauviel A (1993) Cytokine regulation of metalloproteinase gene expression. *J Cell Biochem* 53: 288–295

20 Makela M, Salo T, Larjava H (1998) MMP-9 from TNF-alpha stimulated keratinocytes binds to cell membranes and Type I collagen: A cause for extended matrix degradation in inflammation. *Biochem Biophys Res Commun* 253: 325–335

21 Nagase H (1997) Activation mechanisms of matrix metalloproteinases. *Biol Chem* 378: 151–160

22 Murphy G, Willenbrock F, Crabbe T, O'Shea M, Ward R, Atkinson S, O'Connell J, Docherty A (1994) Regulation of matrix metalloproteinase activity. *Ann NY Acad Sci* 732: 31–41

23 Sato H, Takino T, Okada Y, Cao J, Shinagawa A, Yamamoto E, Seiki M (1994) A matrix metalloproteinase expressed on the surface of invasive tumour cells. *Nature* 370: 61–65

24 Sato H, Takino T, Kinoshita T, Imai K, Okada Y, Stetler Stevenson WG, Seiki M (1996) Cell surface binding and activation of gelatinase A induced by expression of membrane-type-1-matrix metalloproteinase (MT1-MMP). *FEBS Letts* 385: 238–240

25 Knauper V, Cowell S, Smith B, Lopez-Otin C, O'Shea M, Morris H, Zardi L, Murphy G (1997) The role of the C-terminal domain of human collagenase-3 (MMP-13) in the activation of procollagenase-3, substrate specifity, and tissue inhibitor of metalloproteinase interaction. *J Biol Chem* 272: 7608–7616

26 Pei D, Weiss SJ (1995) Furin-dependent intracellular activation of the human stromelysin-3 zymogen. Nature 375: 244–247

27 Sato H, Kinoshita T, Takino T, Nakayama K, Seiki M (1996) Activation of a recombinant membrane type1-matrix metalloproteinase (MT-MMP) by furin and its interaction with tissue inhibitor of metalloproteinases (TIMP)-2. *FEBS Letts* 393: 101–104

28 Hayakawa T, Yamashita K, Ohuchi E, Shinagawa A (1994) Cell growth-promoting activity of tissue inhibitor of metalloproteinases-2 (TIMP-2). *J Cell Sci* 107: 2373–2379

29 Hayakawa T, Yamashita K, Tanzawa K, Uchijima E, Iwata K (1992) Growth-promoting activity of tissue inhibitor of metalloproteinases-1 (TIMP-1) for a wide range of cells. A possible new growth factor in serum. *FEBS Letts* 298: 29–32

30 Thorgeirsson UP, Yoshiji H, Sinha CC, Gomez DE (1996) Breast cancer, tumor neovas-

culature and the effect of tissue inhibitor of metalloproteinases-1 (TIMP-1) on angiogenesis. *In Vivo* 10: 137–144

31 Fata JE, Leco KJ, Voura EB, Yu HY, Waterhouse P, Murphy G, Moorehead RA, Khokha R (2001) Accelerated apoptosis in the Timp-3-deficient mammary gland. *J Clin Invest* 108: 831–841

32 Liu YE, Wang M, Greene J, Su J, Ullrich S, Li H, Sheng S, Alexander P, Sang QA, Shi YE (1997) Preparation and characterization of recombinant tissue inhibitor of metalloproteinase 4 (TIMP-4). *J Biol Chem* 272: 20479–20483

33 Greene J, Wang M, Liu YE, Raymond LA, Rosen C, Shi YE (1996) Molecular cloning and characterization of human tissue inhibitor of metalloproteinase 4. *J Biol Chem* 271: 30375–30380

34 Montfort I, Perez-Tamayo R (1975) The distribution of collagenase in normal rat tissues. *J Histochem Cytochem* 23: 910–920

35 Tyagi SC, Matsubara L, Weber KT (1993) Direct extraction and estimation of collagenase(s) activity by zymography in microquantities of rat myocardium and uterus. *Clin Biochem* 26: 191–198

36 Coker MS, Thomas CV, Doscher MA (1997) Matrix metalloproteinase expression and activity in adult ventricular myocytes: influence of basement membrane adhesion. *Circulation* 96: I–689

37 Tyagi SC, Kumar S, Voelker DJ, Reddy HK, Janicki JS, Curtis JJ (1996) Differential gene expression of extracellular matrix components in dilated cardiomyopathy. *J Cell Biochem* 63: 185–198

38 Spinale FG, Coker ML, Thomas CV, Walker JD, Mukherjee R, Hebbar L (1998) Time-dependent changes in matrix metalloproteinase activity and expression during the progression of congestive heart failure. *Circ Res* 82: 482–495

39 Thomas CV, Coker ML, Zellner JL, Handy JR, Crumbley AJ, Spinale FG (1998) Increased matrix metalloproteinase activity and selective up-regulation in LV myocardium from patients with end-stage dilated cardiomyopathy. *Circulation* 97: 1708–1715

40 Li YY, Feldman AM, Sun Y, McTiernan CF (1998) Differential expression of tissue inhibitors of metalloproteinases in the failing human heart. *Circulation* 98: 1728–1734

41 Coker ML, Thomas CV, Clair MJ, Hendrick JW, Krombach RS, Galis ZS, Spinale FG (1998) Myocardial matrix metalloproteinase activity and abundance with congestive heart failure. *Am J Physiol* 43: H1516–H1523

42 Tyagi SC, Kumar SG, Haas SJ, Reddy HK, Voelker DJ, Hayden MR, Demmy TL, Schmaltz RA, Curtis JJ (1996) Post-transcriptional regulation of extracellular regulation of extracellular matrix metalloproteinase in human heart end-stage failure secondary to ischemic cardiomyopathy. *J Mol Cell Cardiol* 28: 1415–1428

43 Cleutjens JPM, Kandala JC, Guarda E, Guntaka RV, Weber KT (1994) Regulation of collagen degradation in the rat myocardium after infarction. *J Mol Cell Cardiol* 27: 1281–1292

44 Herzog E, Gu A, Kohmoto T, Burkhoff D, Hochman JS (1998) Early activation of met-

alloproteinases after experimental myocardial infarction occurs in infarct and non-infarct zones. *Cardiovasc Pathol* 7: 307–312

45 Carlyle WC, Jacobson AW, Judd DL, Tian B, Chu C, Hauer KM, Hartman MM, McDonald KM (1997) Delayed reperfusion alters matrix metalloproteinase activity and fibronectin mRNA expression in the infarct zone of the ligated rat heart. *J Mol Cell Cardiol* 29: 2451–2463

46 Sato S, Ashraf M, Millard RW, Fujiwara H, Schwartz A (1983) Connective tissue changes in early ischemia of porcine myocardium: An ultrastructural study. *J Mol Cell Cardiol* 15: 261–275

47 Danielsen CC, Wiggers H, Andersen HR (1998) Increased amounts of collagenase and gelatinase in porcine myocardium following ischemia and reperfusion. *J Mol Cell Cardiol* 30: 1431–1442

48 Peterson JT, Li H, Dillon L, Bryant JW (2000) Evolution of matrix metalloprotease and tissue inhibitor expression during heart failure progression in the infarcted rat. *Cardiovasc Res* 46: 307–315

49 Tyagi SC, Campbell SE, Reddy HK, Tjahja E, Voelker DJ (1996) Matrix metalloproteinase activity expression in infarcted, noninfarcted and dilated cardiomyopathic human hearts. *Mol Cell Biochem* 155: 13–21

50 Rohde LE, Ducharme A, Arroyo LH, Aikawa M, Sukhova GH, Lopez-Anaya A, McClure KF, Mitchell PG, Libby P, Lee RT (1999) Matrix metalloproteinase inhibition attenuates early left ventricular enlargement after experimental myocardial infarction in mice. *Circulation* 99: 3063–3070

51 Creemers EEJM, Cleutjens JPM, Smits JFM, Daemen MJAP (1999) Inhibition of matrix metalloproteinase (MMP) activity in mice reduces LV remodeling and depresses cardiac function after myocardial infarction. *Circulation* 100: I–250

52 Lindsey ML, Gannon J, Aikawa M, Schoen FJ, Rabkin E, Lopresti-Morrow L, Crawford J, Black S, Libby P, Mitchell PG et al (2002) Selective matrix metalloproteinase inhibition reduces left ventricular remodeling but does not inhibit angiogenesis after myocardial infarction. *Circulation* 105: 753–758

53 Peterson JT, Hallak H, Johnson L, Li H, O'Brien PM, Sliskovic DR, Bocan TMA, Coker ML, Etoh T, Spinale FG (2001) Matrix metalloproteinase inhibition attenuates left ventricular remodeling and dysfunction in a rat model of progressive heart failure. *Circulation* 103: 2303–2309

54 Spinale FG, Coker ML, Krombach SR, Mukherjee R, Hallak H, Houck WV, Clair MJ, Kribbs SB, Johnson LL, Peterson JT et al (1999) Matrix metalloproteinase inhibition during the development of congestive heart failure: effects on left ventricular dimensions and function. *Circ Res* 85: 364–376

55 Bendeck MP, Irvin C, Reidy MA (1996) Inhibition of matrix metalloproteinase activity inhibits smooth muscle cell migration but not neointimal thickening after arterial injury. *Circ Res* 78: 38–43

56 Strauss BH, Robinson R, Batchelor WB, Chisholm RJ, Ravi G, Natarajan MK, Logan RA, Mehta SR, Levy DE, Ezrin AM, et al. (1996) *In vivo* collagen turnover following

experimental balloon angioplasty injury and the role of matrix metalloproteinases. *Circ Res* 79: 541–550

57 Schonbeck U, Mach F, Libby P (1998) Generation of biologically active IL-1 beta by matrix metalloproteinases: A novel caspase-1-independent pathway of IL-1 beta processing. *J Immunol* 161: 3340–3346

58 Narayanan AS, Page RC, Swanson J (1989) Collagen synthesis by human fibroblasts. Regulation by transforming growth factor-beta in the presence of other inflammatory mediators. *Biochem J* 260: 463–469

59 Heymans S, Luttun A, Nuyens D, Theilmeier G, Creemers E, Moons L, Dyspersin GD, Cleutjens JPM, Shipley M, Angellilo A et al (1999) Inhibition of plasminogen activators or matrix metalloproteinases prevent cardiac rupture but impairs therapeutic angiogenesis and causes cardiac failure. *Nat Med* 10: 1135–1142

60 Przyklenk K, Connelly CM, McLaughlin RJ, Kloner RA, Apstein CS (1987) Effect of myocyte necrosis on strenght, strain, and stiffness of isolated myocardial strips. *Am Heart J* 114: 1349–1359

61 Ducharme A, Frantz S, Aikawa M, Rabkin E, Lindsey M, Rohde LE, Schoen FJ, Kelly RA, Werb Z, Libby P et al (2000) Targeted deletion of matrix metalloproteinase-9 attenuates left ventricular enlargement and collagen accumulation after experimental myocardial infarction. *J Clin Invest* 106: 55–62

62 Lee RT (2001) Matrix metalloproteinase inhibition and the prevention of heart failure. *Trends Cardiovasc Med* 11: 202–205

63 Kim HE, Dalal SS, Young E, Legato MJ, Weisfeldt ML, D'Armiento J (2000) Disruption of the myocardial extracellular matrix leads to cardiac dysfunction. *J Clin Invest* 106: 857–866

64 Roten L, Nemoto S, Simsic J, Coker ML, Rao V, Baicu S, Defreyte G, Soloway PJ, Zile MR, Spinale FG (2000) Effects of gene deletion of the tissue inhibitor of the matrix metalloproteinase-type 1 (TIMP-1) on left ventricular geometry and function in mice. *J Mol Cell Cardiol* 32: 109–120

65 Ye S (2000) Polymorphism in matrix metalloproteinase gene promotors: Implication in regulation of gene expression and susceptibility of various diseases. *Matrix Biol* 19: 623–629

66 Zhang B, Ye S, Herrmann SM, Eriksson P, de Maat M, Evans A, Arveiler D, Luc G, Cambien F, Hamsten A et al (1999) Functional polymorphism in the regulatory region of gelatinase B gene in relation to severity of coronary atherosclerosis. *Circulation* 99: 1788

67 Jormsjo S, Whatling C, Walter DH, Zeiher AM, Hamsten A, Eriksson P (2001) Allele-specific regulation of matrix metalloproteinase-7 promoter activity is associated with coronary artery luminal dimensions among hypercholesterolemic patients. *Arterioscler Thromb Vasc Biol* 21: 1834–1839

68 Hirohata S, Kusachi S, Murakami M, Murakami T, Sano I, Watanabe T, Komatsubara I, Kondo J, Tsuji T (1997) Time dependent alterations of serum matrix metallopro-

teinase-1 and metalloproteinase-1 tissue inhibitor after succesful reperfusion of myocardial infarction. *Heart* 78: 278–284

69   Kai H, Ikeda H, Yasukawa H, Kai M, Seki Y, Kuwahara F, Ueno T, Sugi K, Imaizumi T (1998) Peripheral blood levels of matrix metalloproteinase-2 and -9 are elevated in patients with acute coronary syndromes. *J Am Coll Cardiol* 32: 368–372

70   Carmeliet P, Moons L, Lijnen R, Baes M, Lemaitre V, Tipping P, Drew A, Eeckhout Y, Shapiro S, Lupu F et al (1997) Urokinase-generated plasmin activates matrix metalloproteinases during aneurysm formation. *Nat Gen* 17: 439–444

71   Creemers EEJM, Cleutjens J, Smits J, Heymans S, Moons L, Collen D, Daemen M, Carmeliet P (2000) Disruption of the plasminogen gene in mice abolishes wound healing after myocardial infarction. *Am J Pathol* 156: 1865–1873

72   Keski-Oja J, Lyons RM, Moses HL (1987) Inactive secreted forms of transforming growth factor-beta: activation by proteolysis. *J Cell Biochem* 11a: 60

73   Lijnen HR, Collen D (1989) Congenital and acquired deficiencies of components of the fibrinolytic system and their relation to bleeding and thrombosis. *Fibrinolysis* 3: 67–77

74   Feldman MD, Erikson JM, Mao Y, Korcarz CE, Lang RM, Freeman GL (2000) Validation of a mouse conductance system to determine LV volume: Comparison to echocardiography and crystals. *Am J Physiol Heart Circ Physiol* 279: H1698–H1707

75   Drummond AH, Beckett P, Brown PD, Bone EA, Davidson AH, Galloway WA, Gearing AJH, Huxley P, Laber L, McCourt M et al (1999) Preclinical and clinical studies of MMP inhibitors in cancer. *Ann NY Acad Sci* 878: 228–235

76   Vaalamo M, Mattila L, Johansson N, Kariniemi AL, Karjalainen-Lindsberg ML, Kahari VM, Saarialho-Kere U (1997) Distinct populations of stromal cells express collagenase-3 (MMP-13) and collagenase-1 (MMP-1) in chronic ulcers but not in normally healing wounds. *J Invest Dermatol* 109: 96–101

77   Koivunen E, Arap W, Valtanen H, Rainisalo A, Medina OP, Heikkila P, Kantor C, Gahmberg CG, Salo T, Konttinen YT et al (1999) Tumor targeting with a selective gelatinase inhibitor. *Nature* 17: 768–774

78   Carney DE, Lutz CJ, Picone AL, Gatto LA, Ramamurthy NS, Golub LM, Simon SR, Searles B, Paskanik A, Snyder K et al (1999) Matrix metalloproteinase inhibitor prevents acute lung injury after cardiopulmonary bypass. *Circulation* 100: 400–406

79   Brown PD (1998) Synthetic inhibitors of matrix metalloproteinases. In: Parks WC, Mecham RP (eds): *Matrix metalloproteinases*. Academic Press, San Diego,CA, pp 243–261

80   Jugdutt BI, Khan MI (1992) Impact of increased infarct transmurality on remodeling and function during healing after anterior myocardial infarction in the dog. *Can J Physiol Pharmacol* 70: 949–958

81   Weisman HF, Bush DE, Mannisi JA, Weisfeldt ML, Healy B (1988) Cellular mechanisms of myocardial expansion. *Circulation* 78: 186–201

82   Whittaker P, Boughner DR, Kloner RA (1991) Role of collagen in acute myocardial infarct expansion. *Circulation* 84: 2123–2134

Matrix metalloproteinases in heart failure: evidence from experimental models

Francis G. Spinale

Cardiothoracic Surgery, Room 625, Strom Thurmond Research Building, 770 MUSC Complex, Medical University of South Carolina, 114 Doughty Street, Charleston, SC 29425, USA

Introduction

The LV myocardial remodeling process invariably occurs with the development and progression of congestive heart failure (CHF). LV remodeling is a multi-cellular process that results in abnormalities in LV myocardial wall structure and chamber geometry. It is becoming appreciated that important changes occur within the extra-cellular matrix (ECM) of the myocardium and can contribute to the LV remodeling process. Moreover, it has become increasingly evident that the myocardial ECM is not a static structure, but rather a dynamic entity that may play a fundamental role in myocardial adaptation to a pathological stress and thereby facilitate remodeling. Specifically, in both human and animal studies, it has been reported that alterations in the collagen interface, both in structure and composition, occur within the LV myocardium, which in turn may influence LV geometry [1–5]. The myocardial ECM contains a fibrillar collagen network, a basement membrane, proteoglycans and gly-cosaminoglycans, and bioactive signaling molecules. The myocardial fibrillar collagens such as collagen Types I and III, ensure structural integrity of adjoining myocytes, provide the means by which myocyte shortening is translated into over-all LV pump function and are essential for maintaining alignment of myofibrils within the myocyte through a collagen-integrin-cytoskeletal-myofibril relation. The ECM forms a continuum between different cell types within the myocardium and provides a structural supporting network in order to maintain myocardial geometry during the cardiac cycle. Specific and distinct changes occur within the ECM with each of the three main cardiac disease states which give rise to CHF: Myocardial infarction, severe LV hypertrophy, and the cardiomyopathies. The identification and understanding of the enzyme systems responsible for changes within the ECM with each of these three cardiac disease states would likely yield important insights into the basis for the initiation and progression of CHF. One proteolytic system within the myocardium that likely contributes to ECM remodeling is the matrix metallo-proteinases (MMPs) [6–22]. Changes in MMP abundance and activity have been identified in animal models of MI, hypertrophy, and cardiomyopathy (7–9, 11–24].

Inflammation and Cardiac Diseases, edited by Giora Z. Feuerstein, Peter Libby and Douglas L. Mann
© 2003 Birkhäuser Verlag Basel/Switzerland

A clear cause/effect relationship between MMPs and the LV remodeling process has been demonstrated through the use of animal models of developing CHF, transgenic models, as well as through the use of pharmacological MMP inhibition studies. The purpose of this chapter is to review these studies and place these findings in context with the LV remodeling process and the progression to CHF.

The matrix metalloproteinases and tissue inhibitors

MMP structure and function

The MMPs have been demonstrated to play a pivotal role in normal tissue remodeling processes such as tissue morphogenesis and wound healing [25–30]. This proteolytic system degrades a wide spectrum of ECM proteins and is constitutively expressed in a large number of cell and tissue types. While MMPs likely play important roles in normal tissue remodeling, increased MMP expression has been identified in pathological processes such as tumor angiogenesis and metastasis, rheumatoid arthritis, vascular neointimal hyperplasia, and plaque rupture. The MMPs constitute a family of zinc-dependent enzymes that currently number over 25 species [25–30]. There are two principle types of MMPs; those which are secreted into the extracellular space and those which are membrane bound [25–31]. The secreted MMPs comprise the majority of known MMP species and are released into the extracellular space in a latent or pro-enzyme state (proMMP). Activation of these latent MMPs can be achieved through enzymatic cleavage of the pro-peptide domain. There is a significant degree of homology within the catalytic domain of MMP species, and substrate specificity is determined by the large extracellular binding domain at the C terminus of the enzyme [25, 26]. The classification of MMPs was originally determined by substrate specificity, but as the characterization of this enzyme system has proceeded, a great deal of substrate cross-over between MMP classes and species has been identified. Nevertheless, a general classification and numbering scheme has been developed for the MMPs and a comprehensive table can be consulted from several recent comprehensive reviews [14, 25–32]. Representative MMPs which will be discussed in the context of animal models of heart failure are presented in Table 1.

MMP endogenous inhibitory control

The activated MMPs undergo auto-catalysis resulting in lower molecular weight forms and ultimately inactive protein fragments. Another important control point of MMP activity is through the presence of an endogenous class of low molecular weight molecules called tissue inhibitors of the MMPs (TIMPs). Four different

Table 1 - Classes of MMPs which have been identified within the myocardium
There are over 25 MMPs which have been identified to date and this list is not inclusive. The
MMP numbering and nomenclature is shown along with ECM substrates.

Name	Number	Substrate/Function
Collagenases		
Interstitial collagenase	MMP-1	Collagens I, II, III, VII and basement membrane components
Collagenase 3	MMP-13	Collagens I, II, III
Gelatinases		
Gelatinase A	MMP-2	Gelatins, collagens I, IV, V, VII and basement membrane components
Gelatinase B	MMP-9	Gelatins, collagens IV, V, XIV and basement membrane components
Stromelysins		
Stromelysin 1	MMP-3	Fibronectin, laminin, collagens III, IV, IX, and MMP activation
Membrane-type MMPs		
MT1-MMP	MMP-14	Collagens I, II, III, fibronectin, laminin-1: activates proMMP-2 and proMMP-13

TIMP species have been identified and bind to activated MMPs in a 1:1 stoichio-metric ratio. Furthermore, certain TIMPs bind to proMMPs and thereby form MMP-TIMP complexes. The functional significance of these proMMP-TIMP complexes remains incompletely understood, but may actually facilitate MMP activation [26]. One of the better characterized TIMPs is TIMP-1 which binds with great affinity to activated MMPs. TIMP-4 appears to have a predominant distribution within the myocardium.

Myocardial MMPs in animal models – proof of concept

MMP/TIMPs in models of myocardial infarction

An extensive body of research has been formulated regarding the LV remodeling process through the use of rodent models of myocardial infarction (MI) [3, 4, 9, 12–14, 16, 33]. Most notably are the studies by Pfeffer which demonstrated that inhibition of angiotensin-converting enzyme could modify the extent of LV remodeling following MI induction in rats [33]. These past studies emphasized the importance of identifying cellular and extracellular mechanisms which contribute to the LV remodeling process. Post-MI remodeling comprises a dynamic set of structural events occurring within the MI region as well as in the remote, viable myocardium. Investigators at the Research Institute in Maastricht reported that important changes occurred in the ECM following the induction of MI in rats and mice [3, 12, 14]. In additional studies, this group identified that regional changes in MMP and TIMP levels occurred following MI induction in the rat and that the balance between MMP/TIMP levels likely contribute to the rate and degree of ECM remodeling post-MI [14]. In a study by Peterson and colleagues, it was demonstrated that a temporally distinct set of myocardial MMPs were induced in the post-MI rat model [15]. Early post-MI (less than 14 days), increased myocardial levels of the interstitial collagenases MMP-13 and MMP-8 were observed as well as the gelatinase MMP-9. An important source for MMP-8 and MMP-9 is the neutrophil, and therefore the increased levels of these particular MMPs is likely reflective of the acute inflammatory/wound healing response. With longer post-MI periods, myocardial levels of these particular MMP species returned to relative basal levels, and other MMP species began to emerge. Most notably, MT1-MMP, or MMP-14 was increased late in the post-MI period and was temporally associated with significant LV remodeling. Specifically, the induction of MT1-MMP was associated with adverse remodeling in both the MI zone (expansion) and the viable regions (wall thinning and dilation). These observations suggest that there is temporal pattern of MMPs that are induced in the post-MI period and that the functional role of these MMP profiles with respect to the remodeling process may be distinctly different. Specifically, the increased levels of certain MMPs in the early post-MI period facilitate ECM degradation and initial wound healing, whereas the emergence of other MMPs in the later post-MI period contribute to adverse, or maladaptive LV remodeling.

Using transgenic mouse constructs, the mechanistic importance of MMP activation in the early MI wound healing response has been established [9, 12–14]. For example, in plasminogen-deficient mice, impaired scar formation and alterations in the normal wound healing response was observed following MI when compared to wild-type mice [12]. Since plasmin is a serine protease capable of local activation of MMPs, these investigators postulated that a loss of early MMP activation following MI interfered with ECM degradation and the ingress of inflammatory cells. In fact, it was demonstrated that the degree of cellular infiltrate and ECM degradation was significantly lower in the plasminogen-deficient mice when compared to wild-type mice. Furthermore, the relative degree of angiogenesis within the MI region also appeared impaired in the plasmin deficient mice. In additional studies using this model system, it was observed that plasminogen and MMP-9 were co-expressed in infiltrating neutrophils and lymphocytes [14]. It was also reported that MMP-9 zymographic activity was reduced in plasminogen deficient mice in the early post-MI period when compared to wild type mice. Using a transgenic mouse with targeted gene deletion of MMP-9, Ducharme and colleagues reported alterations in the time-course and composition of the post-MI remodeling process [13]. Specifically, in MMP-9-deficient mice, the relative degree of macrophage deposition and collagen accumulation within the MI region was reduced relative to sibling wild-type mice. These observations suggest that MMP-9 plays an important role in the maturation phase of MI scar formation. Thus, these initial rodent studies demonstrated that early activation of certain MMPs, such as MMP-9 are essential components of the initial reparative response post-MI. Furthermore, these rodent studies have also demonstrated persistent activation of certain myocardial MMPs following resolution of the initial wound healing response, as well as the emergence of other MMP species, particularly in the viable myocardium.

The primary approach for measuring MMP levels and by inference, MMP activity, is by tissue collection and processing. This provides a reasonable assessment of MMP species abundance, but disrupts normal tissue architecture and the interaction of other systems, such as TIMPs. As discussed in a subsequent section, orally-active compounds that inhibit MMP activity have been developed. However, pharmacokinetic studies and the development of proper dosing regimens will require assessment of MMP activity in the intact system. Accordingly, an important avenue of research and development with respect to MMP/TIMP biology is to directly assess proteolytic activity within the interstitium *in vivo*. Accordingly, a micro-dialysis method was developed by this laboratory in order to directly measure myocardial MMP activity in the intact animal [34]. The micro-dialysis probes allow for instillation of a caged fluorogenic "bait" protein into the interstitium and then sample the degree of MMP-dependent fluorescent activity. We deployed this calibrated and validated system to a pig model of acute MI. For the *in vivo* studies, the MMP substrate was infused for 60 minutes in order to reach equilibrium, and baseline interstitial MMP activity determined. A significant increase in myocardial interstitial MMP 2/9 activity was observed after 90 minutes of coronary occlusion within the MI region, but not in the remote region. There are a number of fluorogenic probes being developed that contain recognition sequences for specific MMPs. Thus, it may be possible to directly interrogate the activity of multiple MMPs within the myocardial interstitium. This approach may prove useful in temporally relating the local release of inflammatory mediators into the myocardial interstitium and MMP activation during and following MI.

MMP/TIMPs in models of cardiomyopathy

In a pacing LV failure animal model, a time dependent increase in myocardial MMP levels was demonstrated to accompany the progression of LV dilation and dysfunction [7, 8]. These changes in myocardial MMP levels were accompanied by alterations in ECM structure. Moreover, the increased MMP levels and myocardial remodeling preceded significant changes in isolated myocyte contractile dysfunction. These observations suggested that the induction of myocardial MMPs was an early event in the development of LV remodeling and pump dysfunction with chronic rapid pacing. In the Syrian cardiomyopathy hamster model, *in vitro* MMP activity was increased and noted to be particularly elevated in cardiomyopathic LV samples in which significant cardiac remodeling had occurred [35].

Alterations in MMP/TIMP levels in LV hypertrophy

An important cause of clinical heart failure is diastolic dysfunction secondary to LV hypertrophy. More specifically, LV hypertrophy can cause reduced myocardial compliance and thereby impede adequate filling during diastole. Abnormalities in the structure and the composition of the ECM have been demonstrated to contribute to myocardial compliance and in turn influence specific determinants of diastolic function [4]. Evidence exists to support the concept that diminished myocardial MMP activity can facilitate collagen accumulation in developing hypertrophy [24, 36]. In the Spontaneously Hypertensive Rat (SHR), the development of compensated hypertrophy is associated with increased myocardial TIMP levels; which would imply reduced MMP activity [24]. As the SHR model progresses to decompensation and LV failure, myocardial TIMP levels fall to below normal levels which would favor increased MMP activity [24, 36]. Thus, it is likely that a time-dependent spectrum of myocardial MMP activation occurs with the development of pressure overload hypertrophy and contributes to the overall remodeling process. In support of this postulate, studies completed by this laboratory demonstrated time-dependent changes in myocardial MMP levels following an acute and prolonged pressure overload stimulus [11]. In these studies, acute pressure overload induced myocardial MMP expression and resultant increase in zymographic activity. However, with a prolonged pressure overload, MMP zymographic activity began to normalize and was accompanied by changes in TIMP levels.

In volume overload states such as with mitral regurgitation or aorto-caval fistula, increased myocardial MMP levels and zymographic activity have been reported [11, 24]. For example, in a rat model of volume overload, increased myocardial MMP zymographic activity was associated with changes in LV volumes and mass [24]. These studies would suggest that the early induction of myocardial MMP activity occurs with an overload stimulus which in turn would alter extracellular myocyte support. These changes in extracellular fibrillar support and architecture would in turn facilitate alterations in myocyte size and geometry, which is the structural basis of hypertrophy.

Exogenous MMP inhibition modulates the LV remodeling process

Pharmacological MMP inhibition has been used in several animal models of LV dysfunction [8, 9, 12, 14, 15, 23, 32, 37, 38]. In the mouse MI model, MMP inhibition has been shown to reduce the degree of post-MI LV dilation [9, 14]. For example, Ducharme and colleagues demonstrated that the rate of LV chamber dilation was reduced in mice treated with MMP inhibition (Fig. 1) [14].

More recently, using a pig model of MI, this laboratory examined the effects of MMP inhibition upon regional and global remodeling for up to two months post-MI [37]. This study instituted MMP inhibition at five days post-MI in order to avoid interference with the initial wound healing response and continued treatment for up to two months. Using radio-opaque markers for serial assessment of regional geometry, it was demonstrated that the degree of infarct expansion and chamber dilation was reduced with MMP inhibition (Fig. 2).

These studies, as well as others, have clearly demonstrated that MMP inhibition alters the course of the adverse remodeling which occur post-MI.

In the chronic pacing model, MMP inhibition attenuated the degree of LV dilation that invariably occurs in this model [8]. Moreover, the degree of ECM disruption and disorganization which was observed in the untreated pacing CHF group was attenuated with MMP inhibition. In the Spontaneously Hypertensive Heart Failure (SHHF) rat model, MMP inhibition resulted in an attenuation of LV dilation and improved pump function [15]. In this model, the transition from a compensated LV hypertrophic state to LV dilation and dysfunction occurs during 9–13 months of age. Accordingly, SHHF rats were treated with a broad spectrum MMP inhibitor beginning at nine months of age and compared to age-matched untreated SHHF rats. As expected, significant LV dilation and myocardial remodeling occurred at 13 months of age in the SHHF rats compared to normal rats. However, MMP inhibition significantly attenuated the degree of LV dilation which occurred in this SHHF model. More recently, it has been demonstrated that MMI inhibition reduced the degree of LV dilation which occurred in the aorto-caval fistula model in rats [23]. In these studies, MMP inhibition shifted the LV pressure-volume relationship to the left indicating a movement in the operating volumes towards normal values (Fig. 3).

Thus, using a number of different animal systems of LV remodeling and failure, pharmacological inhibition of MMP activity has uniformly been demonstrated to favorably modify the LV remodeling process. These studies provide clear mechanistic data that myocardial MMP activation contributes to the adverse LV remodeling process in developing CHF. However, there are several critical issues regarding the use of broad-spectrum pharmacological MMP inhibitors. The first generation of MMP inhibitors also appeared to affect other metalloprotease systems such as the ADAMs (a disintegrin and metalloproteinases) that reduced the specificity of these compounds. Another important consideration regarding broad spectrum MMP inhibition is how prolonged treatment may affect endogenous MMP levels.

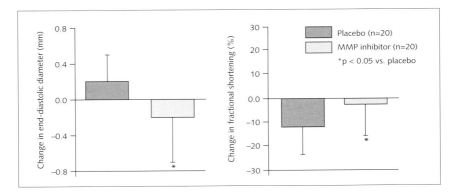

Figure 1
MMP inhibition was instituted in mice following surgical induction of a MI and echocardio-
graphic studies performed at four days post-MI.
The relative degree of LV dilation and decline in ejection performance was attenuated in the
mice treated with MMP inhibition. Adapted from [9].

There is emerging evidence that pharmacological MMP inhibition may increase myocardial MMP levels [8, 38]. This phenomenon may be due to a loss of normal MMP feedback regulation and opens the possibility that prolonged MMP inhibition can cause local MMP levels to rise to such a degree that complete pharmacologic inhibition of certain MMP species may be lost. Results from animal studies in which interruption of MMP activity was instituted early in the post-MI period have also raised some concerning issues. Specifically, in the plasminogen-deficient mouse in which MMP activation is attenuated, the normal MI wound healing response was impaired [12, 14]. In this study, the abnormal MI wound healing response was associated with increased MI rupture and reduced angiogenesis. Additional studies using either MMP-9 knockout mice or MMP inhibition have also reported abnormalities in the normal reparative process early post-MI [13]. Thus, a critical focus for future studies will be to identify optimal timing for the initiation as well as duration of MMP inhibition in the post-MI setting. Therefore, while proof of concept regarding MMP inhibition and the effects on LV remodeling are now established, a number of critical questions remain regarding the basic biologic effects of MMP inhibitory strategies.

Models of inflammation and MMP induction

The inflammatory process is tightly coupled to the induction and release of MMPs within the myocardium. Inflammatory cells such as neutrophils, macrophages and

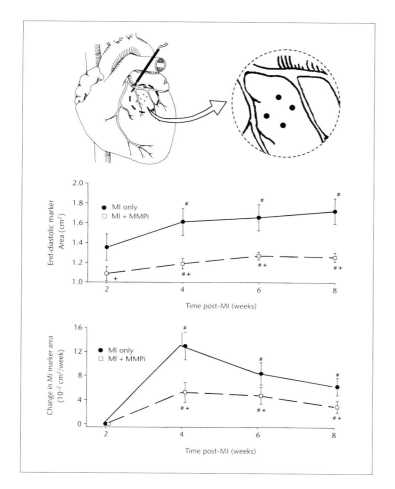

Figure 2

Regional myocardial geometry was serially assessed in pigs following MI.

In these studies, radio-opaque markers were placed within the site of the MI and fluoroscopic quantification of MI geometry was examined in pigs treated with or without an MMP inhibitor (MMPi). The top panel illustrates the location of the occlusion and the markers. MMP inhibition was started at five days post-MI. MMP inhibition significantly attenuated the degree of MI expansion (both absolute size and rate). These effects persisted for up to eight weeks post-MI. (# p < 0.05 baseline, + p < 0.05 versus untreated). Data reproduced from [37].

even platelets contain MMPs that can be released at the site of injury. Moreover, mediators of inflammation such as the cytokines interleukin-1 and TNF-α, can initiate an intracellular signaling cascade that induces MMP transcription [39–41]. A

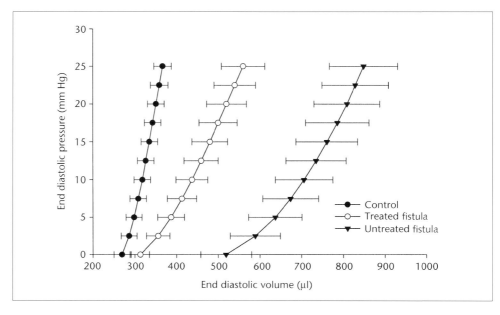

Figure 3
Aorto-caval fistulas were created in rats in order to produce an LV volume overload stimulus. LV pressure-volume curves were generated ex vivo *in order to assess the relative degree of LV chamber remodeling at eight weeks following creation of the volume overload. A significant shift to the right occurred in the fistula rats consistent with LV remodeling and dilation. Treatment with an MMP inhibition from weeks 2–8 resulted in a shift to the left in the LV pressure-volume relation indicating a reduction in the degree of LV remodeling – despite an equivalent volume overload stimulus. Reproduced from [23].*

causative link between myocardial cytokine activation and MMP induction comes from animal models of CHF as well as using transgenic systems [22, 42]. For example, in mice with cardiac restricted over-expression of TNF-α, LV remodeling occurred in conjunction with changes in myocardial MMP levels [22]. In dogs with pacing CHF, treatment with a TNF-α blocking antibody reduced the degree of LV dilation and relative myocardial MMP levels [42]. Thus, a downstream consequence of cytokine activation within the myocardium is the induction and activation of MMPs, which in turn contributes to the LV remodeling process.

Receptor activation by cytokines or bioactive peptides does not result in generic up-regulation of MMPs; rather, it appears that transcription of MMP species is highly tuned to specific extracellular stimuli. A likely mechanism for the differential response to extracellular stimuli with respect to MMP expression is differences in the promoter gene sequence [38–41]. A unique number and type of transcription binding sites exists within the promoter region within each MMP species. For example, several AP-1 sites are present in the promoter region of the MMP-1, -3, and -9 genes, while it is not present in the MMP-2 promoter. Thus, myocardial MMP levels are likely to be differentially regulated based on the summation of distinct extracellular stimuli. Identification of the upstream signals that are critical to the induction of certain MMPs in the LV remodeling process constitutes an important avenue of investigation.

Conclusion and future directions

The goal of this chapter was to review animal data that provides clear evidence that alterations in the normal balance of myocardial MMPs and TIMPs contributes to adverse LV remodeling and the progression to CHF. However, it has also been demonstrated that changes in myocardial MMP levels occur in patients with end-stage CHF which would facilitate adverse LV remodeling [17–21]. Clinical studies have demonstrated that these changes in MMP levels are related to the degree of cytokine activation [43]. In addition, interventional strategies such as mechanical LV unloading have been demonstrated to alter myocardial MMPs towards normal values [22]. Thus, taking the experimental and clinical results together, regulation of myocardial MMP levels and activity constitute a potential approach for interrupting the progression of LV remodeling. However, in addition to the unresolved issues regarding pharmacological MMP inhibition outlined in a previous section, initial clinical trials have raised additional points of concern. The use of broad-spectrum MMP inhibition in patients with metastatic cancer has reported severe musculoskeletal pain necessitating treatment discontinuation [44–46]. In contrast, initial clinical reports suggest that more selective MMP inhibition, in particular sparing MMP-1, was not associated with this musculoskeletal syndrome [44–47]. Thus, an important future direction would be to define the specific portfolio of MMPs which are expressed within the failing myocardium and develop selective targeting strategies to inhibit these MMP species. An important cause of CHF is diastolic dysfunction and a contributory factor may be an imbalance between myocardial collagen synthesis and degradation. In this context, identifying the systems and pathways which regulate myocardial TIMP levels would provide mechanistic insight as well as potential clues for developing therapeutic strategies to reduce the degree of myocardial fibrosis which can occur with severe LV hypertrophy. Finally, future studies which identify the temporal profile of MMP species which are expressed within the myocardium during and following an MI and the functional role of these individual MMPs with respect to the remodeling process needs to be established. Most importantly, the relationship between the inflammatory process post-MI and MMP species induction must be more fully understood. This fundamental information will be necessary in order to develop appropriate pharmacological strategies for targeting the portfolio of MMPs responsible for adverse LV remodeling.

Acknowledgements

Studies cited from the author's laboratory were funded in part by NIH grants HL-45024, HL-97012, and PO1 HL48788.

References

1   Sackner-Bernstein JD (2000) The myocardial matrix and the development and progression of ventricular remodeling. *Curr Cardiol Rep* 2 (2): 112–119

2   Spinale FG (2002) Matrix metalloproteinases; regulation and dysregulation in the failing heart. *Circ Res* 90 (5): 520–530

3   Cluetjens JPM, Verluyten MJA, Smits JFM, Daemen MJAP (1995) Collagen remodeling after myocardial infarction in the rat heart. *Am J Path* 147 (2): 325–338

4   Weber KT, Anversa P, Armstrong PW, Brilla CG, Burnett JC, Cruickshank JM, Devereux, RB, Giles TD, Korsgaard N, Leier CV et al (1992) Remodeling and reparation of the cardiovascular system. *J Am Coll Cardiol* 20: 3–16

5   Cohn JN, Ferrari R, Sharpe N (2000) Cardiac remodeling-concepts and clinical implications: A consensus paper from an international forum on cardiac remodeling. *J Am Coll Cardiol* 35: 569–582

6   Kim HE, Dalal SS, Young E, Legato MJ, Weisfeldt ML, D'Armiento J (2000) Disruption of the myocardial extracellular matrix leads to cardiac dysfunction. *J Clin Invest* 106: 857–866

7   Spinale FG, Coker ML, Thomas CV, Walker JD, Mukherjee R, Hebbar L (1998) Time dependent changes in matrix metalloproteinase activity and expression during the progression of congestive heart failure: Relation to ventricular and myocyte function. *Circ Res* 82: 482–495

8   Spinale FG, Krombach RS, Coker ML, Mukherjee R, Thomas CV, Houck WV, Clair MJ, Kribbs SB, Johnson LL, Peterson JT (1999) Matrix metalloproteinase inhibition during developing congestive heart failure in pigs: Effects on left ventricular geometry and function. *Circ Res* 85: 364–376

9   Rohde LE, Ducharme A, Arroyo LH, Aikawa M, Sukhova GH, Lopez-Anaya A, McClure KF, Mitchell PG, Libby P, Lee RT (1999) Matrix metalloproteinase inhibition attenuates early left ventricular enlargement after experimental myocardial infarction in mice. *Circulation* 99: 3063–3070

10   Roten L, Nemoto S, Simsic J, Coker ML, Rao V, Baicu S, Defreyte G, Soloway PJ, Zile MR, Spinale FG (2000) Effects of gene deletion of the tissue inhibitor of the matrix metalloproteinase-type 1 (TIMP-1) on left ventricular geometry and function in mice. *J Mol Cell Cardiol* 32: 109–120

11 Nagatomo Y, Carabello BA, Coker ML, McDermott PJ, Nemoto S, Hamawaki M, Spinale FG (2000) Differential effects of pressure or volume overload on myocardial MMP levels and inhibitory control. *Am J Physiol* 278: H151–H161

12 Heymans S, Luttun A, Nuyens D, Theilmeier G, Creemers E, Moons L, Dyspersin GD, Cleutjens JP, Shipley M, Angellilo A et al (1999) Inhibition of plasminogen activators or matrix metalloproteinases prevents cardiac rupture but impairs therapeutic angiogenesis and causes cardiac failure. *Nat Med* 5: 1135–1142

13 Ducharme A, Frantz S, Aikawa M, Rabkin E, Lindsey M, Rohde LE, Schoen FJ, Kelly RA, Werb A, Libby P et al (2000) Targeted deletion of matrix metalloproteinase-9 attenuates left ventricular enlargement and collagen accumulation after experimental myocardial infarction. *J Clin Invest* 106: 55–62

14 Creemers EEJM, Cleutjens JPM, Smits JFM, Daemen MJAP (2001) Matrix metalloproteinase inhibition after myocardial infarction. A new approach to prevent heart failure? *Circ Res* 89: 201–210

15 Peterson JT, Hallak H, Johnson L, Li H, O'Brien PM, Sliskovic DR, Bocan TM, Coker ML, Etoh T, Spinale FG (2001) Matrix metalloproteinase inhibition attenuates left ventricular remodeling and dysfunction in a rat model of progressive heart failure. *Circulation* 103: 2303–2309

16 Peterson TJ, Li H, Dillon L, Bryant JW (2000) Evolution of matrix metalloproteinase and tissue inhibitor expression during heart failure progression in the infarcted rat. *Cardiovasc Res* 46: 307–315

17 Thomas CV, Coker ML, Zellner JL, Handy JR, Crumbley AJ, Spinale FG (1998) Increased matrix metalloproteinase activity and selective up-regulation in LV myocardium from patients with end-stage dilated cardiomyopathy. *Circulation* 97: 1708–1715

18 Spinale FG, Coker ML, Heung LJ, Bond BR, Gunasinghe HR, Etoh T, Goldberg AT, Zellner JL, Crumbley AJ (2000) A matrix metalloproteinase induction/activation system exists in the human left ventricular myocardium and is up-regulated in heart failure. *Circulation* 102: 1944–1949

19 Gunja-Smith Z, Morales AR, Romanelli R, Woessner JF (1996) Remodeling of human myocardial collagen in idiopathic dilated cardiomyopathy: Role of metalloproteinases and pyridinoline cross links. *Am J Path* 148:1639–1648

20 Li YY, Feldman AM, Sun Y, McTiernan CF (1998) Differential expression of tissue inhibitors of metalloproteinases in the failing human heart. *Circulation* 98: 1728–1734

21 Li YY, Feng Y, McTiernan CF, Pei W, Moravec CS, Wang P, Rosenblum W, Kormos RL, Feldman AM (2001) Down-regulation of matrix metalloproteinases and reduction in collagen damage in the failing human heart after support with left ventricular assist devices. *Circulation* 104: 1147–1152

22 Sivasubramanian N, Coker ML, Kurrelmeyer KM, MacLellan WR, DeMayo FJ, Spinale FG, Mann DL (2001) Left ventricular remodeling in transgenic mice with cardiac restricted overexpression of tumor necrosis factor. *Circulation* 104: 826–831

23 Chancey AI, Brower GL, Peterson TJ, Janicki JS (2002) Effects of matrix metallopro-

teinase inhibition on ventricular remodeling due to volume overload. *Circulation* 105: 1983–1988

24 Li H, Simon H, Bocan TM, Peterson JT (2000) MMP/TIMP expression in spontaneously hypertensive heart failure rats: The effect of ACE and MMP inhibition. *Cardiovasc Res* 46: 298–306

25 Woessner FJ (1998) The matrix metalloproteinase family. In: Parks WC, Mecham RP (eds): *Matrix metalloproteinases*. Academic Press, San Diego, 1–141

26 Woessner JF, Nagase H (2000) Introduction to the matrix metalloproteinases (MMPs). In: *Matrix metalloproteinases and TIMPs*. Oxford University Press, Oxford, 1–10

27 Vu TH, Werb Z (2000) Matrix metalloproteinases: Effectors of development and normal physiology. *Genes Dev* 14: 2123–2133

28 Nelson AR, Fingleton B, Rotherenberg ML, Matrisian LM (2000) Matrix metalloproteinases: Biological activity and clinical implications. *J Clin Oncol* 18: 1135–1149

29 Hansen-Birkedal H, Moore WGI, Bodden MK, Windsor LJ, Hansen-Birkadal B, DeCarlo A, Engler JA (1993) Matrix metalloproteinases: A review. *Crit Rev Oral Biol Med* 4: 197–250

30 McDonnell S, Morgan M, Lynch C (1999) Role of matrix metalloproteinases in normal and disease processes. *Biochem Soc Trans* 27(4): 734–740

31 Knauper V, Murphy G (1998) Membrane-type matrix metalloproteinases and cell surface-associated activation cascades for matrix metalloproteinases. In: WC Parks and RP Mecham (eds): *Matrix metalloproteinases*. Academic Press, London, 199–218

32 Spinale FG (2002) Matrix metalloproteinases: Regulation and dysregulation in the failing heart. *Circ Res* 90 (5): 520–530

33 Pfeffer MA, Braunwald E (1990) Ventricular remodeling after myocardial infarction. Experimental observations and clinical implications. *Circulation* 81: 1161–1172

34 Etoh T, Joffs C, Deschamps AM, Davis J, Dowdy K, Hendrick J, Baicu S, Mukherjee R, Manhaini M, Spinale FG (2001) Myocardial interstitial matrix metalloproteinase activity following acute myocardial infarction in pigs. *Am J Physiol* 281: H987–994

35 Dixon IMJ, Ju H, Reid NL, Scammell-La Fleur, Werner JP, Jasmin G (1997) Cardiac collagen remodeling in the cardiomyopathic Syrian hamster and the effect of losartan. *J Mol Cell Cardiol* 29: 1837–1850

36 Mujumdar VS, Tyagi SC (1999) Temporal regulation of extracellular matrix components in transition from compensatory hypertrophy to decompensatory heart failure. *J Hyperten* 17: 261–270

37 Mukherjee R, Brinsa TA, Dowdy KB, Scott AA, Baskin JM, Deschamps AM, Lowry AS, Escobar GP, Lucas DG, Yarbrough WM et al (2003) Myocardial infarct expansion and matrix metalloproteinase inhibition. *Circulation* 107 (4): 618–625

38 Lindsey ML, Gannon J, Aikawa M, Schoen FJ, Rabkin E, Lopresti-Morrow L, Crawford J, Black S, Libby P, Mitchell PG, Lee RT (2002) Selective matrix metalloproteinase inhibition reduces left ventricular remodeling but does not inhibit angiogenesis after myocardial infarction. *Circulation* 15: 753–758

39 Fini ME, Cook JR, Mohan R, Brinckerhoff CE (1998) Regulation of matrix metallo-

proteinase gene expression. In: Parks WC, Mecham RP (eds): *Matrix metalloproteinases*. San Diego: Academic, 299–356

40 Vincenti MP (2001) The matrix metalloproteinase (MMP) and tissue inhibitor of metalloproteinase (TIMP) genes. In: Clark I (ed): *Methods in molecular biology, vol 151: Matrix metalloproteinase protocols*. Humana Press Inc., Totawa NJ, 121–148

41 Ries C, Petrides PE (1995) Cytokine regulation of matrix metalloproteinase activity and regulatory dysfunction in disease. *Biol Chem* 376: 345–355

42 Bradham WS, Moe G, Wendt K, Konig A, Romanova M, Naik G, Spinale FG (2002) Tumor necrosis factor-alpha influences myocardial matrix metalloproteinases in experimental heart failure: Relationship to left ventricular remodeling. *Am J Physiol* 282 (4): H1288–1295

43 Wilson EM, Gunasinghe HR, Coker ML, Sprunger P, Lee-Jackson D, Bozkurt B, Deswal A, Mann DL, Spinale FG (2002) Plasma matrix metalloproteinase and inhibitor profiles in patients with heart failure. *J Card Failure* 8 (6): 390–398

44 Drummond AH, Beckett P, Brown PD, Bone EA, Davidson AH, Galloway WA, Gearing AJH, Huxley P, Laber D, McCourt M et al. (1999) Preclinical and clinical studies of MMP inhibitors in cancer. *NY Acad Sci* 878: 228–235

45 Peterson JT, Hua L (2002) Matrix metalloproteinase inhibitor development for the treatment of heart failure. *Drug Devel Res* 55: 29–44

46 Levitt NC, Eskens FALM, O'Byrne KJ, Propper DJ, Denis LJ, Owen SJ, Choi L, Foekens JA, Wilner S, Wood JM et al (2001) Phase I and pharmacological study of the oral matrix metalloproteinase inhibitor, MM1270 (CGS27023A), in patients with advanced solid cancer. *Clin Cancer Res* 7: 1912–1922

47 Brinckerhoff CE, Matrisian LM (2002) Matrix metalloproteinases: A tail of a frog that became a prince. *Nat Rev* 3: 207–214

Inflammatory cytokines in cardiac diseases

The clinical experience with anti-cytokine therapy in heart failure

Anita Deswal, Biykem Bozkurt and Douglas L. Mann

Winters Center for Heart Failure Research, Cardiology Section, Department of Medicine, Veterans Administration Medical Center and Baylor College of Medicine, 6565 Fannin, Houston, TX 77030, USA

Introduction

Recent clinical and experimental studies have identified the importance of classical neurohormones such as angiotensin II and norepinephrine as biological mediators and/or modifiers of left ventricular remodeling and disease progression in the failing heart. This insight has, in turn, provided the rationale basis for antagonizing the activation of these neurohormonal systems (e.g., the renin angiotensin system and the adrenergic system) in the setting of heart failure. In addition to neurohormones, it has become apparent that another portfolio of biologically-active molecules, termed cytokines, is expressed along with the neurohormones in the setting of heart failure. In the present review we will discuss the emerging rationale for studying inflammatory mediators in heart failure, as well as the clinical attempts to antagonize cytokines in the setting of heart failure.

Clinical rationale for studying inflammatory mediators in heart failure

The current interest in understanding the role of pro-inflammatory cytokines in heart failure relates to the observation that many aspects of the syndrome of heart failure can be explained by the *known* biological effects of TNF (Tab. 1). Simply stated, when expressed at sufficiently high concentrations, TNF mimics some aspects of the so-called heart failure phenotype, including (but not limited to) progressive left ventricular (LV) dysfunction, pulmonary edema, LV remodeling, fetal gene expression and cardiomyopathy. Thus the elaboration of TNF, much like the elaboration of neurohormones, may represent a biological mechanism that is responsible for producing symptoms in patients with heart failure.

A second rationale for studying inflammatory mediators in heart failure is that the pattern of expression of cytokines is very similar to that observed with the "classical neurohormones" (e.g., angiotensin II and norepinephrine) that are believed to play an important role in disease progression in heart failure (reviewed in [1]). That

Inflammation and Cardiac Diseases, edited by Giora Z. Feuerstein, Peter Libby and Douglas L. Mann

Table 1 - Deleterious effects of inflammatory mediators in heart failure

Left ventricular dysfunction
Pulmonary edema in humans
Cardiomyopathy in humans
Reduced skeletal muscle blood flow
Endothelial dysfunction
Anorexia and cachexia
Receptor uncoupling from adenylate cyclase experimentally
Activation of the fetal gene program experimentally
Cardiac myocyte apoptosis experimentally

(Modified from [44])

is, inflammatory mediators such as TNF and IL-6 are consistently elevated in patients with heart failure secondary to dilated and/or ischemic cardiomyopathy. Moreover, there is a progressive increase in pro-inflammatory cytokine levels in direct relation to deteriorating New York Heart Association (NYHA) functional class (Fig. 1) [2–5]. Indeed pro-inflammatory cytokines are activated earlier in heart failure (i.e., NYHA Class I and II) than are the classical neurohormones, which tend to be activated in the latter stages of heart failure (i.e., NYHA Class III-IV) [6, 7]. Another clinical similarity between both inflammatory mediators and classical neurohormones is that circulating levels of both families of molecules have prognostic importance in the setting of heart failure [8]. As shown in Figure 2A, data from the multicenter Vesnarinone trial (VEST) showed that there was a significant overall difference in survival as a function of increasing TNF levels, with the worst survival in patients with TNF levels > 75th percentile [5]. Similar findings were observed with respect to the Kaplan-Meier analysis of circulating levels of IL-6 (Fig. 2B). This analysis further showed that levels of soluble TNF receptor type 1 (sTNFR1) and soluble TNF receptor type 2 (sTNFR2) were highly predictive of adverse outcomes, consistent with prior reports (Figs. 2C and 2D) [9, 10]. Indeed, a univariate Cox analysis of the VEST cytokine database showed that TNF (p = 0.01), IL-6 (p = 0.0003), sTNFR1 (p = 0.0001) and sTNFR2 (p = 0.0001) were significant univariate predictors of mortality. Moreover, when the cytokine and/or cytokine receptor were separately entered into a multivariate Cox proportional hazards model that included age, gender, etiology of heart failure, NYHA class, ejection fraction and serum sodium, TNF (p = 0.02), IL-6 (p = 0.002), sTNFR1 (p = 0.0001) and sTNFR2 (p = 0.0001) remained significant independent predictors of mortality; along with NYHA class and ejection fraction [5].

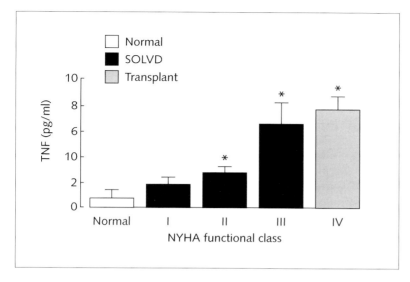

Figure 1
TNF levels in patients with class I–IV heart failure. In comparison to age-matched control subjects (open bar), there was a progressive increase in serum TNF-α levels in direct relation to decreasing functional heart failure classification. The solid bars denote values for patients enrolled in SOLVD [2]; the shaded bar denotes values for NYHA Class IV patients who were undergoing cardiac transplantation [45]. (Reproduced with permission from Seta et al. [46], the Journal of Cardiac Failure.*)*

Inflammatory mediators as therapeutic targets in heart failure

The rationale for employing anti-inflammatory strategies in patients with heart failure is three-fold: First, as noted above, the excessive elaboration of pro-inflammatory cytokines appears to mimic many aspects of the heart failure phenotype; Second, many of the deleterious effects of inflammatory mediators are potentially reversible once inflammation subsides; Third, heart failure remains an ineluctably progressive disease process despite optimal therapy with ACE inhibitors and β-blockers. As shown in Figure 3, the biological effects of pro-inflammatory mediators can be antagonized through transcriptional or translational approaches, or by so-called "biological response modifiers" that bind and/or neutralize soluble mediators (e.g., TNF or IL-1β). In additional there are several novel "immunomodulatory strategies" that alter the levels of inflammatory mediators through multiple mechanisms.

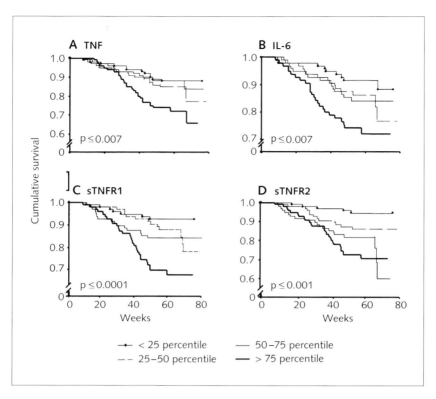

Figure 2
Kaplan Meier survival analysis. The circulating levels of TNF (5A), IL-6 (5B), sTNFR1 (5C) and sTNFR2 (5D) were examined in relation to patient survival during follow-up (mean duration = 55 weeks; maximum duration = 78 weeks). For this analysis the circulating levels of cytokines and cytokine receptors were arbitrarily divided into quartiles. (Reproduced with permission from Deswal et al. [46], the American Heart Association of 2001.)

Transcriptional suppression of pro-inflammatory cytokines

Experimental studies have shown that agents that raise cAMP levels, such as pentoxifylline, dobutamine and milrinone, prevent TNF mRNA accumulation, largely by blocking the transcriptional activation of TNF [11–14]. Whereas, a short-term infusion of dobutamine infusion suppresses TNF production [15], Deng and colleagues reported administration of dobutamine increased IL-6 levels in patients with NYHA Class III-IV heart failure [16]. Thus, it is unclear at the time of this writing whether dobutamine has pro- or anti-inflammatory effects in the setting of heart failure.

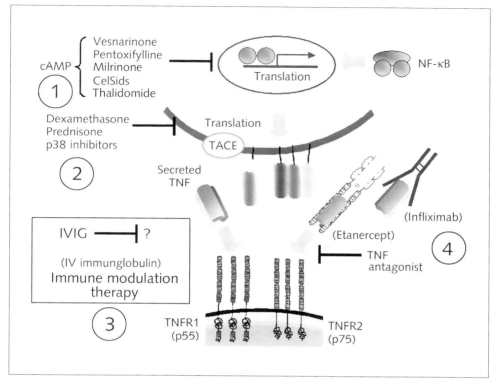

Figure 3

Therapeutic strategies for antagonizing pro-inflammatory mediators. TNF gene transcription is mediated, in part, by activation of nuclear factor- kappa B (NF-κB). Agents that increase intracellular levels of cAMP (1) such as vesnarinone, pentoxifylline, milrinone, thalidomide and thalidomide analogs (Celsius™) decrease the level of inflammatory mediators through transcriptional blockade of inflammatory gene expression. Agents such as dexamethasone and prednisone and some p38 inhibitors suppress inflammation by blocking the translation of inflammatory mediators (2). Secreted TNF can be neutralized (3) by soluble TNF antago-nists (etanercept) or by neutralizing antibodies (infliximab) that prevent TNF from binding to its cognate type 1 (p55) and type 2 (p75) TNF receptors. In addition to these targeted approaches, immunomodulatory strategies have been employed (4) using intravenous immunoglobulin (IVIG) and immune modulation therapy using irradiated whole blood.

More encouraging results with respect to modulating levels of inflammatory mediators through alterations in intracellular cAMP levels have been reported recently by Wagner et al. [17] and Sliwa et al. [18]. Wagner and colleagues showed that adenosine was sufficient to block lipopolysaccharide-induced TNF production in cultured neonatal and adult rat myocytes, as well as in slices of human myocardium obtained from explanted failing human hearts. The effect of adenosine could be mimicked by PD-125944, a selective A_2 receptor agonist (which is known to increase cAMP levels), or forskolin, and antagonized by DPMX, an A_2-selective antagonist. However, adenosine was only able to block TNF production if given before lipopolysaccharide challenge. Adenosine has also been shown to suppress intramyocardial TNF levels in an *ex vivo* model of ischemia reperfusion in the rat, as well as improve post-ischemic myocardial function [19]. More recently, Sliwa and associates studied the effects of pentoxifylline in patients with dilated cardiomyopathy and NYHA Class II-III heart failure. A total of 14 patients received pentoxifylline at a dose of 400 mg three times daily and an equal number received placebo. Four patients died as a result of progressive pump dysfunction during the six month study period, all in the placebo group. At the end of six months there was an improvement in functional class in the pentoxifylline group, whereas there was functional deterioration in the placebo group. At six months there was a significant increase in the ejection fraction (from 22.3 ± 9.0 [S.D.] to 38.7 ± 15.0 [S.D.]) in the pentoxifylline group, whereas there was no significant change in the placebo group. There was, however, no change in the LV end-diastolic dimension in either group. An important observation was that TNF levels fell significantly ($p < 0.002$) from $6.5 \pm$ pg/ml to 2.1 ± 1.0 pg/ml in the pentoxifylline group, whereas there was no significant change in the TNF levels in the placebo group. Thus, it appears that modulation of TNF levels *via* agents that alter intracellular cAMP levels, thus blocking transcriptional activation of TNF, may be a useful strategy for altering cytokine levels in heart failure.

Thalidomide (α-N-phthalimidoglutarimide) is another class of drug that may be useful in suppressing TNF production. Thalidomide selectively inhibits TNF production in monocytes [20], but has no effect on the production of IL-1β, IL-6, or granulocyte/macrophage colony-stimulating factor (GM-CSF). Thalidomide appears to reduce TNF levels by enhancing mRNA degradation [21]. Since the teratogenic and sedative properties of thalidomide may limit its clinical utility, thalidomide analogues which have more potent TNF-lowering properties, and at the same time appear to be non-teratogenic, are being developed.

Translational suppression of pro-inflammatory cytokines

Dexamethasone, which is thought to primarily suppress TNF biosynthesis at the translational level, may also block TNF biosynthesis at the transcriptional level [22]. One of the earliest studies to use this type of approach was performed by Parrillo and colleagues [23], who randomized 102 patients to treatment with prednisone (60 mg per day), or placebo. Following three months of therapy, they observed an increase in ejection fraction of $\geq 5\%$ in 53% of the patients receiving prednisone, whereas only 27% of the controls had a significant improvement in ejection fraction (p = 0.005). Overall, the mean ejection fraction increased $4.3 \pm 1.5\%$ in the prednisone group, as compared with $2.1 \pm 0.8\%$ in the control group (p = 0.054). The patients were then categorized prospectively in two separately randomized subgroups. "Reactive" patients had fibroblastic or lymphocytic infiltration or immunoglobulin deposition on endomyocardial biopsy, a positive gallium scan, or an elevated erythrocyte sedimentation rate. "Non-reactive" patients had none of these features. At three months, 67% of the reactive patients who received prednisone had improvement in LV function, as compared with 28% of the reactive controls (p = 0.004). In contrast, non-reactive patients did not improve significantly with prednisone (p = 0.51). Although specific cytokine levels were not measured in this study, their data suggest that patients with idiopathic dilated cardiomyopathy may have some improvement when given a high dose of prednisone daily.

Targeted anti-cytokine approaches using "biological response modifiers"

Two different targeted approaches have been taken to selectively antagonize pro-inflammatory cytokines in heart failure patients. In the first approach investigators have used recombinant human TNF receptors that act as "decoys" to bind TNF, thereby preventing TNF from binding to TNF receptors on cell surface membranes of target cells. The second approach is to use monoclonal antibodies to bind to and neutralize circulating cytokines.

Soluble TNF receptors

Etanercept (Enbrel™) is a genetically-engineered, dimerized, fusion protein composed of two TNF p75 receptors and an IgG1:Fc portion. Based on early pre-clinical studies which showed that etanercept was sufficient to reverse the deleterious negative inotropic effects of TNF *in vitro* [24] and *in vivo* [25], a series of Phase I clinical studies were performed in patients with moderate to advanced heart failure. Deswal and colleagues reported that a single intravenous infusion of etanercept (4 or 10 mg/m^2) resulted in a significant overall increase in quality of life scores, six minute-walk distance and ejection fraction in patients with moderate heart failure, whereas there was no significant change in these parameters in the placebo group. Bozkurt et al. evaluated the safety of repeated doses of etanercept in a larger Phase I study that was conducted at three different sites. 47 patients with NYHA Class III-IV heart failure were treated with bi-weekly subcutaneous injections of etanercept 5 mg/m^2 (n = 16), etanercept 12 mg/m^2 (n = 15) or placebo (n = 16) in a double-blind, randomized study for three months. They observed that there were improvements in LV ejection fraction and LV volumes measured by echocardiography, whereas there was a trend towards improvement in a clinical composite score. The improvements were more pronounced in the group that received 12 mg/m^2 of etanercept [26].

Following these early encouraging preliminary studies, two multicenter clinical trials were initiated using etanercept in patients with NYHA Class II-IV heart failure. The trial in North America, entitled "Randomized Etanercept North American Strategy to Study AntagoNism of CytokinEs" (RENAISSANCE; n = 900), and the trial in Europe and Australia entitled "Research into Etanercept Cytokine Antagonism in Ventricular Dysfunction" (RECOVER; n = 900), were both quality-of-life trials that used a clinical composite as the primary end-point. The clinical composite score classifies patients as better, worse, or the same after a clinical intervention, based on the patient and the physician's assessment at the end of the study [27]. Both trials had parallel study designs, but differed in the doses of etanercept that were used in the two studies; that is RENAISSANCE employed doses of 25 mg biw and 25 mg tiw, whereas RECOVER employed doses of 25 mg qw and 25 mg biw. A third trial which utilized the pooled data from the RENAISSANCE (biw and tiw dosing) and RECOVER (biw dosing only), termed "Randomized Etanercept Worldwide Evaluation" (RENEWAL; n = 1500), had a primary end-point of all cause mortality and hospitalization for heart failure as the primary end-point. Based upon pre-specified guidelines set forth in the charter of the trials, the trials were stopped prematurely because it was deemed unlikely that, if the two trials were allowed to go to completion, they would show benefit on the primary end-points of the trials [28]. Preliminary analysis of the data showed no benefit for etanercept on the clinical composite end-point in RENAISSANCE and RECOVER, nor a benefit for etanercept on all cause mortality and heart failure hospitalization in RENEWAL [28]. However, in a post-hoc analysis of hazard ratios for death/worsening heart failure, patients taking the biw dose of etanercept appeared to fare slightly better than patients taking the qw dose of etanercept in RECOVER, with hazard ratios for death/heart failure hospitalization of 0.87 and 1.01, respectively. In contrast, RENAISSANCE patients receiving biw etanercept experienced a 1.21 risk of death/heart failure hospitalization compared with placebo, while patients receiving the tiw dose had a slightly worse hazard ratio of 1.23. These disparities in trial findings are likely related to the different length of follow-up in the two trials. Patients in RECOVER received etanercept for a median time of 5.7 months, whereas patients in RENAISSANCE received etanercept for 12.7 months. It bears emphasis that these studies were stopped prematurely; had they been allowed to continue to completion, the hazard ratios may have been worse. On the basis of these findings, the prescribing information for etanercept has been updated, and now suggests that physicians exercise caution in the use of etanercept in patients with heart failure.

Why have targeted anti-TNF therapies failed in heart failure trials?

Given the wealth of pre-clinical data and early clinical studies that suggested a role for TNF antagonism in heart failure, the negative results of the clinical trials have been discouraging. This statement notwithstanding, analysis of the aggregate clinical trial data permits some insight into the potential reasons for why these studies have been negative. It is important to recognize that the long-term trials with etanercept were not neutral (i.e., no effect): That is, there was evidence for dose and time dependent worsening of heart failure and/or worsening outcomes. This in turn suggests that etanercept may have had intrinsic effects, or alternatively that TNF antagonism had an untoward effect in the setting of heart failure. With respect to the first explanation, it bears emphasis that cytokine binding proteins such as etanercept also have intrinsic biological activity and, in certain settings, can act as agonists for the cytokine that they bind [29]. As a case in point, in human studies etanercept acts as a carrier protein that stabilizes TNF and results in the accumulation of high concentrations of immunoreactive TNF in the peripheral circulation (Fig. 4A) [30]. As shown in Figure 4B, TNF complexed to etanercept does not remain tightly bound, but rather dissociates with an extremely fast off-rate (≈ 620 msec) [31]. The increase in the levels of TNF bound to etanercept and the rapid off-rates of TNF from etanercept, can lead to an increase in the duration of TNF bioactivity, as shown in Figure 4C. Thus, in summary, panels 4A–4C show that etanercept can, in certain settings, act as a "stimulating antagonist" [29]. While the aforementioned biological effects of etanercept might not be problematic in rheumatoid arthritis, wherein TNF is encapsulated within a joint space and peripheral circulating TNF levels are relatively low (compared to heart failure) or are non-existent [32], an increase in the circulating levels of biologically active TNF in a patient with heart failure might be expected to produce worsening heart failure, for all of the reasons articulated at the outset of this review (Tab. 1).

With respect to the second explanation for worsening heart failure in the clinical trials, there is a well-established body of literature that suggests that relatively low levels of TNF are cytoprotective in the heart [33–35]. Thus, one potential explanation for the worsening heart failure observed in the anti-TNF trials, albeit speculative, is that our current attempts to antagonize TNF result in the loss of one or more of the beneficial effects of TNF. In our overly simplistic view of heart failure, we tend to view molecules in absolute terms as having either "good" or "bad" effects, with little or no consideration given to the potential for concurrent offsetting biological effects. However, in many instances, molecules such as TNF exert a spectrum of pleiotropic effects in the failing heart: Some beneficial and some potentially deleterious. Accordingly, TNF antagonism might be expected to attenuate both the deleterious and beneficial effects of TNF. The observation that TNF antagonism provides short-term beneficial effects in heart failure patients [26, 36] and yet results in worsening heart failure when used chronically, is entirely consistent with this point of view.

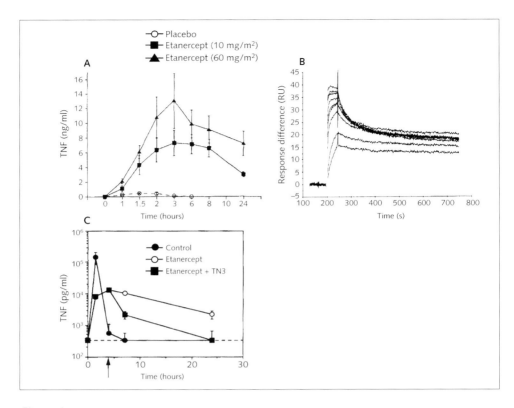

Figure 4

Biological properties of etanercept. (A) Etanercept increases the levels of immunoreactive TNF in the peripheral circulation of human subjects following intravenous endotoxin administration. As shown, high dose etanercept (60 mg/m²) increased immunoreactive TNF levels more than low dose etanercept (10 mg/m²). (Figure modified from [30].) (C) Kinetic analysis of TNF binding to etanercept using surface plasmon resonance biosensor technology (BIAcore assay [47]). Etanercept was exposed to 1000, 500, 250, 125, 62.5, 31.25, 16.63, 3.90 and 1.95 nM of TNF, and the kinetics of TNF binding determined by the decay of the light signal after peak binding to etanercept. The off-rate of TNF from etanercept was determined to be 620 msec. (Reproduced with permission from [31].) (D) Etanercept increases TNF bioactivity. Animals were inoculated with lipopolysaccharide and levels of TNF bioactivity measured at the indicated time points. TNF bioactivity peaked at 90 min after lipopolysaccharide inoculation, but was undetectable at later time points. Mice treated with etanercept after lipopolysaccharide inoculation showed a significant reduction in the level of peak TNF bioactivity; however, as shown TNF bioactivity was significantly prolonged by etanercept. Mice that received etanercept after lipopolysaccharide inoculation followed by an anti-TNF neutralizing antibody (TN3), had a shorter duration of TNF bioactivity. The arrow indicates the timing of the administration of the neutralizing anti-TNF antibody. (Figure modified from [48].)

Immunomodulatory strategies

An alternative approach to targeting specific components of the inflammatory cascade is to use approaches that result in a decrease in the systemic inflammatory response. Thus far, two different approaches have been employed in heart failure studies; intravenous immunoglobulin, and "Immune Modulation Therapy".

Intravenous immunoglobulin

Therapy with intravenous immunoglobulin (IVIG) has been tried in a wide range of immune-mediated disorders, such as Kawasaki's syndrome, dermatomyositis, and multiple sclerosis. Although the exact mechanism of action of IVIG is not known, a number of different mechanisms have been proposed, including Fc receptor blockade, neutralization of auto-antibodies, modulation of cytokine activity, and activation of an inhibitory Fc receptor [37]. Based on an initial report that IVIG was beneficial in acute cardiomyopathy [38], Gullestad and colleagues conducted a double-blind trial with IVIG for 26 weeks in 47 patients with moderate heart failure who were receiving conventional therapy for heart failure, including ACE inhibitors and β-blockers. They observed that, in comparison to placebo, IVIG induced a marked rise in plasma levels of the anti-inflammatory mediators (IL-10, and IL-1 receptor antagonist), and that these changes were accompanied by a significant increase in LV ejection performance by $\approx 10\%$, and a decrease in N-terminal pro-atrial natriuretic peptide levels [39]. Thus, in this small study, immunomodulatory therapy with IVIG was effective in patients with heart failure.

Immune Modulation Therapy

Immune modulation therapy uses a medical device (the VC7000 Blood Treatment System) to expose a sample of blood to a combination of physicochemical stressors *ex vivo*. The treated blood sample is then administered intramuscularly along with local anesthetic into the same patient from whom the sample is obtained. The physicochemical stresses to which the autologous blood sample is subjected are known to initiate or facilitate apoptotic cell death. The uptake of apoptotic cells by macrophages results in a down-regulation of pro-inflammatory cytokines, including TNF, IL-1β, and IL-8, and an increase in production of the anti-inflammatory cytokines, including TGF-β and IL-10 [40, 41]. Recent studies have shown that immune modulation therapy leads to a decrease in the production of pro-inflammatory cytokines and a corresponding increase in anti-inflammatory cytokines in human subjects [42]. Given that an imbalance exists between pro- and anti-inflammatory cytokines in patients with heart failure [4], immune modulation therapy may restore this balance more towards normal. In a recent trial employing immune modulation therapy in 73 patients with moderate heart failure, the investigators noted that, compared to the placebo group, the group receiving immune modulation therapy experienced significantly fewer hospitalizations (24 *versus* 41) or deaths (1 *versus* 7). The decrease in event rate in the treatment arm was also supported by improvements in quality of life and NYHA clinical classification. Based on the line-encouraging results of this pilot trial, a larger pivotal trial with immune modulation therapy is now ongoing [43].

Conclusion

In the present review we have focused on the rationale for studying inflammatory mediators in heart failure, as well as the results of the clinical trials that have been attempted to antagonize inflammatory mediators in heart failure. As noted, patho-physiologically-relevant concentrations of inflammatory mediators mimic many aspects of the so-called heart failure phenotype in experimental animals, including LV dysfunction, LV dilation, activation of fetal gene expression, cardiac myocyte hypertrophy and cardiac myocyte apoptosis (Tab. 1). Thus, analogous to the pro-posed role for neurohormones in heart failure, inflammatory mediators represent another distinct class of biologically-active molecules that may contribute to the progression of heart failure. Nonetheless, the early attempts to translate this infor-mation to the bedside have not only been disappointing, but have in many instances led to worsening heart failure. While one interpretation of these findings is that inflammatory mediators are not viable targets in heart failure, based on the argu-ments delineated above, the counter-veiling point of view is that we simply have not targeted pro-inflammatory mediators with the agents that can be used safely in the context of heart failure, or alternatively, that targeting a single component of the inflammatory cascade is not sufficient in a disease as complex as heart failure. Despite the inauspicious beginning with targeted anti-inflammatory approaches, strategies that use small molecules that have a broad spectrum of anti-inflammato-ry properties (e.g., pentoxifylline and thalidomide [or its analogs]) and immunomodulatory strategies that activate anti-inflammatory pathways (e.g., immune modulation therapy) are currently being evaluated. As with all therapeutic approaches in heart failure, the only way to really answer the question of whether broader spectrum anti-inflammatory strategies will have any added value in heart failure is through well designed clinical trials.

Acknowledgments

The authors would like to thank Ms. Mary Helen Soliz for secretarial support and Dr. Andrew I. Schafer for his past guidance and support. This work was supported, in part, by research funds from the Department of Veterans Affairs and the N.I.H. (P50 HL-O6H and RO1 HL58081-01, RO1 HL61543-01, HL-42250-10/10).

References

1   Mann DL (1999) Mechanisms and models in heart failure: A combinatorial approach. *Circulation* 100: 999–1088

2   Torre-Amione G, Kapadia S, Benedict CR, Oral H, Young JB, Mann DL (1996) Pro-inflammatory cytokine levels in patients with depressed left ventricular ejection fraction: A report from the studies of left ventricular dysfunction (SOLVD). *J Am Coll Cardiol* 27: 1201–1206

3   Testa M, Yeh M, Lee P, Fanelli R, Loperfido F, Berman JW, LeJemtel TH (1996) Circulating levels of cytokines and their endogenous modulators in patients with mild to severe congestive heart failure due to coronary artery disease or hypertension. *J Am Coll Cardiol* 28: 964–971

4   Aukrust P, Ueland T, Lien E, Bendtzen K, Muller F, Andreassen AK, Nordoy I, Aass H, Espevik T, Simonsen S et al (1999) Cytokine network in congestive heart failure secondary to ischemic or idiopathic dilated cardiomyopathy. *Am J Cardiol* 83: 376–382

5   Deswal A, Petersen NJ, Feldman AM, Young JB, White BG, Mann DL (2001) Cytokines and cytokine receptors in advanced heart failure: An analysis of the cytokine database from the Vesnarinone trial (VEST). *Circulation* 103: 2055–2059

6   Benedict CR, Weiner DH, Johnstone DE, Bourassa MG, Ghalli JK, Nicklas J, Kirlin P, Greenberg B, Quinones MA, Yusuf S (1993) Comparative neurohormonal responses in patients with preserved and impaired left ventricular ejection fraction: results of the studies of left ventricular dysfunction (SOLVD) registry. *J Am Coll Cardiol* 22: 146A–153A

7   Benedict CR, Johnstone DE, Weiner DH, Bourassa MG, Bittner V, Kay R, Kirlin P, Nicklas JM, McIntyre K, Quinones MA et al (1994) Relation of neurohormonal activation to clinical variables and degree of ventricular dysfunction: A report from the registry of studies of left ventricular dysfunction. *J Am Coll Cardiol* 23: 1410–1420

8   Cohn JN, Levine TB, Olivari MT, Garberg V, Lura D, Francis GS, Simon AB, Rector T (1984) Plasma norepinephrine as a guide to prognosis in patients with chronic congestive heart failure. *N Engl J Med* 311: 819–823

9   Ferrari R, Bachetti T, Confortini R, Opasich C, Febo O, Corti A, Cassani G, Visioli O (1995) Tumor necrosis factor soluble receptors in patients with various degrees of congestive failure. *Circulation* 92: 1479–1486

10   Rauchhaus M, Doehner W, Francis DP, Davos C, Kemp M, Liebenthal C, Niebauer J, Hooper J, Volk HD, Coats AJ et al (2000) Plasma cytokine parameters and mortality in patients with chronic heart failure. *Circulation* 102: 3060–3067

11   Zabel P, Schade FU, Schlaak M (1993) Inhibition of endogenous TNF formation by pentoxifylline. *Immunbiol* 187: 447–463

12 Zabel P, Greinert U, Entzian P, Schlaak M (1993) Effects of pentoxifylline on circulating cytokines (TNF and IL-6) in severe pulmonary tuberculosis. In: W Fiers, WA Buurman (eds): *Tumor necrosis factor: Molecular and cellular biology and clinical relevance*. S. Karger, Basel, pp 178–181

13 Dezube BJ, Pardee AB, Chapman B, Beckett LA, Korvick JA, Novick WJ, Chiurco J, Kasdan P, Ahlers CM, Ecto LT et al (1993) Pentoxifylline decreases tumor necrosis factor expression and serum triglycerides in people with AIDS. *J Acq Immun Defic Syndrome* 6: 787–794

14 Giroir BP, Beutler B (1992) Effect of amrinone on tumor necrosis factor production in endotoxin shock. *Circ Shock* 36: 200–207

15 Sindhwani R, Yuen J, Hirsch H, Tegguy A, Galvao M, Levato P, LeJemtel TH (1993) *Circulation* 88: I–255 (Abstract)

16 Deng MC, Erren M, Lutgen A, Zimmermann P, Brisse B, Schmitz W, Assman G, Breithardt G, Scheld HH (1996) Interleukin-6 correlates with hemodynamic impairment during dobutamine administration in chronic heart failure. *Int J Cardiol* 57: 129–134

17 Wagner DR, Combes A, McTiernan CF, Sanders VJ, Lemster B, Feldman AM (1998) Adenosine inhibits lipopolysacchide-induced cardiac expression of tumor necrosis factor-α. *Circ Res* 82: 47–56

18 Sliwa K, Skudicky D, Candy G, Wisenbaugh T, Sareli P (1998) Randomized investigation of effects of pentoxifylline on left ventricular performance in idiopathic dilated cardiomyopathy. *Lancet* 351: 1091–1093

19 Meldrum DR, Cain BS, Cleveland JC Jr, Meng X, Ayala A, Banerjee A, Harken AH (1997) Adenosine decreases post-ischemic cardiac TNFα production: Anti-inflammatory implications for preconditioning and transplantation. *Immunology* 92: 472–477

20 Sampaio EP, Sarno EN, Galilly R, Cohn ZA, Kaplan G (1991) Thalidomide selectively inhibits tumor necrosis factor α production by stimulated human monocytes. *J Exp Med* 173: 699–703

21 Moreira AL, Sampaio EP, Zmuidzinas A, Frindt P, Smith KA, Kaplan G (1993) Thalidomide exerts its inhibitory action on tumor necrosis factor-alpha by enhancing messenger RNA degradation. *J Exp Med* 177: 1675–1680

22 Remick DG, Strieter RM, Lynch IJP, Nguyen D, Eskandari M, Kunkel SL (1989) In vivo dynamics of murine tumor necrosis factor-α gene expression. Kinetics of dexamethasone-induced suppression. *Lab Invest* 60: 766–771

23 Parrillo JE, Cunnion RE, Epstein SE, Parker ME, Suffredini AF, Brenner M, Schaer GL, Palmeri ST, Cannon RO, Alling D et al (1989) A prospective randomized controlled trial of prednisone for dilated cardiomyopathy. *N Engl J Med* 321: 1061–1068

24 Kapadia S, Torre-Amione G, Yokoyama T, Mann DL (1995) Soluble tumor necrosis factor binding proteins modulate the negative inotropic effects of TNF-α *in vitro*. *Am J Physiol* 37: H517–H525

25 Bozkurt B, Kribbs S, Clubb FJ Jr, Michael LH, Didenko VV, Hornsby PJ, Seta Y, Oral H, Spinale FG, Mann DL (1998) Pathophysiologically relevant concentrations of tumor

necrosis factor-α promote progressive left ventricular dysfunction and remodeling in rats. *Circulation* 97: 1382–1391

26   Bozkurt B, Torre-Amione G, Warren MS, Whitmore J, Soran OZ, Feldman AM, Mann DL (2001) Results of targeted anti-tumor necrosis factor therapy with etanercept (ENBREL) in patients with advanced heart failure. *Circulation* 103: 1044–1047

27   Packer M (2001) Proposal for a new clinical end-point to evaluate the efficacy of drugs and devices in the treatment of chronic heart failure. *J Card Fail* 7: 176–182

28   Wood S. RENEWAL trial: No benefit for etanercept in CHF. www.theheart.org. August 15, 2002

29   Klein B, Brailly H (1995) Cytokine-binding proteins: Stimulating antagonists. *Immunol Today* 16: 216–220

30   Suffredini AF, Reda D, Banks SM, Tropea M, Agosti JM, Miller R (1995) Effects of recombinant dimeric TNF receptor on human inflammatory responses following intra-venous endotoxin administration. *J Immunol* 155: 5038–5045

31   Frishman JI, Edwards CK III, Sonnenberg MG, Kohno T, Cohen AM, Dinarello CA (2000) Tumor necrosis factor (TNF)-alpha-induced interleukin-8 in human blood cultures discriminates neutralization by the p55 and p75 TNF soluble receptors. *J Infect Dis* 182: 1722–1730

32   Maury CP, Teppo AM (1989) Cachectin/tumour necrosis factor-alpha in the circulation of patients with rheumatic disease. *Int J Tissue React* 11: 189–193

33   Nakano M, Knowlton AA, Dibbs Z, Mann DL (1998) Tumor necrosis factor-α confers resistance to injury induced by hypoxic injury in the adult mammalian cardiac myocyte. *Circulation* 97: 1392–1400

34   Kurrelmeyer K, Michael L, Baumgarten G, Taffet G, Peschon J, Sivasubramanian N, Mann DL (2000) Endogenous myocardial tumor necrosis factor protects the adult cardiac myocyte against ischemic-induced apoptosis in a murine model of acute myocardial infarction. *Proc Natl Acad Sci USA* 290: 5456–5461

35   Lecour S, Smith RM, Woodward B, Opie LH, Rochette L, Sack MN (2002) Identification of a novel role for sphingolipid signaling in TNF alpha and ischemic preconditioning mediated cardioprotection. *J Mol Cell Cardiol* 34: 509–518

36   Deswal A, Bozkurt B, Seta Y, Parilti-Eiswirth S, Hayes FA, Blosch C, Mann DL (1999) A Phase I trial of tumor necrosis factor receptor (p75) fusion protein (TNFR:Fc) in patients with advanced heart failure. *Circulation* 99: 3224–3226

37   Samuelsson A, Towers TL, Ravetch JV (2001) Anti-inflammatory activity of IVIG mediated through the inhibitory Fc receptor. *Science* 291: 484–486

38   McNamara DM, Holubkov R, Starling RC, Dec GW, Loh E, Torre-Amione G, Gass A, Janosko K, Tokarczyk T, Kessler P et al (2001) Controlled trial of intravenous immune globulin in recent-onset dilated cardiomyopathy. *Circulation* 103: 2254–2259

39   Gullestad L, Aass H, Fjeld JG, Wikeby L, Andreassen AK, Ihlen H, Simonsen S, Kjekshus J, Nitter-Hauge S, Ueland T et al (2001) Immunomodulating therapy with intra-venous immunoglobulin in patients with chronic heart failure. *Circulation* 103: 220–225

40   Fadok VA, Bratton DL, Konowal A, Freed PW, Westcott JY, Henson PM (1998) Macrophages that have ingested apoptotic cells *in vitro* inhibit pro-inflammatory cytokine production through autocrine/paracrine mechanisms involving TGF-beta, PGE2, and PAF. *J Clin Invest* 101: 890–898

41   Voll RE, Herrmann M, Roth EA, Stach C, Kalden JR, Girkontaite I (1997) Immunosuppressive effects of apoptotic cells. *Nature* 390: 350–351

42   Babaei S, Stewart DJ, Picard P, Monge JC (2002) Effects of VasoCare therapy on the initiation and progression of atherosclerosis. *Atherosclerosis* 162: 45–53

43   Wood S. Immune modulation for heart failure therapy holds promise, company says. www.theheart.org (August 15, 2002)

44   Kapadia S, Dibbs Z, Kurrelmeyer K, Kalra D, Seta Y, Wang F, Bozkurt B, Oral H, Sivasubramanian N, Mann DL (1998) The role of cytokines in the failing human heart. In: M Crawford (ed): *Cardiology clinics*. WB Saunders, Philadelphia, pp 645–656

45   Torre-Amione G, Kapadia S, Lee J, Durand JB, Bies RD, Young JB, Mann DL (1996) Tumor necrosis factor-α and tumor necrosis factor receptors in the failing human heart. *Circulation* 93: 704–711

46   Seta Y, Shan K, Bozkurt B, Oral H, Mann DL (1996) Basic mechanisms in heart failure: The cytokine hypothesis. *J Cardiac Failure* 2: 243–249

47   Weinberger SR, Morris TS, Pawlak M (2000) Recent trends in protein biochip technology. *Pharmacogenomics* 1: 395–416

48   Evans TJ, Moyes D, Carpenter A, Martin R, Loetscher H, Lesslauer W, Cohen J (1994) Protective effect of 55- but not 75-kD soluble tumor necrosis factor receptor-immunoglobulin G fusion proteins in an animal model of gram-negative sepsis. *J Exp Med* 180: 2173–2179

The role of IL-6 and related cytokines in myocardial remodeling and inflammation – implication for cardiac hypertrophy and heart failure

Antoine Bril[1] and Giora Z. Feuerstein[2]

[1]Institut de Recherches Servier, 11 Rue des Moulineaux, F-92150 Suresnes, France; [2]Pharmacology Department, WP42-209, Merck Research Laboratories, 770 Sumneytown Pike, West Point, PA 19486, USA

Introduction

Cardiac remodeling is a complex dynamic process occurring in reaction to an insult to the myocardium and contributing to the development of congestive heart failure (CHF). Left ventricular remodeling occurs either in response to a loss of cardiac cells as observed after myocardial infarction (MI), or in response to a hemodynamic overload as is the case in patients with chronic hypertension. The remodeling of cardiac tissue is characterized by the presence of hypertrophy, apoptosis and extracellular matrix re-organization and is associated with an inflammatory response [1–3]. Among the different factors involved in the development of cardiac remodeling, recent evidence has suggested a role for various pleiotropic cytokines, including interleukin-6 (IL-6), cardiotrophin-1 (CT-1) and others. Through the stimulation of tyrosine-kinase specific receptors, these cytokines lead to the activation of fetal gene regulatory programs, cardiac cell growth and survival.

The objective of the present chapter is to review the role of interleukin-6 related cytokines in the genesis of cardiac remodeling. After a short summary of the molecular biology of the IL-6 family of cytokines and their receptors, we will identify whether these peptides could be used as markers for cardiac remodeling. Then their involvement in cardiac remodeling process will be analyzed by reviewing the signaling pathways involved in the hypertrophic and survival processes described for these cytokines.

The IL-6 family of cytokines and their receptors

The cytokine super-family is divided into two classes depending on their molecular structure. Class I includes cytokines with four α-helices consisting of two pairs of anti-parallel a helices connected by polypeptides loops. This class of cytokines could be further subdivided into two groups according to the length of the α-helices. "Short chain" cytokines typically have eight to 10 residues and include IL-2, -3 and -4. In contrast, "long chain" cytokines have longer a-helices (between 10 and 20 amino acids) and include growth hormone, granulocyte-colony stimulating factor (G-CSF) and the IL-6 family of cytokines. The second class includes larger proteins such as interferon-gamma with molecular structure that includes eight alpha-helices and could be described as a duplicated version of Class I cytokines [4, 5].

The IL-6 family of cytokines is a family of polypeptides of 180 to 220 amino acids that collectively exhibit a relatively low level of sequence homology (~20%) [4, 6, 7]. Beside IL-6 itself, this family includes leukemia inhibitory factor (LIF), oncostatin M, ciliary neurotrophic factor (CNTF), cardiotrophin-1 (CT-1), IL-11 and the novel neurotrophin-1/B cell-stimulating factor-3 (NNT-1/BSF-3) [8]. X-ray crystallography, nuclear magnetic resonance and molecular modeling studies, reveal typical long-chain four helix structure containing 15–25 amino acid residues connected by three polypeptides loops to form a up-up and down-down (A–B and C–D) configuration.

The cytokine receptor complexes: These different cytokines bind to shared receptors consisting of multi-subunit receptor complexes that all include the glycoprotein 130 (gp130). The interleukin receptors (IL-6 and IL-11) consist of homodimers of gp130 while receptors to the other cytokines (CT-1, LIF, oncostatin M, CNTF and NNT-1/BSF-3) consist of heterodimer of gp130 together with a structurally related protein the LIF receptor (LIFR). Although LIF and oncostatin M appear to bind directly to gp130 and LIFR, IL-6, IL-11, CNTF and CT-1 necessitate binding to a specific receptor called IL-6R, IL-11R, CNTFR and CT-1R, respectively to trigger a signaling cascade [9]. LIFR and gp130 are two structurally related transmembrane proteins [10].

LIFR and gp130 represent the shared signal-transducing receptors and contain three main parts that are a large extracellular domain, a transmembrane domain of ~20 amino acids and a cytoplasmic domain of approximately 250 amino acids.

The molecular structure of the IL-6 receptor complex – which contains IL-6, IL-6R also called Rα, and gp130 – has been investigated using site specific mutagenesis and crystallography studies. Although most studies have been performed using the viral IL-6, vIL-6, which does not need IL-6R to bind to gp130, the results could be used as a template to suggest a molecular structure for human cytokines [11].

Molecular structure of gp130: The extracellular domain of gp130 is made of six different domains, one immunoglobulin domain (D1) and 5 fibronectin III domains (D2–D6). The crystal structure of module D2D3 of gp130, characterizing the "cytokine-binding homology region" (CHR), has been determined and is composed of a tandem of fibronectin-III domains that form a typical and rather rigid elbow [12]. This CHR domain which allows the binding to helices A–C of the cytokine contains the signature WSXWS but is not functional without the D1 immunoglobulin domain. Interestingly, the gp130 cytokine-binding sites are extremely cross-reactive, with the ability to interact with multiple cytokines of low sequence homology. Although this could explain the ability of gp130 to interact with multiple cytokines, the specificity of a given receptor is related to the presence of the third component, a specific, non-signaling receptor, IL-6R. In fact, it is a binary complex of IL-6 and IL-6R which interacts with high affinity to the CHR of gp130.

The IL-6/IL-6R complex: It is established that the activation of the gp130 receptor complex is formed in a hierarchical manner. IL-6 first binds to the CHR domain of the IL-6R through a binding site (Site I) located on helices B–D of the cytokine. The IL-6R-α chain is a protein of 468 amino acids containing a large extracellular domain, a 21 residue transmembrane domain and a 82 residue intracellular domain. The extracellular portion consists of three domains named D1, D2 and D3. In a manner similar to what is described for gp130, D1 domain is an immunoglobulin domain and D2 and D3 are fibronectin III modules that form the CHR and include the recognition site WSXWS [13].

IL-6 can bind to either IL6-R or to a soluble version of the receptor, sIL-6R, and then trigger signaling in cells that do not express the IL-6R-α chain. This complex of IL-6/IL-6R then could interact with the CHR domain of gp130 and form a tri-molecular complex. Interestingly, this complex is not sufficient for signaling and it has been suggested that, in a similar manner to what has been described for vIL-6, a duplication of intermediate complex is required to form the activated receptor leading to a functional hexamer containing two IL-6 molecules, two IL-6R and two gp130 [14, 16]. Alternatively, a tetramer complex has also been described in which the intermediate trimolecular complex would interact with a single molecule of gp130 [14]. It could be suggested that the third binding site of IL-6 (Site III) and the Ig domains (D1) of gp130 play a role in this interaction.

Although the hexamer model appears to be consistent with biochemical studies analyzing IL-6 signaling and recent determination of extracellular architecture [15, 16], the stoichiometry of receptor complexes in which gp130 required LIFR to be activated such as for LIF or CT-1, is not defined yet and both hexamer and tetramer models could be envisaged. The recent description of an interaction between D4–D6 domains of gp130 with LIFR could suggest a basis for the formation of the heterodimerization of gp130 and LIFR at a site remote from the Site III of the cytokine. Indeed, the deletion of each of the membrane-proximal fibronectin domains (D4–D6) of gp130 inhibits LIF response toward heterodimerization between gp130 and LIFR [17]. These data suggest that whereas the membrane distal domains D1–D3) of gp130 and LIFR are involved in recognition of the ligand, membrane proximal domains would be required for heterodimerization and signal transduction.

Signaling pathway involved in the effect of IL-6/CT-1 on cardiac myocyte

Upon activation, the IL-6 cytokine receptors stimulate the gp130 signaling pathway involving routes such as the Janus kinase/signal transducer and activator of transcription (JAK/STAT) pathway. However, the downstream effects to JAK are more complex and also involve the mitogen activated protein kinase (MAPK) and phosphatidylinositol-3 kinase (PI3K) pathways.

All these pathways are involved in the pathophysiologic process induced by these cytokines which manifest as cardiac hypertrophy and protection against apoptosis [18–21].

The gp130 signaling pathway

Role of JAK/STAT

The binding of the IL-6 cytokine ligand (IL-6, CT-1, LIF) induces homo- or heterodimerization of the receptor subunits and activates JAK tyrosine kinase. This activation induces the phosphorylation of specific tyrosine residues located at the cytoplasmic tail of the receptor which then serve as docking site for STAT. The STAT proteins are then phosphorylated and form homodimeric or heterodimeric complexes that can translocate to the nucleus, where they bind to specific DNA sequences and induce nuclear transcription activity [22, 23]. The JAK family of protein consists of four members three of which are expressed in cardiac tissue (Tyk2, JAK1, and JAK2) and the STAT family consists of seven members (STAT1, STAT2, STAT3, STAT4, STAT5A, STAT5B, and STAT6) that have all been reported to be expressed in cardiac tissue [24]. Beside the IL-6 family of cytokines other stimuli, including the angiotensin II receptor, mechanical stress, pressure overload, insulin, ischemia/reperfusion, have been shown to activate the JAK/STAT pathway and are suggested to induce opposite downstream effects. Indeed, whereas angiotensin II, mechanical stress and pressure overload induce hypertrophy and apoptosis, IL-6, LIF and CT-1 would be rather responsible for a survival effect. All these different effects could, at least in part, be explained as the result of the activation of different isoforms of JAK/STAT. Cytokines of the IL-6 family are more potent inducers of STAT3 than other STAT member and are also more potent than other stimuli such as angiotensin II [24]. Importantly it has been shown that several regulatory feedback mechanisms can turn off the JAK/STAT signaling [25]. Among those negative feedbacks, dephosphorylation of tyrosine 759 of gp130 by a SH2-containing phosphatases, SHP-2, allows a rapid control of cytokine activation.

Beside such phosphorylation-dependent feedback mechanisms, families of proteins such as suppressor of cytokine signaling, SOCS, proteins have been shown to play a major role in regulating the activity of most cytokines [26]. The SOCS family is comprised of eight members, SOCS-1 to SOCS-7 and cytokine inducible SH2-containing protein (CIS), and many of them are induced in response to cytokines [23]. It has been shown that the expression of SOCS-3 mRNA is induced by a variety of cytokines including IL-6, LIF and CT-1 [27, 28]. When over expressed, SOCS-3 binds to JAK and/or gp130 probably through binding to Tyr-759, but in contrast to SOCS-1, SOCS-3 does not prevent the kinase activity of JAK1 or JAK2 [23].

Role of ERK

Regulation of the cytokine activity could also be achieved *via* cross-talk with other signaling mechanisms such as the mitogen activated protein kinase (MAPK) pathway. The MAP kinase family comprised three main groups of kinases, the extracellular signal regulated kinases (ERKs, p42/44), c-Jun N-terminus kinases (JNKs) and p38 kinases, that all have been involved in the remodeling process [29, 30]. These enzymatic pathways consist of MAP kinase kinase kinase (MEKKs), dual specific MAP kinase kinase (MKKs) and MAP kinases and are activated through G-protein coupled receptors, mechanical stretch, or pressure overload [31]. In the case of IL-6 related cytokines, the activation of JAK has been shown to activate RAS, an upstream mediator of the MAPK cascades, as the ratio of GTP-bound RAS to GDP-bound RAS increases in response to IL-6 [5]. Although the mechanism linking gp130 stimulation to GTP-modifications of RAS is not clearly defined, the effects of cytokines such as CT-1, IL-6 are blocked by compounds inhibiting the MAP kinase pathway such as PD98059 which inhibits MEK-1, the MAP kinase upstream of p42/44 MAPK [32].

Role of Akt

IL-6-related cytokines such as LIF or CT-1 have been shown to activate phosphatidylinositol 3-kinase (PI3K) through the activation of gp130 and thus to stimulate Akt/PKB phosphorylation in cardiac myocytes [33]. The phosphorylation of Akt is a critical event in cardiac remodeling process as this pathway interacts with both the hypertrophic signaling through phosphorylation of GSK-3 but could also interact with an anti-apoptotic pathway through phosphorylation of BAD. When unphosphorylated BAD associates with Bcl-Xl. In contrast, the phosphorylation of BAD relieves this association and released Bcl-Xl inhibits apoptotic pathways and promotes cell survival. This signaling pathway has been demonstrated in isolated cardiac myocytes upon stimulation with CT-1 [34]. However, whether this is a general pathway for the downstream effect of IL-6-related cytokines in cardiac tissue remains to be determined. Indeed, it has been suggested that in the presence of a constitutive activation of PI3K as well as with the insulin-like growth factor, activation of PI3K is shown not to be linked with a phosphorylation of BAD but with an inhibition of caspases-3 [35].

Glycogen synthase kinase 3 (GSK-3) is a well defined target of Akt and the activity of GSK-3 is negatively regulated by Akt. Indeed, upon phosphorylation by Akt,

GSK-3 becomes inactive [36]. The role of GSK-3 is involved in many cell regulation systems and has been shown to play a role in hypertrophy, cell cycle, metabolism, apoptosis [36, 37].

Hypertrophic action of IL-6/CT-1

The identification of IL-6 producing myxoma in a patient with left ventricular hypertrophy suggested that IL-6 could represent a key factor in the pathogenesis of ventricular hypertrophy [38]. However, although in isolated cardiac myocytes, IL-6 itself does not induce hypertrophy presumably because cardiac myocytes do not express IL-6R, in the presence of the sIL-6R, a hypertrophic phenotype could be observed [39]. In contrast, several lines of evidence also demonstrated the role of IL-6-related cytokines in mediating cardiac hypertrophy through the stimulation of gp130.

By using a high throughput screen in isolated cardiac myocytes, Pennica and colleagues isolated novel cardiac growth factors among which cardiotrophin-1 was responsible for an increase in cell size [40, 41]. In isolated neonatal cardiac myocytes, CT-1 and LIF induce dose dependent increase in cell size, reorganization of sarcomere organization, activation of gene transcription and secretion of atrial natriuretic peptide (ANP) [39, 40, 42]. Interestingly, it has been shown that CT-1 and LIF, *via* the activation of the gp130 signaling pathway, induce a distinct form of myocardial hypertrophy [43, 44]. When added to cardiac myocytes in culture, CT-1 and LIF promote sarcomere assembly in series and thus increase cell length rather than cell width. CT-1-induced stimulation of JAK/STAT3 has been shown to increase angiotensinogen expression and hypertrophic phenotype due to CT-1 appears to be blunted by the specific angiotensin-II receptor antagonist, losartan [45] suggesting a close interaction between both the IL-6 related cytokines and neuroendocrine pathways in cardiac remodeling. Interestingly, it has also been shown that angiotensin II can induce IL-6, CT-1 and LIF in cardiac fibroblasts and that these released cytokines could, at least in part, contribute to the cardiac myocyte hypertrophy induced by angiotensin-II [46].

Similar to *in vitro* studies, several *in vivo* experiments have provided compelling evidence for a role of IL-6 related cytokines in cardiac remodeling. The chronic administration of CT-1 to mice by intraperitoneal injection for 14 days induce an increase in heart weight and ventricular weight to body weight ratio providing confirmation of its hypertrophic action but also induce structural changes of organs such as liver, kidneys, spleen [47]. Additional evidence for the role of IL-6-related cytokine came from the use of genetically engineered mice. Although mice over expressing either IL-6 or IL-6R alone did not show any evidence of cardiac abnormality, mice over expressing both IL-6 and IL-6R showed constitutively active gp130, as evidenced by tyrosine phosphorylation, associated with a pronounced cardiac hypertrophy due to a wall thickening of the heart [48]. However, mice in which the gp130 is inactivated in cardiac myocytes specifically, by using the cre-LoxP technology, developed normally [48]. However when subjected to pressure overload induced by transverse aortic constriction, these mice were unable to activate the JAK/STAT signaling pathway and showed no evidence of concentric cardiac hypertrophy.

In contrast, they presented a rapid-onset dilated cardiomyopathy associated to a massive myocyte apoptosis suggesting that balance between hypertrophic and apoptotic pathways is tightly controlled in cardiac remodeling [18]. Additional evidence for a role of IL-6-related cytokines in cardiac remodeling has been obtained in transgenic mice expressing a dominant-negative mutant of gp130. In these mice, the pressure overload-induced increases in the heart weight/body weight ratio, ventricular wall thickness, and cross-sectional areas of cardiac myocytes were significantly smaller than in wild type mice [49]. Although the stimulation of gp130/JAK signaling pathway could be beneficial, negative feedback has been described to tightly regulate the appropriate duration and intensity of the action IL-6-related cytokines. One of such feedback mechanisms, the suppressor of cytokine signaling 3 (SOCS3), has been shown to be induced by chronic pressure overload in mice [50]. In this study, adenovirus-mediated gene transfer of SOCS to ventricular myocytes completely suppressed the phenotypic features of cardiomyocytes hypertrophy due to CT-1 [50]. Among the signaling pathways downstream gp130/JAK, the activation of Akt/protein kinase B could play a major role in the hypertrophic effect of IL-6-related cytokines. By using constitutively active forms of Akt to generate transgenic mice, it is demonstrated that Akt is sufficient to induce a marked increase in heart size [51] similar to the hypertrophic effect induced by PI3K activation [52]. Taken altogether these results suggest that the activation of the PI3K-Akt pathway through the stimulation of gp130 receptors could be a critical mechanism for protective hypertrophy since this signaling pathway has been shown is several systems to mediate beneficial growth. However, it should be noted that in mice in which a constitutively activated form of Akt is over expressed the occurrence of fibrosis and cardiac failure increases with age [51]. This result reinforces the need for feedback mechanisms, such as the SOCS signaling, to modulate the activity of hypertrophic cytokines.

Protection against apoptosis by IL-6/CT-1

Another consequence of gp130 stimulation by IL-6-related cytokines is the protection against cardiac apoptosis that has been demonstrated both in isolated myocytes and in animal models of cardiac remodeling and failure.

In isolated neonatal rat cardiac myocytes in culture, it has been shown that cellular apoptosis induced by serum deprivation [32], ischemia [53] or doxorubicin [54] is prevented by IL-6 cytokines such as cardiotrophin and LIF. The mechanism involved in this protective effect is related to the stimulation of the gp130 signaling mechanism and could also be associated with an up-regulation of bcl-X [55] or with the activation of Akt which is a well established survival pathway in many cell types [56]. *In vivo*, the most compelling evidence demonstrating the role of gp130 in protecting against apoptosis comes from a study in mice harboring a cardiac specific inactivation of the gp130 gene [48]. Indeed, in contrast to control mice which present concentric hypertrophy after aortic banding, gp130 knockout mice exhibit a rapid onset cardiac dilatation associated with a high mortality rate. In these mice it is shown that apoptosis is dramatically activated compared to control mice suggesting the protective role of IL-6-related cytokines in the setting of cardiac remodeling. Additional evidence was obtained in rats subjected to coronary artery occlusion and myocardial infarction [57]. In these rats, administration of a JAK2 inhibitor to inhibit the gp130 signaling pathway by blocking the JAK/STAT enzymes, results in a deterioration of myocardial viability and an increase in apoptosis during myocardial infarction. Similarly, mice with cardiac-specific over expression of the STAT3 gene exhibit myocardial hypertrophy with increased expression of the atrial natriuretic factor (ANF), beta-myosin heavy chain (MHC), and cardiotrophin (CT)-1 genes but when they were injected with doxorubicin, an anti-neoplastic drug with restricted use because of its cardiotoxicity, the survival rates were dramatically improved [58].

Beside studies in which IL-6 related cytokines were administered exogenously or in which the gp130 signaling pathway is activated using genetic methods, evidence for the involvement of these inflammatory cytokines has been obtained using models of cardiac remodeling, pressure-overload in various animal species.

IL-6/CT-1 and the risk of myocardial remodeling

Myocardial remodeling occurring after an ischemic insult or a pressure overload is associated with cardiac cell hypertrophy, neuroendocrine stimulation, fibrosis and apoptosis together with evidence of inflammation. Therefore the role of inflammatory cytokines in the genesis of cardiac remodeling has been suggested and could be due to altered expression tissue level. Similarly, a modification in the plasma level of these inflammatory cytokines and/or evidence of polymorphism could represent critical markers of the physiopathologic process.

Plasma IL-6/CT-1 as marker of ischemic heart disease

Only few studies have investigated the expression level of IL-6-related cytokines such as cardiotrophin in the plasma of patients with heart failure on in animal models of cardiac remodeling. In patients with dilated cardiomyopathy classified according to their left ventricular mass index and the ejection fraction as marker of severity of CHF, a positive correlation is observed with the plasma level of cardiotrophin [59]. Several other studies have shown that plasma levels of cardiotrophin and other cytokines are increased in heart failure [60–64]. However, it could be concluded from these studies that plasma level in itself may not be informative regarding the role of the gp130 signaling pathway in the progression of cardiac remodeling since the activity of the various effectors involved in the signaling cascade need also to be determined [65].

IL-6/CT-1 expression in myocardial infarction and heart failure

The IL-6 cytokine family such as IL-6, CT-1 and LIF is widely expressed and the expression patterns of these inflammatory cytokines show detectable levels not only in heart but also in skeletal muscle, lung, kidney, prostate and many other organs. However in the heart the expression level of IL-6 and CT-1 have been shown to be altered by myocardial infarction, pressure overload and remodeling. In isolated cardiac myocytes, mechanical stretch augments the mRNA expression of cardiotrophin-1, IL-6, and leukemia inhibitory factor and activates the JAK/STAT pathway suggesting that myocytes can produce cytokines [66]. In experimental studies performed in dogs or in rats subjected to coronary artery occlusion, the cardiac expression level of IL-6 is shown to be increased shortly after coronary occlusion but not after long term occlusion in contrast to the atrial natriuretic peptide (ANP) whose expression progressively increased with time after coronary artery occlusion [67, 68]. However, it appears that the myocardial expression of IL-6 is stimulated by reperfusion [67]. Similarly, pressure overload induced over expression of both IL-6 and CT-1 was detected in cardiac tissue [69]. Interestingly, it has been shown that cardiotrophin-1 mRNA, but not LIF which is not detectable, is increased at an early stage of hypertrophy in spontaneously hypertensive rats stroke prone (SHR-SP) and remains elevated when hypertrophy is established [70]. It should also be noted that fibrosis which is commonly observed in remodeled hearts post-myocardial infarction or after long term hypertension, could be associated with an increased expression of cytokines. Indeed, norepinephrine and isoproterenol increase IL-6 expression in cardiac fibroblasts [71] and cardiotrophin-1 as well as endothelin-1 can promote fibroblast proliferation [72].

In human the expression pattern of IL-6-related cytokines and their receptor is controversial In a study comparing the expression pattern of IL-6, IL-6 receptor and gp130 in non-failing and failing hearts no major difference was observed while LIF mRNA levels were increased in failing hearts [73]. In contrast, when investigating the expression level in control and donor hearts, a difference in IL-6 and IL-6 receptor is observed. In this study the expression levels of cytokines and their receptors are similar in failing and donor hearts but are increased compared to normal tissue [74].

Although these findings need to be confirmed in other groups of patients, the myocardial expression level of cardiotrophin has been shown recently to be increased in patients with either ischemic or dilated cardiac myopathy [75]. However, this study showed that mRNA and protein expression levels of gp130 are reduced in patients and suggested that the gp130 signaling down-regulation or the increase in SOCS-3/gp130 ratio may compensate the cardiotrophin-induced increase in heart size [75]. This study tends to confirm experimental data suggesting that SOCS-3 proteins could modulate the effect of cardiotrophin in inducing cardiac hypertrophy [50]. Interestingly, it could be suggested that both fibroblasts and cardiac myocytes could produce IL-6 cytokines as well as the soluble receptors, sIL-6R and sgp130 since they were identified in human cardiac myocyte and fibroblast cultures and in pericardial fluids [76, 77].

IL-6 polymorphism as risk for cardiac disorders

Polymorphisms for IL-6 have been demonstrated to be a possible biological candidate for involvement in the regulation of the inflammatory response. The IL-6 −174C polymorphism is located in the IL-6 promoter region and influences IL-6 gene transcription and therefore has been suggested to be associated with plasma level of inflammatory markers. The −174C allele was claimed to be associated with a significant effects on systolic blood pressure and a higher risk of coronary heart disease [78, 79] suggesting a role for inflammatory system in determining the risk of coronary heart disease. Interestingly an association between plasma levels of C-reactive protein and the genotype at the -G174C polymorphism has been demonstrated in a large population of 98 families [79]. However previous studies in which the vascular phenotype and the IL-6 promoter genotype were investigated provided rather discrepant findings. In some studies, the C allele is associated with a reduced IL-6 plasma level [80], in some others it is associated with an increased concentration of IL-6 in plasma [81] while others found no effect of the polymorphism on baseline plasma IL-6 levels [82–84].

Such a discrepancy is also observed when the endpoint measure is mortality or severity or aortic atherothrombosis therefore suggesting that additional studies in which large cohorts of patients are included are required to provide a definitive evidence for a role of inflammatory cytokines in the genesis of coronary heart diseases. Furthermore, beside IL-6 polymorphisms in other cytokines such as cardiotrophin or LIF remain to be investigated.

Conclusion

This brief review summarizes some recent information regarding the role of inflammatory cytokines in cardiac remodeling. It is indeed well established that cardiac myocytes and fibroblasts can produce cytokines locally. Experimental studies suggest that several cytokines such as LIF or cardiotrophin-1 represent a mechanism of adaptation of the conditions of stress overload. The molecular mechanism involved in this beneficial effect has been widely recognized to be due to the activation of the gp130 signaling pathway which probably through a combined activation of MAP kinases and PI3K/Akt would promote myocyte survival. However it should be noted that recent studies have shown that mice harboring a constitutively active form of Akt a phenotype of hypertrophied heart associated with interstitial fibrosis and a rather high incidence of heart failure [51]. This data suggest that the beneficial effect of cytokine activation in the heart might be offset by non-myocyte cell proliferation and activation (e.g., fibroblasts) leading to stiffness of the ventricle wall and arrhythmogenic predisposition. Cytokines are also known to activate MAP kinase pathways downstream of gp130. Through this mechanism also a beneficial survival effect could be considered and it has been recently shown that urocortin, a peptide hormone that shares 45% amino acid homology with the hypothalamic peptide Corticotrophin Releasing Hormone (CRH), can also induce a protective hypertrophy through the stimulation of the MAP kinase p42/44 signaling cascade combined with an activation of the mitochondrial ATP sensitive potassium channel [85, 86]. Further studies, including clinical investigations, will therefore be required to determine the effect of the interventions limiting hypertrophic mechanism but favoring the protection against apoptosis in situation where neuro-hormonal therapies are administered.

With the launch of large-scale collaborations such as the Alliance for Cellular Signaling [87, 88], it could be hypothesized that relationship and connectivity between the various signaling pathways involved in cardiac remodeling will be identified leading to novel specific therapeutic approaches to improve survival in patients in whom cardiac remodeling remains a critical issue.

References

1   Blum A, Miller H (2001) Pathophysiological role of cytokines in congestive heart failure. *Annu Rev Med* 52: 15–27

2   Frangogiannis NG, Smith CW, Entman ML (2002) The inflammatory response in myocardial infarction. *Cardiovasc Res* 53: 31–47

3   Mann DL (2002) Inflammatory mediators and the failing heart. Past, present, and the foreseeable future. *Circ Res* 91: 988–998

4   Bravo J, Heath JK (2000) Receptor recognition by gp130 cytokines. *Embo J* 19; 2399–2411

5   Taga T, Kishimoto (1997) T gp130 and the interleukin-6 family of cytokines. *Ann Rev Immunol* 15: 797–819

6   Hinds MG, Maurer T, Zhang JG, Nicola NA, Norton RS (1998) Solution structure of leukemia inhibitory factor. *J Biol Chem* 273: 13738–13745

7   Hill CP, Osslund TD, Eisenberg D (1993) The structure of granulocyte-colony-stimulat-

ing factor and its relationship to other growth factors. *Proc Natl Acad Sci USA* 90: 5167–5171

8   Senaldi G, Varnum BC, Sarmiento U, Starnes C, Lile J, Scully S, Guo J, Elliott G, McNinch J, Shaklee CL (1999) Novel neurotrophin-1/B cell-stimulating factor-3: A cytokine of the IL-6 family. *Proc Natl Acad Sci USA* 96: 11458–11463

9   Robledo O, Fourcin M, Chevalier S, Guillet C, Auguste P, Pouplard-Barthelaix A, Pennica D, Gascan H (1997) Signaling of the cardiotrophin-1 receptor. Evidence for a third receptor component. *J Biol Chem* 272: 4855–4863

10   Gearing DP, Thut CJ, VandeBos T, Gimpel SD, Delaney PB, King J, Price V, Cosman D, Beckmann MP (1991) Leukemia inhibitory factor receptor is structurally related to the IL-6 signal transducer, gp130. *Embo J* 10: 2839–2848

11   Chow D, Brevnova L, He X, Martick MM, Bankovich A, Garcia KC (2002) A structural template for gp130-cytokine signaling assemblies. *Biochim Biophys Acta* 1592: 225–235

12   Chow D, He X, Snow AL, Rose-John S, Garcia KC (2001) Structure of an extracellular gp130 cytokine receptor signaling complex. *Science* 291: 2150–2155

13   Ozbek S, Grotzinger J, Krebs B, Fischer M, Wollmer A, Jostock T, Mullberg J, Rose-John S (1998) The membrane proximal cytokine receptor domain of the human interleukin-6 receptor is sufficient for ligand binding but not for gp130 association. *J Biol Chem* 273: 21374–21379

14   Chow D, Ho J, Nguyen Pham TL, Rose-John S, Garcia KC (2001) *In vitro* reconstitution of recognition and activation complexes between interleukin-6 and gp130. *Biochemistry* 40: 7593–7603

15   Somers W, Stahl M, Seehra JS (1997) 1.9A crystal structure of interleukin 6: Implications for a novel mode of receptor dimerization and signaling. *Embo J* 16: 989–997

16   Varhese JN, Moritz RL, Lou MZ, van Donkelaar A, Ji H, Ivancic N, Branson KM, Hall NE, Simpson RJ (2002) Stucture of the extracellular domains of the human interleukin-6 receptor alpha-chain. *Proc Natl Acad Sci USA* 99: 15959–15964

17   Timmermann A, Kuster A, Kurth I, Heinrich PC, Muller-Newen G (2002) A functional role of the membrane-proximal extracellular domains of the signal transducer gp130 in heterodimerization with the leukemia inhibitory factor receptor. *Eur J Biochem* 269: 2716–2726

18   Hunter JJ, Chien KR (1999) Signaling pathways for cardiac hypertrophy and failure. *N Eng J Med* 341: 1276–1283

19   Yamauchi-Takihara K, Kishimoto T (2000) A novel role for STAT3 in cardiac remodeling. *Trends Cardiovasc Med* 10: 298–303

20   Wollert KC, Drexler H (2001) The role of interleukin-6 in the failing heart. *Heart Failure Rev* 6: 95–103

21   Kallen KJ (2002) The role of trans-signalling *via* the agonistic soluble IL-6 receptor in human diseases. *Biochim Biophys Acta* 1592: 323–343

22   Touw IP, De Koning JP, Ward AC, Hermans MH (2000) Signaling mechanisms of cytokine receptors and their perturbances in disease. *Mol Cell Endocrinol* 160: 1–9

23 Ishihara K, Hirano T (2002) Molecular basis of the cell specificity of cytokine action. *Biochim Biophys Acta* 1592: 281–296

24 Booz GW, Day JNE, Baker KM (2002) Interplay between the cardiac renin angiotensin system and JAK-STAT signaling: Role in cardiac hypertrophy, ischemia/reperfusion dysfunction, and failure. *J Mol Cell Cardiol* 34: 1443–1453

25 Yasukawa H, Sasaki A, Yoshimura A (2000) Negative regulation of cytokine signaling pathways. *Annu Rev Immunol* 18: 143–164

26 Starr R, Willson TA, Viney EM, Murray LJ, Rayner JR, Jenkins BJ, Gonda TJ, Alexander WS, Metcalf D, Nicola NA et al (1997) A family of cytokine-inducible inhibitors of signalling. *Nature* 387: 917–921

27 Bousquet C, Susini C, Melmed S (1999) Inhibitory roles for SHP-1 and SOCS-3 following pituitary pro-opiomelanocortin induction by leukemia inhibitory factor. *J Clin Invest* 104: 1277–1285

28 Hamanaka I, Saito Y, Yasukawa H, Kishimoto I, Kuwahara K, Miyamoto Y, Harada M, Ogawa E, Kajiyama N, Takahashi N et al (2001) Induction of JAB/SOCS-1/SSI-1 and CIS3/SOCS-3/SSI-3 is involved in gp130 resistance in cardiovascular system in rat treated with cardiotrophin-1 *in vivo*. *Circ Res* 88: 727–732

29 Sugden PH (1999) Signaling in myocardial hypertrophy: Life after calcineurin? *Circ Res* 84: 633–646

30 Sugden PH, Clerk A (1998) Cellular mechanisms of cardiac hypertrophy. *J Mol Med* 76: 725–746

31 Sugden PH (2001) Signalling pathways in cardiac myocyte hypertrophy. *Ann Med* 33: 611–622

32 Sheng Z, Knowlton K, Chen J, Hoshijima M, Brown JH, Chien KR (1997) Cardiotrophin 1 (CT-1) inhibition of cardiac myocyte apoptosis *via* a mitogen-activated protein kinase-dependent pathway. Divergence from downstream CT-1 signals for myocardial cell hypertrophy. *J Biol Chem* 272: 5783–5791

33 Oh H, Fujio Y, Kunisada K, Hirota H, Matsui H, Kishimoto T, Yamauchi-Takihara K (1998) Activation of phosphatidylinositol 3-kinase through glycoprotein 130 induces protein kinase B and p70 S6 kinase phosphorylation in cardiac myocytes. *J Biol Chem* 273: 9703–9710

34 Kuwahara K, Saito Y, Kishimoto I, Miyamoto Y, Harada M, Ogawa E, Hamanaka I, Kajiyama N, Takahashi N, Izumi T et al (2000) Cardiotrophin-1 phosphorylates akt and BAD, and prolongs cell survival *via* a PI3K-dependent pathway in cardiac myocytes. *J Mol Cell Cardiol* 32: 1385–1394

35 Wu W, Lee WL, Wu YY, Chen D, Liu TJ, Jang A, Sharma PM, Wang PH (2000) Expression of constitutively active phosphatidylinositol 3-kinase inhibits activation of caspase 3 and apoptosis of cardiac muscle cells. *J Biol Chem* 275: 40113–40119

36 Hardt SE, Sadoshima J (2002) Glycogen synthase kinase-3 beta: A novel regulator of cardiac hypertrophy and development. *Circ Res* 90: 1055–1063

37 Antos CL, McKinsey TA, Frey N, Kutschke W, McAnally J, Shelton JM, Richardson JA,

Hill JA, Olson EN (2002) Activated glycogen synthase-3 beta suppresses cardiac hypertrophy *in vivo*. *Proc Natl Acad Sci USA* 99: 907–912

38 Kanda T, Nakajima T, Sakamoto H, Suzuki T, Murata K (1994) An interleukin-6 secreting myxoma in a hypertrophic left ventricle. *Chest* 105: 962–963

39 Hirota H, Yoshida K, Kishimoto T, Taga T (1995) Continuous activation of gp130, a signal-transducing receptor component for interleukin 6-related cytokines, causes myocardial hypertrophy in mice. *Proc Natl Acad Sci USA* 92: 4862–4866

40 Pennica D, King KL, Shaw KJ, Luis E, Rullamas J, Luoh SM, Darbonne WC, Knutzon DS, Yen R, Chien KR et al (1995) Expression cloning of cardiotrophin 1, a cytokine that induces cardiac myocyte hypertrophy. *Proc Natl Acad Sci USA* 92: 1142–1146

41 Pennica D, Wood WI, Chien KR (1996) Cardiotrophin-1: A multifunctional cytokine that signals *via* LIF receptor-gp130 dependent pathways. *Cytokine Growth Factor Rev* 7: 81–91

42 Kodama H, Fukuda K, Pan J, Makino S, Baba A, Hori S, Ogawa S (1997) Leukemia inhibitory factor, a potent cardiac hypertrophic cytokine, activates the JAK/STAT pathway in rat cardiomyocytes. *Circ Res* 81: 656–663

43 Wollert KC, Taga T, Saito M, Narazaki M, Kishimoto T, Glembotski CC, Vernallis AB, Heath JK, Pennica D, Wood WI et al (1996) Cardiotrophin-1 activates a distinct form of cardiac muscle cell hypertrophy. Assembly of sarcomeric units in series *via* gp130/ leukemia inhibitory factor receptor-dependent pathways. *J Biol Chem* 271: 9535–9545

44 Wollert KC, Chien KR (1997) Cardiotrophin-1 and the role of gp130-dependent signaling pathways in cardiac growth and development. *J Mol Med* 75: 492–501

45 Tone E, Kunisada K, Fujio Y, Matsui H, Negoro S, Oh H, Kishimoto T, Yamauchi-Takihara K (1998) Angiotensin II interferes with leukemia inhibitory factor-induced STAT3 activation in cardiac myocytes. *Biochem Biophys Res Commun* 253: 147–150

46 Sano M, Fukuda K, Kodama H, Pan J, Saito M, Matsuzaki J, Takahashi T, Makino S, Kato T, Ogawa S (2000) Interleukin-6 family of cytokines mediate angiotensin II-induced cardiac hypertrophy in rodent cardiomyocytes. *J Biol Chem* 275: 29717–29723

47 Jin H, Yang R, Keller GA, Ryan A, Ko A, Finkle D, Swanson TA, Li W, Pennica D, Wood WI et al (1996) *In vivo* effects of cardiotrophin-1. *Cytokine* 8: 920–926

48 Hirota H, Chen J, Betz UA, Rajewsky K, Gu Y, Ross J Jr, Muller W, Chien KR (1999) Loss of a gp130 cardiac muscle cell survival pathway is a critical event in the onset of heart failure during biomechanical stress. *Cell* 97: 189–198

49 Uozumi H, Hiroi Y, Zou Y, Takimoto E, Toko H, Niu P, Shimoyama M, Yazaki Y, Nagai R, Komuro I (2001) gp130 plays a critical role in pressure overload-induced cardiac hypertrophy. *J Biol Chem* 276: 23115–23119

50 Yasukawa H, Hoshijima M, Gu Y, Nakamura T, Pradervand S, Hanada T, Hanakawa Y, Yoshimura A, Ross J Jr, Chien KR (2001) Suppressor of cytokine signaling-3 is a biomechanical stress-inducible gene that suppresses gp130-mediated cardiac myocyte hypertrophy and survival pathways. *J Clin Invest* 108: 1459–1467

51 Shioi T, McMullen JR, Kang PM, Douglas PS, Obata T, Franke TF, Cantley LC, Izumo

S (2002) Akt/protein kinase B promotes organ growth in transgenic mice. *Mol Cell Biol* 22: 2799–2809

52   Shioi T, Kang PM, Douglas PS, Hampe J, Yballe CM, Lawitts J, Cantley LC, Izumo S (2000) The conserved phosphoinositide 3-kinase pathway determines heart size in mice. *Embo J* 19: 2537–2548

53   Stephanou A, Brar B, Heads R, Knight RD, Marber MS, Pennica D, Latchman DS (1998) Cardiotrophin-1 induces heat shock protein accumulation in cultured cardiac cells and protects them from stressful stimuli. *J Mol Cell Cardiol* 30: 849–855

54   Negoro S, Oh H, Tone E, Kunisada K, Fujio Y, Walsh K, Kishimoto T, Yamauchi-Taki-hara K (2001) Glycoprotein 130 regulates cardiac myocyte survival in doxorubicin-induced apoptosis through phosphatidylinositol 3-kinase/Akt phosphorylation and Bcl-xL/caspase-3 interaction. *Circulation* 103: 555–561

55   Fujio Y, Kunisada K, Hirota H, Yamauchi-Takihara K, Kishimoto T (1997) Signals through gp130 upregulate bcl-x gene expression *via* STAT1-binding cis-element in cardiac myocytes. *J Clin Invest* 99: 2898–2905

56   Shiojima I, Walsh K (2002) Role of Akt signaling in vascular homeostasis and angiogenesis. *Circ Res* 90: 1243–1250

57   Negoro S, Kunisada K, Tone E, Funamoto M, Oh H, Kishimoto T, Yamauchi-Takihara K (2000) Activation of JAK/STAT pathway transduces cytoprotective signal in rat acute myocardial infarction. *Cardiovasc Res* 47: 797–805

58   Kunisada K, Negoro S, Tone E, Funamoto M, Osugi T, Yamada S, Okabe M, Kishimo-to T, Yamauchi-Takihara K (2000) Signal transducer and activator of transcription 3 in the heart transduces not only a hypertrophic signal but a protective signal against doxorubicin-induced cardiomyopathy. *Proc Natl Acad Sci USA* 97: 315–319

59   Tsutamoto T, Wada A, Maeda K, Mabuchi N, Hayashi M, Tsutsui T, Ohnishi M, Fujii M, Matsumoto T, Yamamoto T et al (2001) Relationship between plasma level of cardiotrophin-1 and left ventricular mass index in patients with dilated cardiomyopathy. *J Am Coll Cardiol* 38: 1485–1490

60   Ng LL, O'Brien RJ, Demme B, Jennings S (2002) Non-competitive immunochemiluminometric assay for cardiotrophin-1 detects elevated plasma levels in human heart failure. *Clin Sci (Lond)* 102: 411–416

61   Talwar S, Squire IB, O'Brien RJ, Downie PF, Davies JE, Ng LL (2002) Plasma cardiotrophin-1 following acute myocardial infarction: relationship with left ventricular systolic dysfunction. *Clin Sci (Lond)* 102: 9–14

62   Talwar S, Squire IB, Downie PF, O'Brien RJ, Davies JE, Ng LL (2000) Elevated circulating cardiotrophin-1 in heart failure: Relationship with parameters of left ventricular systolic dysfunction. *Clin Sci (Lond)* 99: 83–88

63   Talwar S, Squire IB, Downie PF, Davies JE, Ng LL (2000) Plasma N terminal pro-brain natriuretic peptide and cardiotrophin-1 are raised in unstable angina. *Heart* 84: 421–424

64   Hojo Y, Ikeda U, Takahashi M, Shimada K (2002) Increased levels of monocyte-related cytokines in patients with unstable angina. *Atherosclerosis* 161: 403–408

65 Bristow MR, Long CS (2002) Cardiotrophin-1 in heart failure. *Circulation* 106: 1430–1432

66 Pan J, Fukuda K, Saito M, Matsuzaki J, Kodama H, Sano M, Takahashi T, Kato T, Ogawa S (1999) Mechanical Stretch Activates the JAK/STAT Pathway in Rat Cardiomyocytes. *Circ Res* 84: 1127–1136

67 Kukielka GL, Smith CW, Manning AM (1995) Induction of IL-6 synthesis in the myocardium. *Circulation* 92: 1866–1875

68 Deten A, Volz HC, Briest W, Zimmer HG (2002) Cardiac cytokine expression is up-regulated in the acute phase after myocardial infarction. Experimental studies in rats. *Cardiovasc Res* 55: 329–340

69 Pan J, Fukuda K, Kodama H, Sano M, Takahashi T, Makino S, Kato T, Manabe T, Hori S, Ogawa S (1998) Involvement of gp130-mediated signaling in pressure overload-induced activation of the JAK/STAT pathway in rodent heart. *Heart Vessels* 13: 199–208

70 Ishikawa M, Saito Y, Miamoto Y, Harada M, Kuwahara K, Ogawa E, Nakagawa O, Hamanaka I, Kajiyama N, Tkahashi N (1999) A heart-specific increase in carditrophin-1 gene expression precedes the establishment of ventricular hypertrophy in genetically hypertensive rats. J Hypertens 17: 807–816

71 Burger A, Benicke M, Deten A, Zimmer HG (2001) Catecholamines stimulate interleukin-6 synthesis in rat cardiac fibroblasts. *Am J Physiol* 281: H14–H21

72 Tsuruda T, Jougasaki M, Boerrigter G, Huntley BK, Chen HH, D'Assoro AB, Lee SC, Larsen AM, Cataliotti A, Burnett JC Jr (2002) Cardiotrophin-1 stimulation of cardiac fibroblast growth. Roles for glycoprotein 130/leukemia inhibitory factor receptor and the endothelin type A receptor. *Circ Res* 90: 128–134

73 Eiken HG, Oie E, Damas JK, Yndestad A, Bjerkeli V, Aass H, Simonen S, Geiran OR, Tonnessen T, Christensen G et al (2001) Myocardial gene expression of leukaemia inhibitory factor, interleukin-6 and glycoprotein 130 in end-stage human heart failure. Eur *J Clin Invest* 31: 389–397

74 Plenz G, Eschert H, Erren M, Wichter T, Bohm M, Flesch M, Scheld HH, Deng MC (2002) The interleukin-6/interleukin-6-receptor system is activated in donor hearts. *J Am Coll Cardiol* 39: 1508–1512

75 Zolk O, Ng LL, O'Brien RJ, Weyand M, Eschenhagen T (2002) Augmented expression of cardiotrophin-1 in failing human hearts is accompanied by diminished glycoprotein 130 receptor protein abundance. *Circulation* 106: 1442–1446

76 Menet E, Corbi P, Ancey C, Morel F, Delwail A, Garcia M, Osta AM, Wijdenes J, Potreau D, Lecron JC (2001) Interleukin-6 (IL-6) synthesis and gp130 expression by human pericardium. *Eur Cytokine Netw* 12: 639–646

77 Ancey C, Corbi P, Froger J, Delwail A, Wijdenes J, Gascan H, Potreau D, Lecron JC (2002) Secretion of IL-6, IL-11 and LIF by human cardiomyocytes in primary culture. *Cytokine* 18: 199–205

78 Humphries SE, Luong LA, Ogg MS, Hawe E, Miller GJ (2001) The interleukin-6-174

G/C promoter polymorphism is associated with risk of coronary heart disease and systolic blood pressure in healthy men. *Eur Hear J* 22: 2243–2252

79   Vickers MA, Green FR, Terry C, Mayosi BM, Julier C, Lathrop M, Ratcliffe PJ, Watkins HC, Keavney B (2002) Genotype at a promoter polymorphism of the interleukin-6 gene is associated with baseline levels of plasma C-reactive protein. *Cardiovasc Res* 53: 1029–1034

80   Fishman D, Faulds G, Jeffery R, Mohaned-Ali V, Yudkin JS, Humphries S, Woo P (1998) The effect of novel polymorphisms in the interleukin-6 (IL-6) gene on IL-6 transcription and plasma IL-6 levels, and association with systemic-onset juvenile chronic arthritis. *J Clin Invest* 102: 1369–1376

81   Jones KG, Brull DJ, Brown LC, Sian M, Greenhalgh RM, Humphries SE, Powell JT (2001) Interleukin-6 (IL-6) and the prognosis of abdominal aortic aneurisms. *Circulation* 103: 2260–2265

82   Brull DJ, Montgomery HE, Sanders J, Dhamrait S, Luong L, Rumley A, Lowe GD, Humphries SE (2001) Interleukin-6 gene-174G/C and −572G/C promoter polymorphisms are strong predictors of plasma interleukn-6 levels after coronary artery bypass surgery. *Atherioscler Thromb Vasc Biol* 21: 1458–1463

83   Rauramaa R, Vaisanen SB, Luong LA, Schmidt-Trucksass A, Penttila IM, Bouchard C, Toyry J, Humphries SE (2000) Stromelysin-1 and interleukin-6 gene promoter polymorphisms are determinants of asymptomatic carotid artery atherosclerosis. *Atherioscler Thromb Vasc Biol* 20: 2657–2662

84   Margaglione M, Bossone A, Cappucci G, Colaizzo D, Grandone E, Di Minno G (2001) The effect of interleukin-6 C/G-174 polymorphism and circulating interleukin-6 on fibrinogen plasma level. *Haematologica* 86: 199–204

85   Railson JE, Liao Z, Brar BK, Buddle JC, Pennica D, Stephanou A, Latchman DS (2002) Cardiotrophin-1 and urocortin cause protection by the same pathway and hypertrophy *via* distinct pathways in cardiac myocytes. *Cytokine* 17: 243–253

86   Lawrence KM, Chanalaris A, Scarabelli T, Hubank M, Pasini E, Townsend PA, Comini L, Ferrari R, Tinker A, Stephanou A et al (2002) KATP channel gene expression is induced by urocortin and mediates its cardioprotective effect. *Circulation* 106: 1556–1562

87   Participating investigators and scientists of the alliance for cellular signaling (2002) Overview of the alliance for cellular signaling. *Nature* 420: 703–706

88   Sambrano GR, Fraser I, Han H, Ni Y, O'Connell T, Yan Z, Stull JT (2002) Navigating the signalling network in mouse cardiac myocytes. *Nature* 420: 712–714

Toll-like receptors and the cardiovascular system

Stefan Frantz[1], Ralph A. Kelly[2] and Todd Bourcier[3]

[1]Medizinische Universitätsklinik Würzburg, Josef-Schneider-Str. 2, 97080 Würzburg, Germany; [2]Genzyme Corporation, 15 Pleasant St, Connector, P.O. Box 9322, Framingham, MA 01701-9322, USA; [3]Cardiovascular Division, Brigham and Women's Hospital, 75 Francis Street, Boston, MA 02115, USA

Introduction

Most micro-organisms that are encountered daily by a healthy individual are detected initially by defense mechanisms that are not antigen-specific, a response that is mediated by the innate immune system. In contrast to the adaptive immunity, where specific antigen receptors are generated by somatic hypermutation and selection, the innate immune systems uses germline encoded proteins that recognize specific patterns shared by groups of pathogens, but not the host. These receptors are called "pattern recognition receptors" ("PRRs") and recognize largely invariant "pathogen-associated molecular patterns" ("PAMPs"), as for example lipopolysaccharides of bacteria or double-stranded RNA of viruses [1]. This review will focus on the toll-like receptor (TLR) family, a class of pattern recognition receptors of major importance [2].

A total of ten human and nine murine transmembrane proteins of the TLR family have been identified to date [3–7]. They are dispersed throughout the genome [8] and are characterized by an extracellular leucine-rich repeat domain and an intracytoplasmic toll/interleukin-1 receptor homology (TIR) domain [9]. The TLR family members are classic pattern recognition receptors, exhibiting relatively low affinity ligand binding [10]. Upon binding of their specific ligands, TLRs can rapidly initiate an immune response: First, as an innate immune response, macrophages are activated by induction of pro-inflammatory cytokines and antimicrobial molecules such as nitric oxide. This enables macrophages to eliminate invading micro-organisms. Secondly, TLRs can activate dendritic cells. Dendritic cells can stimulate T-cell expansion and differentiation and thereby initiate an adaptive immune response. Thirdly, TLRs provide the necessary co-stimulatory molecules necessary for sustained activation of adaptive immunity.

Inflammation and Cardiac Diseases, edited by Giora Z. Feuerstein, Peter Libby and Douglas L. Mann
© 2003 Birkhäuser Verlag Basel/Switzerland

Toll-like receptors and their ligands

A growing list of subclass-specific TLR ligands has been identified to date (Tab. 1) and many more will likely be identified. The best characterized ligands to date are those for TLRs 2, 3, 4, and 9.

TLR2

TLR2 recognizes a variety of pathogens (Tab. 1). Most important is its activation by peptidoglycans (PGN) found in the cell walls of gram-positive bacteria. Indeed, TLR2-deficient mice do not respond to PGN, whereas the response to LPS is preserved [11]. TLR2 can also recognize mycoplasma, bacteria that lack a cell wall. Bacterial lipoproteins, such as MALP-2 (macrophage activating lipopeptide 2), also serve as activators of TLR-2 [12].

In order to activate an immune response to such a variety of structurally different pathogen-associated molecular patterns, TLR2 also forms heterodimers with other TLRs. This concept has been introduced by the observation that co-expression of TLR 2 and 6 confers responsiveness to gram-positive bacteria [13] as well as MALP-2 [14], whereas cells expressing TLR2 alone could not. Another functional heterodimer, consisting of TLR1 and 2, is also required for the recognition of *Neisseria* [15].

TLR3

The intracellular replication of some viruses results in the generation of double-stranded RNA that is obviously not produced by the host. Indeed, TLR3-deficient animals showed decreased responses to polyinosine-polycytidylic acid (poly(I:C)), a synthetic analogue of viral RNA. Therefore, TLR3 appears to be the pattern recognition receptor for viral double-stranded RNA.

TLR4

Human TLR4 was the first mammalian TLR described [16] and is the best characterized receptor of the TLR family so far, and recognizes a variety of PAMPs. Importantly, TLR4 functions as the long sought pattern recognition receptor for lipopolysaccharides (LPS). LPS is the major component of the outer membrane of gram-negative bacteria, and is composed of polysaccharides extending outward from bacterial cell surface and a lipid portion, called lipid A. LPS is first bound to a serum protein called LPS binding protein (LBP), which transfers LPS to CD14, which is both secreted in the serum and expressed on the plasma membranes of macrophages. After association with MD2 [17], the CD14 and LPS complex can activate TLR4.

The function of TLR4 as signal transducing receptor for LPS has been confirmed by several TLR4 deficient murine models. It had been known for some time that two spontaneous mutant mouse strains, C3H/HeJ and C57BL/10ScCr, were resistant to LPS [18, 19]. After the first description of TLR4, both strains were shown to carry mutations in the TLR4 gene. Furthermore, mice with targeted disruption of TLR4 (KO) were confirmed to exhibit a defect in the response to LPS [20], as expected. Initial reports had also suggested TLR2 as a LPS receptor [21]. However, in TLR2 KO animals LPS signaling was not found to be compromised, and the apparent activation of TLR2 by LPS was eventually attributed to contaminants which could also function as TLR2 agonist [22].

Interestingly, TLR4 does not only recognize PAMPs from invading pathogens, but several other ligands as well. For example, paclitaxol, a well-known chemotherapeutic agent, is recognized by TLR4 [23]. Moreover, TLR4 also appears to be involved in the recognition of host-derived inflammatory products. For example, heat shock protein 60 (HSP60) is a molecular chaperone that is conserved in both invertebrates and vertebrates, and can activate NF-κB through both TLR2 and TLR4 [24]. As expected, HSP60 did not cause an inflammatory response in the TLR4 deficient C3H/HeJ mice [25]. Finally, degradation products of fibronectin and collagen can exert their pro-inflammatory activity through TLR4 signaling [26].

TLR9

Utilizing TLR9 KO mice, TLR9 is able to recognize all unmethylated CpG motifs in bacterial DNA [4]. Bacteria lack cytosine methylation while most of the CpG is methylated in the mammalian genome. Thus unmethylated CpG motifs are an ideal pathogen-associated pattern. Finally, TLR9 could also be implicated in the recognition of autoimmune antigens and subsequent activation of B cells. TLR9 could therefore play an important role in autoimmune diseases [27].

In summary, different TLRs can discriminate among specific molecular patterns associated with pathogens and therefore participate in triggering a specific adaptive immune response. Moreover, several additional features enable the TLR system to initiate a cell and pathogen specific immune response. First, TLR family members are differentially expressed among immune and parenchymal cells. Second, several TLRs will often be activated by more than one class of PAMPs. For example, zymosan, a PAMP found in yeast, activates TLR signaling by utilizing functional heterodimers of TLR2 and 6 [13]. Third, different classes of TLRs trigger distinct cell signaling pathways. For example, TLR4 responses include secretion of IL-10, IFN-β and IL-12, whereas TLR2 responses include IL-8, IL-12, and IL-23 [28]. Thus

Table 1

TLR	Origin of ligand	Ligand	Comments
1	*Neisseria meningitides*	Soluble factors [15]	Functional heterodimer with TLR2 [15]
2	Gram-positive bacteria	Lipoprotein [29, 30] Peptidoglycan [11, 31] Lipoteichic acids [31, 32]	Functional heterodimer with TLR6 [13]
	Staphylococcus	Modulin [33]	
	Mycoplasma, mycobacteria, spirochetes	Lipopeptides, lipopeptides [34–37]	
	Mycoplasma	MALP-2 [14]	Functional heterodimer with TLR6 [14]
	Spirochetes	Glycolipids [32]	
	Listeria	Heat killed bacteria [38]	
	Mycobacteria	Lipoarabinomannan [39, 40]	
	Porphyromonas, spirochetes (leptospira)	LPS [41, 42]	
	Yeast	Zymosan [13]	Functional heterodimer with TLR6 [13]
	Trypanosoma cruzi	GPI anchor [43]	
	Klebsiella	Outer membrane protein A [44]	
	Neisseria meningitides	Soluble factors [15]	
	Borellia burgdorferi	Lipopeptides [37]	
	Treponema pallidum	Lipopeptides [37]	
3	Virus	Double stranded RNA [45]	
4	Gram-negative bacteria	LPS [18–20]	
	Gram-positive bacteria	Lipoteichic acid [11]	
	Plant	Taxol [23]	
	RSV (respiratory syncytial virus)	F protein [46]	
	Host	*HSP 60* [25]	
		Fibronectin EDA domain [26]	

Table 1 - continued

TLR	Origin of ligand	Ligand	Comments
5	Bacteria with flagella	Flagellin [47]	
6	Mycoplasma	MALP-2 [14]	Functional heterodimer with TLR2 [14]
	Gram-positive bacteria		Functional heterodimer with TLR2 [13]
	Yeast	Zymosan [13]	Functional heterodimer with TLR2 [13]
9	Bacteria	Unmethylated CpG DNA [4]	Potential role in autoimmune diseases
	Host	IgG2a [27]	

Modified after [10]

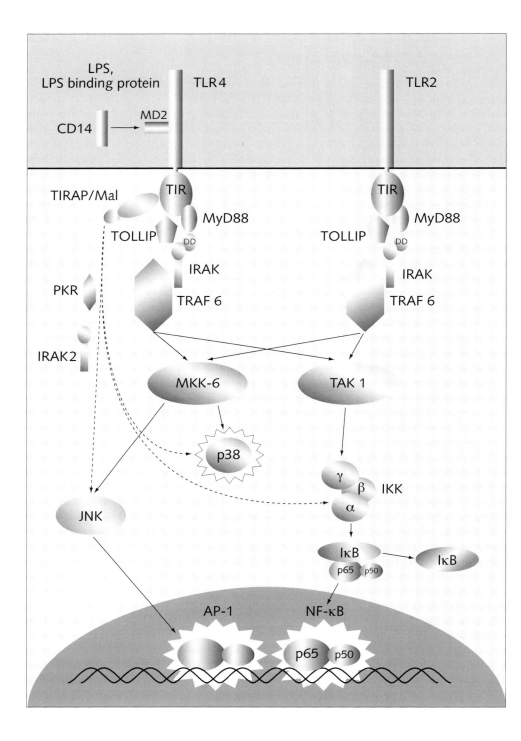

TLR-dependent innate immunity signaling pathways do trigger responses with some degree of specificity, allowing specific immune responses for specific PAMPs.

Toll-like receptor signaling pathways

TLRs are type 1 membrane-spanning receptors, with an extracellular leucine-rich repeat (LRR) motif and an intracellular signaling motif similar to those of the inter-leukin-1 (IL-1R) and interleukin-18 receptor (IL-18R) (i.e., the toll-interleukin 1 receptor or TIR homology domain) [48, 49]. TLR signaling (Fig. 1) is similar to that mediated by IL-1. After recruiting the cytoplasmic adapter protein MyD88 and IRAK (interleukin receptor associated kinase), which is associated with TOLLIP (toll interacting protein) [50], MKK6 (mitogen activated protein kinase kinase 6) or TAK1 (TGF-β activated kinase) is activated through TRAF6 (tumor necrosis factor receptor-activated factor-6). TAK1 activates subsequently an IκB kinase which results in phosphorylation of IκB, thereby promoting NF-κB translocation to the nucleus, and gene transcription [51, 52]. MKK6 can activate p38 MAPK or JNK (c-Jun-N-terminal kinase).

However, a MyD88 independent pathway also exists for TLR4. Upon activation with LPS, MyD88 deficient cells could not induce the production of cytokines and co-stimulatory molecules, as expected, but these cells did exhibit delayed activation of NF-κB and MAPK [53]. This observation was eventually attributed to a new TLR4 specific adapter protein, termed TIRAP (TIR containing adapter protein) or Mal (MyD88 adapter link) [54, 55]. NF-κB can be activated by formation of TIRAP/Mal hetero- or homodimers including IRAK-2 and PKR (dsRNA-dependent protein kinase). In addition, there is good evidence that several other, as yet unidentified, pathways may exist as well [56].

Toll-like receptors in the cardiovascular system

Toll-like receptors are expressed by virtually all cells of the heart. In the vasculature, TLRs 1–6 are expressed in macrophages, smooth muscle cells, and endothelial cells.

Figure 1

Toll signaling pathway. A white star marks activation. Abbreviations: LPS, lipopolysaccharide; TIR, toll-interleukin-1 receptor homology domain; IRAK, interleukin receptor associated kinase; TOLLIP, toll interacting protein; MKK6, mitogen activated protein kinase kinase; TAK1, TGFβ activated kinase; TRAF6, tumor necrosis factor receptor-activated factor-6; NF-κB, nuclear factor κB; MAPK, mitogen activated protein kinase; JNK, c-Jun-N-terminal kinase; TIRAP, TIR containing adapter protein; Mal, MyD88 adapter link.

When compared to normal vessels, expression of TLRs 1, 2, and 4 are markedly enhanced in human atherosclerosis plaques [57]. Moreover, TLR4 can be up-regulated in macrophages by oxidized LDL suggesting that TLR4 might provide one link between lipids, inflammation and atherosclerosis [58].

In the myocardium TLRs 1 and 5 cannot be detected by RT-PCR. However, TLRs 2, 3, 4, and 6 are readily detectable [59]. Moreover, there is evidence linking TLR signaling with the pathogeneses of the cardiomyopathy associated with systemic sepsis, and in several forms of congestive heart failure (CHF). In our current understanding of sepsis, bacteria or bacterial related products activate pro-inflammatory cytokines, including TNF and IL-1β among others, leading to multiple-organ failure including myocardial depression. To date, cardiac dysfunction in septic shock has been mainly attributed to direct effects of several cytokines on cardiac function. However, TLR4 might also be of major importance and be upstream of the pro-inflammatory response. Indeed, C3H/HeJ mice, which do not have any functioning TLR4 receptors, following challenge with LPS have a significantly lower induction of pro-inflammatory markers, as for example IL-1β, iNOS, and NF-κB, when compared to mice with intact TLR4 signaling [60]. Moreover, following LPS injection the cardiac contractility of control mice was depressed, whereas the contractility of TLR4-deficient mice was preserved as measured by echocardiography and *in vivo* hemodynamics [61]. This suggests that TLR4 is involved in mediating LPS induced negative inotropic effects in septic cardiomyopathy *in vivo*.

TLRs might also be involved in another cardiac disease not directly related to sepsis or infection. In congestive heart failure (CHF) a number of inflammatory cytokines, including TNF, IL-1β, IL-6 and IL-8, as well as iNOS, have been implicated in myocardial depression and myocardial remodelling characteristic of CHF. Since there is no evidence for an infectious pathogen in most causes of heart failure, with the exception of infectious myocarditis, the proximal events triggering cytokine and iNOS expression are not well understood. However, the majority of cytokines associated with CHF, as well as iNOS, are part of the innate immune response. Indeed, several innate immune receptors appear to be highly expressed and activated in CHF. TLR4 expression, for example, is increased in the myocardium of humans and experimental animals with CHF. In addition to increased expression of TLR4, there is also a change in its expression pattern. Whereas in normal murine and human myocardium TLR4 expression is diffuse and predominantly expressed in cardiac myocytes, myocardium from patients with advanced heart failure showed focal areas of intense TLR4 staining. The reason for this change in TLR4 expression in the "remodelling" failing myocardium is not yet known [52]. Furthermore, a potential role of TLR2 in the response to oxidative stress could be demonstrated in neonatal rat cardiac myocytes. Blockade of TLR2 by an antibody was also able to inhibit hydrogen peroxide induced NF-κB activation and to increase cytotoxicity and apoptosis [59]. Considering that TLR4 is most highly up-regulated in the failing heart following myocardial infarction in the border zone between viable and damaged myocardium, one might speculate that activation of TLRs could play a role in the protection of ischemic but viable cardiac myocytes. Conversely, if TLR4 triggers an excessive inflammatory response, one might speculate that TLR4 could exacerbate types of myocardial injury. Recent results from our laboratory support the latter scenario in a murine model of myocardial ischemia/reperfusion injury (I/R). Following one hour ischemia and 24 hours reperfusion, hearts from TLR4-deficient C57/BL10 ScCr mice (Cr) sustained smaller infarctions compared to the parental C57/BL10 ScSn mice or C57/BL6 mice that express TLR4 normally, despite all strains having similar areas at risk of infarction. Smaller infarct size in TLR4-deficient Cr mice was associated with less lipid peroxidation, fewer infiltrating neutrophils, and less myocardial deposition of complement factor-3. Of particular interest, all three murine strains exhibited the same degree of leukocyte infiltration in a model of thioglycollate-induced peritonitis, suggesting that TLR4 is involved in some, but not all types of inflammation.

In summary, toll-like receptors are an important family of innate pattern recognition receptors that both trigger innate immune effector proteins and provide essential co-stimulatory signals for adaptive immunity. TLRs are readily detectable in the cardiovascular system and up-regulated in cardiovascular diseases such as atherosclerosis, septic cardiomyopathy and heart failure. Although there is not yet a consensus as to the specific role played by the innate immune system in these diseases, a growing understanding of the innate immune system in the heart could lead to novel therapeutic strategies.

References

1   Janeway CA Jr (1989) Approaching the asymptote? Evolution and revolution in immunology. *Cold Spring Harb Symp Quant Biol* 54 Pt 1: 1–13

2   Medzhitov R (2001) Toll-like receptors and innate immunity. *Nature Rev Immunol* 1: 135–145

3   Chuang T, Ulevitch RJ (2001) Identification of hTLR10: A novel human Toll-like receptor preferentially expressed in immune cells. *Biochim Biophys Acta* 1518: 157–161

4   Hemmi H, Takeuchi O, Kawai T, Kaisho T, Sato S, Sanjo H, Matsumoto M, Hoshino K, Wagner H, Takeda K et al (2000) A Toll-like receptor recognizes bacterial DNA. *Nature* 408: 740–745

5   Du X, Poltorak, A, Wei Y, Beutler B (2000) Three novel mammalian toll-like receptors: Gene structure, expression, and evolution. *Eur Cytokine Netw* 11: 362–371

6   Takeuchi O, Kawai T, Sanjo H, Copeland NG, Gilbert DJ, Jenkins NA, Takeda K, Akira S (1999) TLR6: A novel member of an expanding toll-like receptor family. *Gene* 231: 59–65

7   Rock FL, Hardiman G, Timans JC, Kastelein RA, Bazan JF (1998) A family of human receptors structurally related to drosophila toll. *Proc Natl Acad Sci USA* 95: 588–593

8   Akira S, Takeda K, Kaisho T (2001) Toll-like receptors: Critical proteins linking innate and acquired immunity. *Nat Immunol* 2: 675–680

9   Means TK, Golenbock DT, Fenton MJ (2000) Structure and function of toll-like receptor proteins *Life Sci* 68: 241–258

10 Kaisho T, Akira S (2002) Toll-like receptors as adjuvant receptors. *Biochim Biophys Acta* 1589: 1–13

11 Takeuchi O, Hoshino K, Kawai T, Sanjo H, Takada H, Ogawa T, Takeda K, Akira S (1999) Differential roles of TLR2 and TLR4 in recognition of gram-negative and gram-positive bacterial cell wall components. *Immunity* 11: 443–451

12 Takeuchi O, Kaufmann A, Grote K, Kawai T, Hoshino K, Morr M, Muhlradt PF, Akira S (2000) Cutting edge: Preferentially the R-stereoisomer of the mycoplasmal lipopeptide macrophage-activating lipopeptide-2 activates immune cells through a toll-like receptor 2- and MyD88-dependent signaling pathway. *J Immunol* 164: 554–557

13 Ozinsky A, Underhill DM, Fontenot JD, Hajjar AM, Smith KD, Wilson CB, Schroeder L, Aderem A (2000) The repertoire for pattern recognition of pathogens by the innate immune system is defined by co-operation between toll-like receptors. *Proc Natl Acad Sci USA* 97: 13766–13771

14 Takeuchi O, Kawai T, Muhlradt PF, Morr M, Radolf JD, Zychlinsky A, Takeda K, Akira S (2001) Discrimination of bacterial lipoproteins by toll-like receptor 6. *Int Immunol* 13: 933–940

15 Wyllie DH, Kiss-Toth E, Visintin A, Smith SC, Boussouf S, Segal DM, Duff GW, Dower SK (2000) Evidence for an accessory protein function for toll-like receptor 1 in anti-bacterial responses. *J Immunol* 165: 7125–7132

16 Medzhitov R, Preston-Hurlburt P, Janeway CA Jr. (1997) A human homologue of the *Drosophila* toll protein signals activation of adaptive immunity. *Nature* 388: 394–397

17 Shimazu R, Akashi S, Ogata H, Nagai Y, Fukudome K, Miyake K, Kimoto M (1999) MD-2, a molecule that confers lipopolysaccharide responsiveness on toll-like receptor 4. *J Exp Med* 189: 1777–1782

18 Poltorak A, He X, Smirnova I, Liu MY, Huffel CV, Du X, Birdwell D, Alejos E, Silva M, Galanos C et al (1998) Defective LPS signaling in C3H/HeJ and C57BL/10ScCr mice: Mutations in tlr4 gene. *Science* 282: 2085–2088

19 Qureshi ST, Larivire L, Leveque G, Clermont S, Moore KJ, Gros P, Malo D (1999) Endotoxin-tolerant mice have mutations in toll-like receptor 4 (Tlr4). *J Exp Med* 189: 615–625

20 Hoshino K, Takeuchi O, Kawai T, Sanjo H, Ogawa T, Takeda Y, Takeda K, Akira S (1999) Cutting edge: Toll-like receptor 4 (TLR4)-deficient mice are hyporesponsive to lipopolysaccharide: Evidence for TLR4 as the Lps gene product. *J Immunol* 162: 3749–3752

21 Yang RB, Mark MR, Gray A, Huang A, Xie MH, Zhang M, Goddard A, Wood WI, Gurney AL, Godowski PJ (1998) Toll-like receptor-2 mediates lipopolysaccharide-induced cellular signaling. *Nature* 395: 284–288

22 Hirschfeld M, Ma Y, Weis JH, Vogel SN, Weis JJ (2000) Cutting edge: Repurification of

lipopolysaccharide eliminates signaling through both human and murine toll-like receptor 2. *J Immunol* 165: 618–622

23 Kawasaki K, Akashi S, Shimazu R, Yoshida T, Miyake K, Nishijima M (2000) Mouse toll-like receptor 4.MD-2 complex mediates lipopolysaccharide-mimetic signal transduction by taxol. *J Biol Chem* 275: 2251–2254

24 Vabulas RM, Ahmad-Nejad P, da Costa C, Miethke T, Kirschning CJ, Hacker H, Wagner H (2001) Endocytosed HSP60s use toll-like receptor 2 (TLR2) and TLR4 to activate the toll/interleukin-1 receptor signaling pathway in innate immune cells. *J Biol Chem* 276: 31332–31339

25 Ohashi K, Burkart V, Flohe S, Kolb H (2000) Cutting edge: Heat shock protein 60 is a putative endogenous ligand of the toll-like receptor-4 complex. *J Immunol* 164: 558–561

26 Okamura Y, Watari M, Jerud ES, Young DW, Ishizaka ST, Rose J, Chow JC, Strauss JF 3rd (2001) The extra domain A of fibronectin activates toll-like receptor 4. *J Biol Chem* 276: 10229–10233

27 Leadbetter EA, Rifkin IR, Hohlbaum AM, Beaudette BC, Shlomchik MJ, Marshak-Rothstein A (2002) Chromatin-IgG complexes activate B cells by dual engagement of IgM and toll-like receptors. *Nature* 416: 603–607

28 Re F, Strominger JL (2001) Toll-like receptor 2 (TLR2) and TLR4 differentially activate human dendritic cells. *J Biol Chem* 276: 37692–37699

29 Yoshimura A, Lien E, Ingalls RR, Tuomanen E, Dziarski R, Golenbock D (1999) Cutting edge: Recognition of gram-positive bacterial cell wall components by the innate immune system occurs *via* toll-like receptor 2. *J Immunol* 163: 1–5

30 Underhill DM, Ozinsky A, Hajjar AM, Stevens A, Wilson CB, Bassetti M, Aderem A (1999) The toll-like receptor 2 is recruited to macrophage phagosomes and discriminates between pathogens. *Nature* 401: 811–815

31 Schwandner R, Dziarski R, Wesche H, Rothe M, Kirschning CJ (1999) Peptidoglycan- and lipoteichoic acid-induced cell activation is mediated by toll-like receptor 2. *J Biol Chem* 274: 17406–17409

32 Opitz B, Schroder NW, Spreitzer I, Michelsen KS, Kirschning CJ, Hallatschek W, Zahringer U, Hartung T, Gobel UB, Schumann RR (2001) Toll-like receptor-2 mediates treponema glycolipid and lipoteichoic acid-induced NF-kappa-B translocation. *J Biol Chem* 276: 22041–22047

33 Hajjar AM, O'Mahony DS, Ozinsky A, Underhill DM, Aderem A, Klebanoff SJ, Wilson CB (2001) Cutting edge: Functional interactions between toll-like receptor (TLR) 2 and TLR1 or TLR6 in response to phenol-soluble modulin. *J Immunol* 166: 15–19

34 Aliprantis AO, Yang RB, Mark MR, Suggett S, Devaux B, Radolf, JD, Klimpel GR, Godowski P, Zychlinsky A (1999) Cell activation and apoptosis by bacterial lipoproteins through toll-like receptor-2. *Science* 285: 736–739

35 Brightbill HD, Libraty DH, Krutzik SR, Yang RB, Belisle JT, Bleharski JR, Maitland M, Norgard MV, Plevy SE, Smale ST et al (1999) Host defense mechanisms triggered by microbial lipoproteins through toll-like receptors. *Science* 285: 732–736

36   Hirschfeld M, Kirschning CJ, Schwandner R, Wesche H, Weis JH, Wooten RM, Weis JJ (1999) Cutting edge: Inflammatory signaling by *Borrelia burgdorferi* lipoproteins is mediated by toll-like receptor 2 [In Process Citation]. *J Immunol* 163: 2382–2386

37   Lien E, Sellati TJ, Yoshimura A, Flo TH, Rawadi G, Finberg RW, Carroll JD, Espevik T, Ingalls RR, Radolf JD et al (1999) Toll-like receptor 2 functions as a pattern recognition receptor for diverse bacterial products. *J Biol Chem* 274: 33419–33425

38   Flo TH, Halaas O, Lien E, Ryan L, Teti G, Golenbock DT, Sundan A, Espevik T (2000) Human toll-like receptor 2 mediates monocyte activation by listeria monocytogenes, but not by group B streptococci or lipopolysaccharide. *J Immunol* 164: 2064–2069

39   Means TK, Wang S, Lien E, Yoshimura A, Golenbock DT, Fenton MJ (1999) Human toll-like receptors mediate cellular activation by mycobacterium tuberculosis. *J Immunol* 163: 3920–3927

40   Means TK, Lien E, Yoshimura A, Wang S, Golenbock DT, Fenton MJ (1999) The CD14 Ligands lipoarabinomannan and lipopolysaccharide differ in their requirement for toll-like receptors. *J Immunol* 163: 6748–6755

41   Werts C, Tapping RI, Mathison JC, Chuang TH, Kravchenko V, Saint Girons I, Haake DA, Godowski PJ, Hayashi F, Ozinsky A et al (2001) Leptospiral lipopolysaccharide activates cells through a TLR2-dependent mechanism. *Nat Immunol* 2: 346–352

42   Hirschfeld M, Weis JJ, Toshchakov V, Salkowski CA, Cody MJ, Ward DC, Qureshi N, Michalek SM, Vogel SN (2001) Signaling by toll-like receptor 2 and 4 agonists results in differential gene expression in murine macrophages. *Infect Immun* 69: 1477–1482

43   Campos MA, Almeida IC, Takeuchi O, Akira S, Valente EP, Procopio DO, Travassos LR, Smith JA, Golenbock DT, Gazzinelli RT (2001) Activation of toll-like receptor-2 by glycosylphosphatidylinositol anchors from a protozoan parasite. *J Immunol* 167: 416–423

44   Jeannin P, Renno T, Goetsch L, Miconnet I, Aubry JP, Delneste Y, Herbault N, Baussant T, Magistrelli G, Soulas C et al (2000) OmpA targets dendritic cells, induces their maturation and delivers antigen into the MHC Class I presentation pathway. *Nat Immunol* 1: 502–509

45   Alexopoulou L, Holt AC, Medzhitov R, Flavell RA (2001) Recognition of double-stranded RNA and activation of NF-kappa-B by toll-like receptor 3. *Nature* 413: 732–738

46   Kurt-Jones EA, Popova L, Kwinn L, Haynes LM, Jones LP, Tripp RA, Walsh EE, Freeman MW, Golenbock DT, Anderson LJ et al (2000) Pattern recognition receptors TLR4 and CD14 mediate response to respiratory syncytial virus. *Nat Immunol* 1: 398–401

47   Hayashi F, Smith KD, Ozinsky A, Hawn TR, Yi EC, Goodlett DR, Eng JK, Akira S, Underhill DM, Aderem A (2001) The innate immune response to bacterial flagellin is mediated by toll-like receptor 5. *Nature* 410: 1099–1103

48   Medzhitov R, Janeway CA Jr (1998) An ancient system of host defense. *Curr Opin Immunol* 10: 12–15

49   Kopp EB, Medzhitov R (1999) The toll-receptor family and control of innate immunity. *Curr Opin Immunol* 11: 13–18

50 Burns K, Clatworthy J, Martin L, Martinon F, Plumpton C, Maschera B, Lewis A, Ray K, Tschopp J, Volpe F (2000) Tollip, a new component of the IL-1RI pathway, links IRAK to the IL-1 receptor. *Nat Cell Biol* 2: 346–351

51 Medzhitov R, Preston-Hurlburt P, Kopp E, Stadlen A, Chen C, Ghosh S, Janeway CA Jr. (1998) MyD88 is an adaptor protein in the htoll/IL-1 receptor family signaling pathways. *Mol Cell* 2: 253–258

52 Frantz S, Kobzik L, Kim YD, Fukazawa R, Medzhitov R, Lee RT, Kelly RA (1999) Toll4 (TLR4) expression in cardiac myocytes in normal and failing myocardium. *J Clin Invest* 104: 271–280

53 Kawai T, Adachi O, Ogawa T, Takeda K, Akira S (1999) Unresponsiveness of MyD88-deficient mice to endotoxin. *Immunity* 11: 115–122

54 Horng T, Barton GM, Medzhitov R (2001) TIRAP: An adapter molecule in the toll signaling pathway. *Nat Immunol* 2: 835–841

55 Fitzgerald KA, Palsson-McDermott EM, Bowie AG, Jefferies CA, Mansell AS, Brady G, Brint E, Dunne A, Gray P, Harte M.T et al (2001) Mal (MyD88-adapter-like) is required for toll-like receptor-4 signal transduction. *Nature* 413: 78–83

56 Underhill DM, Ozinsky A (2002) Toll-like receptors: Key mediators of microbe detection. *Curr Opin Immunol* 14: 103–110

57 Edfeldt K, Swedenborg J, Hansson GK, Yan ZQ (2002) Expression of toll-like receptors in human atherosclerotic lesions: A possible pathway for plaque activation. *Circulation* 105: 1158–1161

58 Xu XH, Shah PK, Faure E, Equils O, Thomas L, Fishbein MC, Luthringer D, Xu XP, Rajavashisth TB, Yano J et al (2001) Toll-like receptor-4 is expressed by macrophages in murine and human lipid-rich atherosclerotic plaques and up-regulated by oxidized LDL. *Circulation* 104: 3103–3108

59 Frantz S, Kelly RA, Bourcier T (2001) Role of TLR-2 in the activation of nuclear factor-kappa-B by oxidative stress in cardiac myocytes. *J Biol Chem* 276: 5197–5203

60 Baumgarten G, Knuefermann P, Nozaki N, Sivasubramanian N, Mann DL, Vallejo JG (2001) *In vivo* expression of pro-inflammatory mediators in the adult heart after endotoxin administration: The role of toll-like receptor-4. *J Infect Dis* 183: 1617–1624

61 Nemoto S, Vallejo JG, Knuefermann P, Misra A, Defreitas G, Carabello BA, Mann DL (2002) Escherichia coli LPS-induced LV dysfunction: Role of toll-like receptor-4 in the adult heart. *Am J Physiol Heart Circ Physiol* 282: H2316–2323

The role of IL-6 in experimental and clinical heart failure

Elaine J. Tanhehco and Hani N. Sabbah

Departments of Medicine, Division of Cardiovascular Medicine, Henry Ford Heart and Vascular Institute, 2799 West Grand Boulevard, Detroit, MI 48202, USA

Introduction

In the United States alone, nearly five million people carry the diagnosis of heart failure (HF) with approximately 550,000 new cases diagnosed each year and 250,000 deaths attributed to the disease. The early stages of HF are often clinically asymptomatic due to physiological compensatory mechanisms. However, these same mechanisms can precipitate the ventricular dysfunction and remodeling that ultimately culminate in overt intractable HF. The cause of the progressive deterioration of left-ventricular (LV) function in HF remains unknown. Factors such as ongoing intrinsic contractile dysfunction of residual viable cardiocytes [1], progressive LV remodeling manifested by progressive LV dilation, cardiocyte hypertrophy and interstitial fibrosis [2, 3] and ongoing loss of residual viable cardiocytes [4, 5] have been implicated as contributors to the progression of LV dysfunction in HF. In addition, enhanced activation of several neurohumoral systems, including sustained elevation of plasma norepinephrine, increased levels of plasma angiotensin-II, and down-regulation of cardiac β-adrenergic receptors [6] are observed in HF. Inflammatory cytokines are also thought to contribute to LV dysfunction in HF, including interleukin–6 (IL-6) and members of the IL-6 family [7]. Clinically, plasma levels of IL-6 have been shown to be inversely correlated to LV function in HF patients [8–11]. Growing experimental evidence also points to a role for IL-6 in mediating some of the detrimental cardiovascular changes that occur during HF.

IL-6

IL-6 is a ubiquitously expressed inflammatory cytokine produced in response to infection and injury, and is induced by factors such as other cytokines, hormones and microbial products [12, 13]. IL-6 is a member of a family of structurally related cytokines including IL-11, cardiotrophin-1 (CT-1), oncostatin M, ciliary neurotrophic factor, leukemia inhibitory factor (LIF), and novel neurotrophin-1/B cell stimulatory factor-3 [14–19]. In addition to sharing a similar structure, these

Inflammation and Cardiac Diseases, edited by Giora Z. Feuerstein, Peter Libby and Douglas L. Mann
© 2003 Birkhäuser Verlag Basel/Switzerland

cytokines also appear to be functionally redundant in a wide variety of cell types. The IL-6 receptor complex consists of an IL-6 receptor (IL-6R) and the signal transducing subunit, glycoprotein (gp) 130. The IL-6 related cytokines also signal *via* gp130 and this may account for their overlapping functions [20, 21]. After binding to its receptor, IL-6 triggers homodimerizaton of gp130, which then leads to the activation of the Jak/STAT pathway and ultimately affects transcription of a variety of genes, including those for acute phase proteins [22, 23]. The other members of the IL-6 family operate through heterodimerization of gp130 with the LIF-receptor (except for IL-11, which, like IL-6, relies on gp130 homodimerization) [7]. The actions of IL-6 are pleiotropic, affecting several aspects of the inflammatory response such as B-cell terminal differentiation, activation of T-cells, initiation of acute phase protein synthesis and stimulation of hemopoietic progenitors [23]. The inflammatory cytokines IL-1 and tumor necrosis factor (TNF)-α both increase IL-6 expression [23, 24], and all three cytokines together induce the production of acute phase proteins [23]. The complexity of the inflammatory response requires the coordinated efforts of several key factors, with IL-6 being one of the pivotal components.

IL-6 in clinical heart failure

Circulating IL-6 levels have been found to be inversely correlated with myocardial function in patients with HF [8–11]. In addition, levels of soluble gp130 are also increased in HF patients and reflect New York Heart Association (NYHA) functional class (25). Interestingly, enhanced IL-6 bioactivity has been observed in the HF state, suggesting augmentation of the inflammatory response [25]. Plasma IL-6 levels have been deemed as an independent prognostic indicator of adverse outcomes in patients with HF regardless of etiology [10, 26]. The database of the Vesnarinone trial (VEST) was analyzed for levels of cytokines and cytokine receptors in 1,200 patients with advanced HF and determined that circulating IL-6 levels correlated with worsening LV function and predicted incidence of mortality [27]. The study revealed that IL-6 levels were significantly greater in NYHA Class III *versus* Class IV patients and significantly higher in ischemic compared to dilated cardiomyopathy [27]. IL-6 levels were also significantly increased in patients that died during follow up (mean = 55 weeks) [27]. In addition, expression of the IL-6 related protein, CT-1, has been found to be elevated in HF [28]. However, the same study found a concomitant decrease in gp130 protein, suggesting a counter-regulatory mechanism.

Sustained activation of the sympathetic nervous system and of the renin-angiotensin-aldosterone system, occurs during the progression of HF and is thought to directly contribute to the progression of LV dysfunction. IL-6 spillover has been positively and independently correlated with a rise in plasma norepinephrine in HF patients [10]. The β-blocker carvedilol, but not metoprolol, was shown to decrease IL-6 in HF patients [29–31]. Beta-blockers are known to significantly improve morbidity and mortality in HF [32, 33]. Unlike metoprolol, carvedilol is a non-selective adrenoceptor antagonist and possesses antioxidant effects, which may account for the differential effects of these agents on circulating IL-6 levels [34–36]. Angiotensin converting enzyme (ACE) inhibitors also appear to alter IL-6 in HF. It was reported that enalapril decreases IL-6 bioactivity [37]. The angiotensin-II AT-1 receptor antagonist, candesartan, was shown to decrease plasma IL-6 (38) in HF patients. Diminished IL-6 bioactivity was also found to be significantly correlated to a decrease in interventricular septum thickening in HF patients treated with enalapril [37]. Finally, in the Prospective Randomized Amlodipine Survival Evaluation (PRAISE) trial, treatment with the calcium channel blocker, amlodipine, was associated with decreased circulating IL-6 in HF patients [39]. These results suggest that the beneficial effects of these drugs in HF may, in part, be explained by reducing IL-6 production and bioactivity but a cause-effect relation has yet to be demonstrated.

Experimental evidence for the role of IL-6 in heart failure

Increased IL-6 generation has also been shown in experimental animal models of HF. In rats with post-infarction LV dysfunction and failure, IL-6 mRNA is increased, indicating that the cytokine may act in an autocrine manner [31, 40]. Humoral mediators that adversely impact LV function in HF, including TNF-α, angiotensin-II and norepinephrine increase IL-6 expression in cardiomyocytes [24, 41]. Angiotensin-II also raises expression of IL-6, CT-1 and LIF in cardiac myocytes, fibroblasts and vascular smooth muscle cells [42–45]. These data suggest that IL-6 may arise from a variety of cell types in the setting of HF. In addition, adrenergic stimulation increases CT-1 in cardiac myocytes [46], suggesting that locally produced IL-6 related cytokines also participate in the pathophysiology of HF.

Both LV dilation and hypertrophy are distinguishable features of HF. IL-6 related cytokines have been shown to induce cardiomyocyte hypertrophy in several animal models of HF. In dogs with pacing-induced HF and hypertensive rats, myocardial CT-1 expression was found to be elevated in the myocardium [47, 48]. Though the role of CT-1 in the development of ventricular hypertrophy was questionable in the hypertension model, its expression appeared to be directly related to LV mass index in the HF dogs [47, 48]. In murine cardiomyocytes, exposure to CT-1 increases angiotensinogen mRNA as well as induces cellular hypertrophy [49]. The angiotensin-II AT-1 receptor blocker losartan attenuates this effect, illustrating the potential interplay between IL-6 related cytokines and activation of the renin-angiotensin system [49]. LIF also produces hypertrophy in isolated rat ventricular cardiomyocytes in a similar manner compared to CT-1, namely by activating the same immediate early genes, inducing an increase in cell size and sarcomere organization and increasing atrial natriuretic peptide transcription [50]. The overloaded failing myocardium is also subject to stretch, which can activate several genes. Isolated cardiomyocytes exhibit rapid phosphorylation of gp130 and STAT3 when stretched [51], while over-expression of STAT3 leads to hypertrophy [52]. Stretch also increases IL-6, CT-1, and LIF transcription in cardiomyocytes [51]. Together, these data suggest that IL-6 and IL-6 related cytokines may contribute to cellular hypertrophy induced by stretch*via* activation of the STAT pathway. A lesser degree of hypertrophy is noted in pressure overloaded gp130 knockouts, further supporting this action of IL-6 related cytokines [53]. Double transgenic over-expressing IL-6 and IL-6R show constitutive phosphorylation of gp130 with an accompanying increase in cardiac weights, LV wall thickness and size, while mice over-expressing IL-6 alone do not exhibit and detectable cardiovascular abnormalities, indicating the importance of gp130 signaling [54].

Protective effects of IL-6

Though the effects of IL-6 appears to be primarily detrimental in HF, this cytokine also exerts actions that may be cardioprotective. Both IL-6 and CT-1 have been shown to prevent apoptosis [55, 56], which has been proposed as a mechanism of myocyte cell loss in HF [4, 5]. This can possibly be explained by the ability of IL-6 and LIF to increase expression of the anti-apoptotic gene, bcl-XL [57]. LIF also protects serum-starved cardiomyocytes from cell death [57]. In addition, gp130 knockout mice display an increase in the incidence of myocyte apoptosis, indicating that the same signaling molecule that induces hypertrophy may also affect cell survival [58]. IL-6 also decreases TNF-α generation [59], and thus may serve as both a propagator and a regulatory factor in the inflammatory response.

Conclusion

Even though there appears to be an association between increased activity and expression of IL-6 and worsening of the HF state, the importance of this in the pathophysiology of HF remains to be fully explored. Several studies have shown that circulating IL-6 could serve as an independent prognostic indicator for HF. However, clear evidence that IL-6 directly contributes to the progressive worsening of LV function and remodeling in HF is yet to be established.

Acknowledgement

The Study was supported, in part, by a grant from the National Heart, Lung, and Blood Institute HL 49090-07.

References

1   Spinale FG, Holzgrefe HH, Mukherjee R, Hird R, Walker JD, Arnim-Barker A, Powell JR, Joster WH (1995) Angiotensin-converting enzyme inhibition and the progression of congestive cardiomyopathy. Effects on left ventricular and myocyte structure and function. *Circulation* 92: 562–578

2   Sabbah HN, Sharov VG, Lesch M, Goldstein S (1995) Progression of heart failure: A role for interstitial fibrosis. *Mol Cell Biochem* 147: 29–34

3   Sabbah HN, Goldstein S (1993) Ventricular remodeling: Consequences and therapy. *Eur Heart J* 14 (Supplement C): 24–29

4   Narula J, Haider N, Virmani R, DiSalvo TG, Kolodgie FD, Hajjar RJ, Schmidt U, Semigran MJ, Dec GW, Khaw BA (1996) Apoptosis in myocytes in end-stage heart failure. *N Engl J Med* 335: 1182–1189

5   Olivetti G, Abbi R, Quaini F, Kajstura J, Cheng W, Nitahara JA, Quaini E, Di Loreto C, Beltrami CA, Krajewski S et al (1996) Apoptosis in the failing human heart. *N Engl J Med* 336: 1131–1141

6   Fowler MB, Laser JA, Hopkins GL, Minobe W, Bristow MR (1986) Assessment of the beta-adrenergic receptor pathway in the intact failing human heart: Progressive receptor down-regulation and sub-sensitivity to agonist response. *Circulation* 74: 1290–1302

7   Wollert KC, Drexler H (2001) The role of interleukin-6 in failing heart. *Heart Failure Rev* 6: 95–103

8   Torre-Amione G, Kapadia S, Benedict C, Oral H, Young JB, Mann DL (1996) Proinflammatory cytokine levels in patients with depressed left ventricular ejection fraction: A report from the studies of left ventricular dysfunction (SOLVD). *J Am Coll Cardiol* 27: 1201–1206

9   MacGowan GA, Mann DL, Kormos RL, Feldman AM, Murali S (1997) Circulating interleukin-6 in severe heart failure. *Am J Cardiol* 79: 1128–1131

10   Tsutamoto T, Wada A, Maeda K, Mabuchi N, Hayashi M, Tsutsui T, Ohnishi M, Sawaki M, Fujii M, Matsumoto T et al (2000) Angiotensin II Type 1 receptor antagonist decreases plasma levels of tumor necrosis factor alpha, interleukin-6 and soluble adhesion molecules in patients with chronic heart failure. *J Am Coll Cardiol* 35: 714–721

11   Raymond RJ, Dehmer GJ, Theoharides TC, Deliargyris EN (2001) Elevated interleukin-6 levels in patients with asymptomatic left ventricular systolic dysfunction. *Am Heart J* 141: 435–438

12   Barton BE (1997) IL-6: Insights into novel biological activities. *Clin Immunol Immunopathol* 85: 16–20

13   Hirano T (1992) The biology of interleukin-6. *Chem Immunol* 51: 153–180

14   Paul SR, Bennett F, Calvetti JA, Kelleher K, Wood CR, O'Hara RM Jr, Leary AC, Sibley B, Clark SC, Williams DA et al (1990) Molecular cloning of a cDNA encoding interleukin 11, a stromal cell-derived lymphopoietic and hematopoietic cytokine. *Proc Natl Acad Sci USA* 87: 7512–7516

15   Gearing DP, Gouch NM, King JA, Hilton DJ, Nicola NA, Simpson RJ, Nice EC, Kelso

A, Metcalf D (1987) Molecular cloning and expression of cDNA encoding a murine myeloid leukaemia inhibitory factor (LIF). *EMBO J* 6: 3995–4002

16 Malik N, Kallestad JC, Gunderson NL, Austin SD, Neubauer MG, Ochs V, Marquardt H, Zarling JM, Shoyab M, Wei CM et al (1989) Molecular cloning, sequence analysis, and functional expression of a novel growth regulator, oncostatin M. *Mol Cell Biol* 9: 2847–2853

17 Stockli KA, Lottspeich F, Sendtner M, Masiakowski P, Carroll P, Gotz R, Lindholm D, Thoenen H (1989) Molecular cloning, expression and regional distribution of rate ciliary neurotrophic factor. *Nature* 342: 920–923

18 Pennica D, King KL, Shaw KJ, Luis E, Rullamas J, Luoh SM, Darbonne WC, Knutzon DS, Yen R, Chien KR et al (1995) Expression cloning of cardiotrophin-1, a cytokine that induces cardiac myocyte hypertrophy. *Proc Natl Acad Sci USA* 93: 1142–1146

19 Senaldi G, Varnum BC, Sarmiento U, Starnes C, Lile J, Scully S, Guo J, Elliott G, McNinch J, Shaklee CL et al (1999) Novel neurotropin-1/B cell stimulating factor-3: A cytokine of the IL-6 family. *Proc Natl Acad Sci USA* 96: 11458–11463

20 Taga T (1997) The signal transducer gp130 is shared by interleukin-6 family of haematopoietic and neurotrophic cytokines. *Ann Med* 29: 63–72

21 Taga T, Kishimoto T (1997) Gp130 and the interleukin-6 family of cytokines. *Annu Rev Immunol* 15: 797–819

22 Zhong Z, Wen Z, Darnell JE Jr (1994) Stat3: A STAT family member activated by tyrosine phosphorylation in response to epidermal growth factor and interleukin-6. *Science* 264: 95–98

23 Wang H, Tracey KJ (1999) Tumor necrosis factor, interleukin-6, macrophage migration inhibitory factor, and macrophage inflammatory protein-1 in inflammation. In: JI Gallin, R Synderman (eds): *Inflammation: basic principles and clinical correlates*. Lippincott, Williams and Wilkins, Philadelphia, 471–486

24 Gwechenberger M, Mendoza LH, Youker KA, Frangogiannis NG, Smith CW, Michael LH, Entman ML (1999) Cardiac myocytes produce interleukin-6 in culture and in viable border zone of reperfused infarctions. *Circulation* 99: 546–551

25 Aukrust P, Ueland T, Lien E, Bendtzen K, Muller F, Andreassen AK, Nordoy I, Aass H, Espevik T, Simonsen S et al (1999) Cytokine network in congestive heart failure secondary to ischemic or idiopathic dilated cardiomyopathy. *Am J Cardiol* 83: 376–382

26 Orus J, Roig E, Perez-Villa F, Pare C, Azqueta M, Filella X, Heras M, Sanz G (2000) Prognostic value of serum cytokines in patients with congestive heart failure. *J Heart Lung Transplant* 19: 419–425

27 Deswal A, Petersen NJ, Feldman AM, Young JB, White BG, Mann DL (2001) Cytokines and cytokine receptors in advanced heart failure. An analysis of the cytokine database from the Vesnarinone trial (VEST). *Circulation* 103: 2055–2059

28 Zolk O, Ng LL, O'Brien RJ, Weyand M, Eschenhagen T (2002) Augmented expression of cardiotrophin-1 in failing human hearts is accompanied by diminished glycoprotein 130 receptor protein abundance. *Circulation* 106: 1442–1446

29 Ohtsuka T, Hamada M, Saeki H, Ogimoto A, Hiasa G, Hara Y, Shigematsu Y, Hiwada

K (2002) Comparison of effects of carvedilol *versus* metoprolol on cytokine levels in patients with idiopathic dilated cardiomyopathy. *Am J Cardiol* 89: 996–999

30 Matsumura T, Tsushima K, Ohtaki E, Misu K, Tohbaru T, Asano R, Nagayama M, Kitahara K, Umemura J, Sumiyoshi T et al (2002) Effects of carvedilol on plasma levels of interleukin-6 and tumor necrosis factor-alpha in nine patients with dilated cardiomyopathy. *J Cardiol* 39: 253–257

31 Prabhu SD, Chandrasekar B, Murray DR, Freeman GL (2000) β-adrenergic blockade in developing heart failure: Effects on myocardial inflammatory cytokines, nitric oxide and remodeling. *Circulation* 102: 2103–2109

32 Goldstein S, Fagerberg B, Hjalmarson A, Kjekshus J, Waagstein F, Wedel H, Wikstrand J, The MERIT-HF study group (2001) Metoprolol controlled release/extended release in patients with severe heart failure: Analysis of the experience in the MERIT-HF study. *J Am Coll Cardiol* 38: 932–938

33 Packer M, Fowler MB, Roecker EB, Coats AJ, Katus HA, Krum H, Mohacsi P, Rouleau, Tendera M, Staiger C et al (2002) Effect of carvedilol on the morbidity of patients with severe chronic heart failure: results of the carvedilol prospective randomized cumulative survival (COPERNICUS) study. *Circulation* 106: 2194–2199

34 Ohlstein EH, Douglas SA, Sung CP, Yue T-L, Louden C, Arleth A, Poste G, Ruffolo RR, Feuerstein GZ (1993) Carvedilol, a cardiovascular drug, prevents vascular smooth muscle cell proliferation, migration, and neointimal formation following vascular injury. *Proc Natl Acad Sci USA* 90: 6189–6193

35 Sung CP, Arleth AJ, Ohlstein EH (1993) Carvedilol inhibits vascular smooth muscle cell proliferation. *Proc Natl Acad Sci USA* 21: 221–227

36 Yue TL, Cheng HY, Lysko PG, McKenna PJ, Feuerstein R, Gu JL, Lysko KA, Davis LL, Feuerstein G (1992) Carvedilol, a new vasodilator and beta adrenoceptor antagonist, is an antioxidant and free radical scavenger. *J Pharmacol Exp Therapeut* 263: 92–98

37 Gullestad L, Aukrust P, Ueland T, Espevik T, Yee G, Vagelos R, Froland SS, Fowler M (1999) Effect of high-versus low-dose angiotensin converting enzyme inhibition on cytokine levels in chronic heart failure. *J Am Coll Cardiol* 34: 2061–2067

38 Tsutamoto T, Hisanaga T, Wada A, Maeda K, Ohnishi M, Fukai D, Mabuchi N, Sawaki M, Kinoshita M (1998) Interleukin-6 spillover in the peripheral circulation increases with the severity of heart failure, and the high plasma level of interleukin-6 is an important prognostic predictor in patients with congestive heart failure. *J Am Coll Cardiol* 31: 391–398

39 Mohler ER 3rd, Sorenson LC, Ghali JK, Schocken DD, Willis PW, Bowers JA, Cropp AB, Pressler ML (1997) Role of cytokines in the mechanism of action of amlodipine: The PRAISE heart failure trial. Prospective randomized amlodipine survival evaluation. *J Am Coll Cardiol* 30: 35–41

40 Ono K, Matsumori A, Shioi T, Furukawa Y, Sasayama S (1998) Cytokine gene expression after myocardial infarction in rat hearts: Possible implication in left ventricular remodeling. *Circulation* 98: 149–156

41 Burger A, Benicke M, Deten A, Zimmer HG (2001) Catecholamines stimulate inter-

leukin-6 synthesis in rat cardiac fibroblasts. *Am J Physiol Heart Circ Physiol* 381: H14–H21

42 Sano M, Fukuda K, Kodoma H, Takahashi T, Kato T, Hakuno D, Sato T, Manabe T, Tahara S, Ogawa S (2000) Autocrine/paracrine secretion of IL-6 family cytokines causes angiotensin II-induced delayed STAT3 activation. *Biochem Biophys Res Commun* 269: 798–802

43 Sano M, Fukuda K, Kodama H, Pan J, Saito M, Matsuzaki J, Takahashi T, Makino S, Kato T, Ogawa S (2000) Interleukin-6 family of cytokines mediate angiotensin II-induced cardiac hypertrophy in rodent cardiomyocytes. *J Biol Chem* 275: 29717–29723

44 Han Y, Runge MS, Brasier AR (1999) Angiotensin II induces interleukin-6 transcription in vascular smooth muscle cells through pleiotropic activation of nuclear factor-kappa-B transcription factors. *Circ Res* 84: 695–703

45 Schieffer B, Schieffer E, Hilfiker-Kleiner D, Hilfiker A, Kovanen PT, Kaartinen M, Nussberger J, Harringer W, Drexler H (2000) Expression of angiotensin II and interleukin 6 in human coronary atherosclerotic plaques: Potential implications for inflammation and plaque instability. *Circulation* 101: 1372–1378

46 Funamoto M, Hishinuma S, Fujio Y, Matsuda Y, Kunisada K, Oh H, Negoro S, Tone E, Kishimoto T, Yamauchi-Takihara K (2000) Isolation and characterization of the murine cardiotrophin-1 gene: Expression and norepinephrine-induced transcriptional activation. *J Mol Cell Cardiol* 32: 1275–1284

47 Jougasaki M, Tachibana I, Luchner A, Leskinen H, Redfield MM, Burnett JC Jr (2000) Augmented cardiac cardiotrophin-1 in experimental congestive heart failure. *Circulation* 101: 14–17

48 Ishikawa M, Saito Y, Miyamoto Y, Harada M, Kuwahara K, Ogawa E, Nakagawa O, Hamanaka I, Kajiyama N, Takahashi N (1999) A heart-specific increase in cardiotrophin-1 gene expression precedes the establishment of ventricular hypertrophy in genetically hypersensitive rats. *J Hypertens* 17: 807–816

49 Fukuzawa J, Booz GW, Hunt RA, Shimizu N, Karoor V, Baker KM, Dostal DE (2000) Cardiotrophin-1 increases angiotensinogen mRNA in rat cardiac myocytes through STAT3: An autocrine loop for hypertrophy. *Hypertension* 35: 1191–1196

50 Wollert KC, Taga T, Saito M, Narazaki M, Kishimoto T, Glembotski CC, Vernallis AB, Heath JK, Pennica D, Wood WI et al (1996) Cardiotrophin-1 activates a distinct form of cardiac muscle hypertrophy. Assembly of sarcomeric units in series *via* gp130/leukemia inhibitory factor receptor-dependent pathways. *J Biol Chem* 271: 9535–9545

51 Pan J, Fukuda K, Saito M, Matsuzaki J, Kodama H, Sano M, Takahashi T, Kato T, Ogawa S (1999) Mechanical stretch activates the JAK/STAT pathway in rat cardiomyocytes. *Circ Res* 84: 1127–1136

52 Kunisada K, Tone E, Fujio Y, Matsui H, Yamauchi-Takihara K, Kishimoto T (1998) Activation of gp130 transduces hypertrophic signals*via* STAT3 in cardiac myocytes. *Circulation* 98: 346–352

53 Uozomi H, Hiroi Y, Zhou Y, Takimoto E, Toko H, Niu P, Shimoyama M, Yazaki Y,

Nagai R, Komuro I (2001) gp130 plays a critical role in pressure overload-induced cardiac hypertrophy. *J Biol Chem* 276: 23115–23119

54 Hirota H, Yoshida K, Kishimoto T, Taga T (1995) Continuous activation of gp130, a signal-transducing receptor component for interleukin 6-related cytokines, causes myocardial hypertrophy in mice. *Proc Natl Acad Sci USA* 92: 4862–4866

55 Craig R, Larkin A, Mingo AM, Thuerauf DJ, Andrews C, McDonough PM, Glembotski CC (2000) p38 MAPK and NF-kappa-B collaborate to induce interleukin-6 gene expression and release. Evidence for a cytoprotective autocrine signaling pathway in a cardiac myocyte model system. *J Biol Chem* 275: 23814–23824

56 Sheng Z, Knowlton K, Chen J, Hoshijima M, Brown JH, Chien KR (1997) Cardiotrophin 1 (CT-1) inhibition of cardiac myocyte apoptosis *via* a mitogen-activated protein kinase-dependent pathway. Divergence from downstream CT-1 signals for myocardial cell hypertrophy. *J Biol Chem* 272: 5783–5791

57 Fujio Y, Kunisada K, Hirota H, Yamauchi-Takihara K, Kishimoto T (1997) Signals through gp130 up-regulate bcl-x gene expression *via* STAT1-binding cis-element in cardiac myocytes. *J Clin Invest* 99: 2898–2905

58 Hirota H, Chen J, Betz UA, Rajewsky K, Gu Y, Ross J Jr, Muller W, Chien KR (1999) Loss of a gp130 cardiac muscle cell survival pathway is a critical event in the onset of heart failure during biomechanical stress. *Cell* 97: 189–198

59 Aderka D, Le JM, Vilcek (1989) IL-6 inhibits lipopolysaccharide-induced tumor necrosis factor production in cultured human monocytes, U937 cells, and in mice. *J Immunol* 143: 3517–3523

Oxygen and nitrogen reactive radicals in cardiac inflammation and disease

Myocardial nitric oxide in cardiac remodeling

Flora Sam, Douglas B. Sawyer and Wilson S. Colucci

Myocardial Biology Unit, Boston University School of Medicine, Cardiovascular Division, Department of Medicine, Boston University Medical Center, 88 East Newton Street, D-8, Boston, MA 02118, USA

Introduction

Evidence has emerged that nitric oxide (NO) plays a role in the pathogenesis of myocardial failure. The effects of NO in heart failure, as in other clinical situations, may be either beneficial or deleterious. It has been hypothesized that NO at relatively low levels appears to modulate the response of the myocardium to potentially deleterious stimuli, and thus in some situations may offset the progression of myocardial failure. On the other hand, at higher levels NO has the ability to impair normal myocardial function and to exert direct toxic effects in the myocardium, as it can in other tissues. The effects of higher levels of NO may be relevant to a variety of situations in which myocardial NO is increased. These include conditions in which there is a clear inflammatory reaction such as sepsis, myocarditis, transplant rejection or acute infarction. There is also evidence that NO production is increased above physiologic levels in the myocardium of patients with chronic heart failure. These observations have led to the concern that with increasing levels, NO may contribute to the pathogenesis of myocardial failure, and thus change from a friend to a foe.

Nitric oxide synthases in the myocardium

Constitutive NOS in the myocardium

NO is a ubiquitous signaling molecule synthesized in the conversion of L-arginine to L-citrulline by a family of nitric oxide synthases [1]. In the heart, there are at least three different nitric oxide synthase (NOS) isoforms: NOS1 in neurons, cardiac myocytes, vascular smooth muscle [2, 3], NOS2 expressed in almost any cell type

Inflammation and Cardiac Diseases, edited by Giora Z. Feuerstein, Peter Libby and Douglas L. Mann

upon appropriate stimulation such as bacterial endotoxin or pro-inflammatory cytokines and NOS3 in endothelial cells and myocytes. Recently, Elfering and colleagues reported the presence of mitochondrial NOS (mtNOS) which is constitutively expressed and membrane bound [4]. MtNOS is the same as NOS1 but differ in localization and post-translational modification. Both constitutive (NOS1 and NOS3) and inducible (NOS2) are present in the myocardium, and there appear to be changes in the activity of all of these enzymes in the setting of myocardial failure. There is spatial confinement of these isoforms in the myocyte, thus allowing NO to have independent and even counter-regulatory effects in the heart [5].

Under normal circumstances, myocardial NO is produced only by NOS1 and NOS3, both of which are regulated predominantly at the post-translational level. The activity of this enzyme, which is present constitutively in virtually all cell types in the myocardium including cardiac myocytes, fibroblasts and endothelial cells, is regulated by a calcium-sensitive interaction with calmodulin in response to signals that increase intracellular calcium. Malinski and colleagues have used a porphyrinic NO-sensitive micro-electrode in the intact normal heart and found that there are beat-to-beat changes in the amount of NO present [6]. These changes in NO on a short time-scale may work to control energy utilization and instantaneous myocardial function. It has been hypothesized that post-nitrosylational modification of transcription factors regulates target genes [7]. Each redox-related modification may have its own functional consequences. Using the same technique in isolated ventricular myocytes, Malinski and colleagues [8] were able to demonstrate a transient increase in NO after stimulation with a β-adrenergic agonist. However longer periods of exposure to elevated levels of cAMP or phosphodiesterase inhibitors decrease the expression of NOS3 mRNA as well as the activity of the enzyme in isolated cardiac myocytes [9].

Inducible NOS in the myocardium

In the presence of hypoxia or increased levels of inflammatory cytokines, endothelial cells, myocytes and infiltrating macrophages can markedly increase their production of NO *via* the induction of NOS2. This enzyme is not expressed in the myocardium under normal conditions. However, after exposure to cytokines, hypoxia, ischemia-reperfusion and perhaps other stimuli there is rapid expression of NOS2 in the myocardium due to activation of specific transcription factors [10] such as NF-κB [11]. Although NOS2 can produce low levels of NO that may exert a modulatory function, when fully induced NOS2 more typically produces much higher "pathologic" levels of NO that may be deleterious. This capacity to damage cells should come as no surprise, since it is presumed by the generation of high levels of NO that NOS2 serves as the effector arm of the immunologic response to certain pathogens [12, 13].

NO and human heart failure

Some investigators have found that the expression and activity of NOS2 are increased in the myocardium of patients with both idiopathic and ischemic dilated cardiomyopathies [14, 15]. However, this finding has not been universal, and other studies have found elevations of NOS2 only in patients with sepsis [16]. Several animal models of heart failure show elevations of NOS2 activity, including models of myocardial infarction [17] and autoimmune myocarditis [18]. The mediators of the increase in NOS2 expression appear to include a combination of factors, including cytokines and adrenergic agonists. The levels of circulating pro-inflammatory cytokines are elevated systemically [19, 20] and in the myocardium [21] of patients with idiopathic and ischemic dilated cardiomyopathies, as is the level of adrenergic agonists [22]. Pro-inflammatory cytokines including interleukin-1β and tumor necrosis factor-α have been shown to induce the expression of NOS2 in isolated cardiac myocytes, as well as microvascular endothelial cells from the heart [23]. Although norepinephrine does not directly induce NOS2, it potentiates the expression of cytokine-stimulated NOS2 by stabilizing its mRNA [24]. Thus, increased NO production in failing myocardium is most likely due to the expression of NOS2.

Recently, Heymes and colleagues showed that NOS2 and NOS3 gene expression in LV endomyocardial biopsies varied with the severity of LV dysfunction in patients with dilated, non-ischemic cardiomyopathy. There was a good correlation with NOS2 and NOS3 gene expression with LV stroke volume and stroke work suggesting that there is a beneficial effect of NO on LV function [25].

Effects of nitric oxide on myocardial function

NO and myocardial contractility

NO appears to play an important role in determining the myocardial response to both sympathetic and parasympathetic stimulation. In particular, the increase in myocardial NO may account, in part, for the blunted adrenergic responsiveness that occurs in heart failure. Gulick et al. showed that in isolated cardiac myocytes the contractile response to isoproterenol was attenuated by exposure to media conditioned by monocytes activated by lipopolysaccharide [26]. Balligand et al. [27] showed that inhibitors of NOS potentiate the positive inotropic response to β-adrenergic stimulation in single myocytes treated with inflammatory cytokines. These investigators and others have gone on to show that conditioned media and cytokines can induce the expression of NOS2 in myocytes [28, 29] with an increase in NO produced by single myocytes as detected by a NO sensitive microelectrode [23].

Similar observations have been made in the intact heart. We found that in closed chest dogs the intracoronary infusion of NOS inhibitors had no effect on basal contractility (as assessed by measurement of +dP/dt), but significantly augmented the positive inotropic response to β-adrenergic stimulation [29]. Likewise, in patients with various degrees of left ventricular dysfunction we found that the intracoronary infusion of the NOS inhibitor L-NMMA potentiated the positive inotropic response to dobutamine [30]. We have also found that intracoronary infusion of L-NMMA potentiated the positive inotropic response to dobutamine in patients with clinical heart failure due to systolic LV dysfunction, but had no effect in subjects with normal LV function [31]. These results are consistent with the *in vitro* experiments showing that NO impairs β-adrenergic responsiveness. NO from NOS2 is increased in the failing human heart.

Heart failure is associated with expression of the NOS2 in the LV myocardium and that NO generated by this enzyme modulates cardiac relaxation and contraction in the failing heart. High cardiac NOS2 activity in failing left ventricles is associated with shortening of relaxation and an attenuated positive inotropic response to β-adrenergic stimulation.

NO inhibits the positive inotropic response in patients with severe heart failure *in vitro* [32]. Inhibition of NO synthesis by N^G-monomethyl-L-arginine (L-NMMA) recovers β-stimulation responsiveness in patients with high levels of myocardial NOS2 activity, suggesting that the response to β-adrenergic stimulation is related to the endogenous cardiac generation of nitric oxide by NOS2 (rather than NOS3). Thus, NOS2 activity attenuates responsiveness to β-adrenergic stimulation.

It is unclear whether this inhibitory effect of NO on the inotropic responses to β-adrenergic stimulation in patients with heart failure is adaptive or maladaptive. Since β-adrenergic stimulation is a short-term adaptation that serves to support cardiac function, a negative inotropic action of myocardial NO might promote further LV dysfunction and thereby worsen the severity of heart failure. However, there is also evidence that chronic β-adrenergic activation may be deleterious by causing progression of myocardial failure. This view is supported by the demonstration that β-blockers can decrease the rate of disease progression and improve functional class and survival in patients with chronic stable heart failure [33, 34]. In this context, inhibition of β-adrenergic responsiveness by NO could be considered adaptive. NO might thus have beneficial effects similar to β-adrenergic receptor blockade. Some of these beneficial effects are possibly due to inhibition of adverse effects of adrenergic over-activity on remodeling. Gealekman et al. [35] recently showed that myocardial NOS2 is activated in rats with volume-overload HF and suggest that increased NOS2 activity contributes to depressed myocardial contractility and β-adrenergic hypo-responsiveness.

Recently functional expression of β_3-adrenergic receptors has been shown in the human heart. Their stimulation, in marked contrast with that of β_1- and β_2-adrenergic receptors, induces a decrease in contractility through presently unknown mechanisms. There is activation of NOS3 in human myocardium to the β_3 adrenergic receptor family, in extracts of endomyocardial biopsies. Exposure of these LV fragments to norepinephrine in the presence of full α_1, β_1 and β_2-adrenoceptor blockade induced an increase in the intracellular concentration of cyclic GMP that was abolished by inhibitors of NO synthase. These effects were reproduced with preferential β_3-adrenoceptor agonists, that also elicited increases in NO production directly measurable with a porphyrinic electrode [36].

Role of NO in mediating parasympathetic actions

The negative chronotropic and inotropic effects of parasympathetic stimulation may be mediated, in part, *via* NO. In isolated spontaneously-beating ventricular myocytes, inhibition of NOS prevents the negative chronotropic action of muscarinic cholinergic stimulation [37]. This effect of NO appears to be mediated by activation of guanylate cyclase resulting in cGMP-dependent phosphorylation of the L-type calcium channel [38]. Likewise, the effects of vagal stimulation on cardiac function *in vivo* are attenuated by inhibition of NOS. For example, in closed-chest dogs muscarinic cholinergic actions caused by direct stimulation of the vagus nerve attenuate the positive inotropic effect of dobutamine [39]. We found that this inhibitory effect of vagal stimulation depends, in part, on NO, since the intracoronary infusion of L-NMMA reduced the inhibitory effect of vagal stimulation by 60%, and the subsequent infusion of L-arginine restored the inhibitory effect. Thus, NO plays an important modulatory role in the myocardium by inhibiting the response to sympathetic stimulation and mediating the action of parasympathetic stimulation.

Direct negative inotropic effects of NO

There is evidence, both *in vitro* and *in vivo*, that cytokine-induced increases in NO production by NOS2 may be sufficient to decrease basal ventricular contractile function (i.e., in the unstimulated state). For example, Finkel et al. showed that inflammatory cytokines cause direct negative inotropic effects in isolated papillary muscles that are prevented by NOS inhibition [40]. Similarly, Brady et al. found that basal contractile function was reduced in myocytes exposed to systemic endotoxin for four hours [41]. Inhibition of NOS with L-NMMA in the media caused an improvement in myocyte function that was overcome by L-arginine, suggesting that the negative inotropic effect of endotoxemia was mediated by NO. In intact animals, Pagani et al. found that infusion of TNF-α in dogs for 24–48 hours caused a decrease in left ventricular systolic and diastolic function over 24–48 hours that was prevented by inhibitors of NOS [42].

The mechanism by which NO can depress basal contractile function is not fully understood, but may simply reflect a more profound inhibition of voltage-dependent calcium channels by high levels of cGMP. Alternatively, it might be due to inhibition of mitochondrial respiration resulting in reduced ATP availability. In cultured rat ventricular myocytes, stimulation with the cytokine interleukin-1β caused a reversible decrease in mitochondrial respiration that was prevented by a NOS inhibitor [43]. It is also possible that reduced contractility is due to the modification of thiol groups on proteins involved in excitation-contraction coupling, with subsequent alteration in protein function [44, 45]. Funakoshi and colleagues showed that in genetically modified mice over-expressing TNF-α, disruption of NOS2 increased the response to β-adrenergic stimulation [46].

Effects on nitric oxide on ventricular remodeling

Myocyte protective effects of NO *in vitro*

The modulatory or beneficial effects of NO on adrenergic responses in the heart go beyond their effects on contractility. Chronic adrenergic stimulation has been implicated in ventricular remodeling and the progression of myocardial failure. In animal models, chronic adrenergic stimulation leads to myocardial hypertrophy [47, 48], altered gene expression with down-regulation of genes involved in excitation-contraction coupling [49], and programmed cell death of cardiac myocytes [50]. In cardiac myocytes and fibroblasts *in vitro*, we found that many of the effects of adrenergic stimulation can be attenuated with NO donors in a concentration-dependent manner [51]. For example, in cardiac myocytes the NO donor S-nitroso-N-acetyl-D,L-penicillamine (SNAP) attenuated the ability of norepinephrine to stimulate protein synthesis, whereas addition of a NOS inhibitor augmented the response to norepinephrine. The effects of NO were mimicked by cGMP, indicating that this action of NO is likely mediated *via* a cGMP-dependent pathway. NO through a cGMP-dependent pathway stimulates mitochondrial biogenesis [52].

Cytokines such as interleukin-1β (IL-1β) can also induce hypertrophy and altered gene expression in isolated cardiac myocytes [53]. Although cytokines are potent stimulators of NOS2 expression and activity [28], the hypertrophic response of myocytes to IL-1β appears not to be attenuated by NO, perhaps reflecting differences in the signaling pathways used by norepinephrine and IL-1β.

NO attenuates stretch-induced apoptosis in cardiac myocytes

A variety of exogenous stimuli, including mechanical stretch and norepinephrine, have been found to increase the rate of apoptosis in cardiac myocytes *in vitro*.

Cheng et al. stretched isolated papillary muscles by 20% for four hours [54]. Under these conditions, mechanical stretch induced apoptosis in myocytes, and this effect was inhibited completely by the addition of an NO donor. The mechanism by which NO protects myocytes remains to be elucidated. However, in other cell types, it appears that NO can inhibit apoptosis by inhibiting specific enzymes in the programmed cell death pathway [55]. Of note, Cheng et al. [54] found that the protective effect of NO correlated with its ability to decrease the level of superoxide in the myocardium, suggesting that it might exert its beneficial action by scavenging superoxide generated by mechanical stretch.

Myocardial toxicity of NO and the role of NO in apoptosis

Experiments *in vitro* show direct toxic effects of high concentrations of NO on cardiac myocytes. Pinsky et al. demonstrated that adult rat ventricular myocytes in culture died in response to stimulation with cytokines (IL-1β, interferon-γ, and tumor necrosis factor-α) [56]. This effect of the cytokines could be prevented by inhibition of NOS with L-NMMA, suggesting that NO played an important role. Bishopric and colleagues showed that induction of apoptosis in cardiac myocytes by inflammatory cytokines requires NO by exposure to an NO donor that directly induces cardiac myocyte apoptosis in a dose-dependent and antioxidant-sensitive manner [57]. Conversely Li et al., showed that lipopolysaccharide-induced apoptosis in myocytes was not NO-mediated [58]. The induction was through activation of cardiac AT-1 receptors. We have found that NO donors that result in high levels of NO cause apoptosis of cardiac myocytes *in vitro* [59]. This observation raises the intriguing possibility that in failing myocardium, high levels of NO produced by NOS2 may contribute to progressive myocardial failure by causing apoptosis [60].

The mechanism by which NO causes myocyte apoptosis remains to be elucidated. One possibility is the formation of reactive oxygen and nitrogen species when NO is produced at extremely high levels. NO is a free radical gas that is buffered in the cell by reactions with glutathione. Through chemical reactions with other oxygen species, NO can either decrease or increase the oxidative state of a cell or tissue. On the one hand, NO may reduce the level of oxidative stress by buffering low levels of reactive oxygen species (ROS). Alternatively, higher levels of NO may increase oxidative stress by, among other means, reacting with superoxide anion (O_2^-) to generate peroxynitrite ($ONOO^-$), a free radical which may be more toxic and long-lived than either NO or O_2^- [61]. $ONOO^-$ can react with tyrosine residues of susceptible proteins, in some cases causing irreversible inactivation [62].

Based on the relative rate constants of O_2^- with superoxide dismutase (SOD) and NO, the formation of $ONOO^-$ is favored when the levels of O_2^- or NO are high, or the level of SOD is low [63]. Moreover, Wang and Zweier have shown that under appropriate conditions of substrate deficiency NOS2 is capable of directly catalyzing the formation of O_2^- [64]. Interestingly, Singal and colleagues have shown that the activity of antioxidant enzymes, including SOD, is reduced in two models of heart failure [65, 66], and might thus account for increased levels of O_2^- and $ONOO^-$. It is therefore interesting that myocardial $ONOO^-$ formation is increased in autopsy samples of patients who died of sepsis or myocarditis, as evidenced by increased staining for nitrotyrosine [53].

Animal models implicating a role of NO in left ventricular (LV) remodeling

Animal models of autoimmune and viral myocarditis implicate a direct toxic effect of NO and $ONOO^-$ *in vivo*. In these models there is massive inflammation in the heart that results in overt myocyte necrosis. Ishiyama et al. were able to reduce the amount of necrotic myocardium as well as the elevation of creatine kinase in rats with experimental autoimmune myocarditis using aminoguanidine, an inhibitor of NOS2 [18]. Interestingly, in that system treatment with aminoguanidine also decreased the amount of superoxide anion formed. The source of superoxide anion in that model was not determined. While it is possible that superoxide anion was formed by NOS2 in this system, equally likely is that an increase in superoxide anion resulted from the inactivation of MnSOD by $ONOO^-$.

We studied the role of NOS2 in LV remodeling one month and six months after Myocardial Infarction (MI) in mice lacking NOS2 [67]. In this model NOS2 contributes to decreased contractility, increased myocyte apoptosis in the remote, non-infarcted myocardium, and reduced survival late after MI. NOS2 expression is clearly associated with TUNEL positivity, a modest decrease in systolic function, and an increased mortality rate late after MI. Feng and colleagues findings were similar to ours in that they showed that in a LV infarcted mouse-model, NOS2 contributes to increased LV dysfunction and mortality.

Other have shown that in a transgenic mouse model conditionally targeting the over expression of human NOS2 cDNA to myocardium led to increased production of peroxynitrite [68]. This was associated with a mild inflammatory cell infiltrate, cardiac fibrosis, hypertrophy, and dilatation. NOS2-overexpressing mice infrequently developed overt heart failure, but displayed a high incidence of sudden cardiac death due to bradyarrhythmia. This dramatic cardiac phenotype was rescued by specific attenuation of transgene activity.

Interestingly others have suggested that this is not the case. Heger et al. generated transgenic mice over-expressing NOS2 under the alpha-myosin heavy chain promoter [69]. They showed that cardiac-specific over-expression of NOS2 did not result in severe cardiac dysfunction despite increase *in vitro*, NOS2 activity in TG hearts by 260- to 400-fold above controls.

NOS3 limits LV dysfunction and remodeling by an afterload-independent mechanism, in part by decreasing myocyte hypertrophy in the remote myocardium [70].

Mikama et al. were able to reveal both protective and toxic effects of NO when they examined the effect of inhibition of NO synthesis with L-NAME on the mortality and the extent of myocardial injury in a murine model of viral myocarditis [55]. Mice were infected with Coxsackie virus B3 in the presence of increasing doses of L-NAME. At the highest dose of L-NAME, survival was markedly worse in the infected but untreated mice. At a low dose, however, L-NAME improved survival, and reduced the severity of heart failure and area of myocardial necrosis. This is consistent with a dual action of NO, where some NO (low concentrations of L-NAME) is better than too much NO (no L-NAME), and no NO (high concentrations of L-NAME) is worst of all. Further insight into the mechanisms by which NO exerts these opposing actions will be needed before rational therapies can be designed.

It is unlikely that NO and reactive nitrogen species can explain all of the effects of the inflammatory cytokines in the heart. For example, in the murine model of cardiac myosin-induced autoimmune myocarditis, Bachmaier et al. were able to show that NOS2 expression was present in the heart in both inflammatory macrophages as well as cardiomyocytes [71]. Autoimmune heart disease was accompanied by formation of the $ONOO^-$ reaction product nitrotyrosine in inflammatory macrophages as well as in cardiomyocytes. Mice defective for the interferon regulatory transcription factor-1 ($IRF-1^{-/-}$) after gene targeting failed to induce NOS2 expression and nitrotyrosine formation in the heart, but developed cardiac myosin-induced myocarditis at prevalence and severity similar to those of heterozygous littermates.

Humans and NO in left ventricular (LV) remodeling

In human studies, Kalra and colleagues provide evidence that tumor necrosis factor-α (TNF-α) and NOS2 play a role in mediating myocardial hibernation [72]. There observations support the notion that TNF-α and NOS2 cause dose-dependent changes in myocardial dysfunction, with moderate increases leading to reversible myocardial dysfunction, and greater increases contributing to irreversible injury.

Conclusions

NO plays a central role in normal myocardial physiology. In addition, NO has the ability to exert either beneficial or deleterious effects on the myocardium. At lower concentrations, NO may protect from deleterious stimuli such as mechanical stress and norepinephrine. At higher concentrations, NO may change to a pathogen capable of stimulating the loss of myocytes and affecting myocyte function. The mechanism by which NO exerts these contrasting effects may involve decreases and

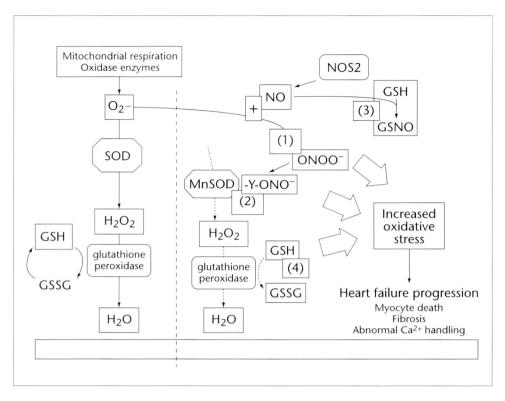

Figure 1

Mechanisms of NO induced increases in oxidative stress. The normal handling of reactive oxygen species (left) can be altered by large increases in NO that may occur in heart failure due to induction of NOS2 activity, leading to increases in oxidative stress. NO can react directly with O_2^- directly to form the $ONOO^-$ (1). ONOO- formation may lead to inactivation of MnSOD through nitrotyrosine formation (2), thus further increasing the levels of O_2^-. NO reacts with glutathione (GSH) to form GSNO (3), thus depleting reduced glutatione, an important cellular antioxidant. GSH is a necessary cofactor for the activity of glutathione peroxidase, and thus depletion of GSH will lead to increased levels of peroxides, with increased formation of hydroxyl radicals as well (4).

increases in oxidative stress, respectively (Fig. 1). The use of genetically-modified mice has led to an improved understanding of the physiological and pathophysiological roles of NO. A better understanding of the role that NO plays in the development and progression of myocardial failure may lead to new treatment strategies.

References

1   Nathan C (1995) Natural resistance and nitric oxide. *Cell* 82 (6): 873–876

2   Boulanger CM, Heymes C, Benessiano J, Geske RS, Levy BI, Vanhoutte PM (1998) Neuronal nitric oxide synthase is expressed in rat vascular smooth muscle cells: Activation by angiotensin II in hypertension. *Circ Res* 83 (12): 1271–1278

3   Xu KY, Huso DL, Dawson TM, Bredt DS, Becker LC (1999) Nitric oxide synthase in cardiac sarcoplasmic reticulum. *Proc Natl Acad Sci USA* 96 (2): 657–662

4   Elfering SL, Sarkela TM, Giulivi C (2002) Biochemistry of mitochondrial nitric-oxide synthase. *J Biol Chem* 277 (41): 38079–38086

5   Barouch LA, Harrison RW, Skaf MW, Rosas GO, Cappola TP, Kobeissi ZA, Hobai IA, Lemmon CA, Burnett AL, O'Rourke B et al (2002) Nitric oxide regulates the heart by spatial confinement of nitric oxide synthase isoforms. *Nature* 416 (6878): 337–339

6   Pinsky DJ, Patton S, Mesaros S, Brovkovych V, Kubaszewski E, Grunfeld S, Malinski T (1997) Mechanical transduction of nitric oxide synthesis in the beating heart. *Circ Res* 81(3): 372–379

7   Marshall HE, Merchant K, Stamler JS (2000) Nitrosation and oxidation in the regulation of gene expression. *FASEB J* 14 (13): 1889–1900

8   Kanai AJ, Mesaros S, Finkel MS, Oddis CV, Birder LA, Malinski T (1997) Beta-adrenergic regulation of constitutive nitric oxide synthase in cardiac myocytes. *Am J Physiol* 273 (4 Pt 1): C1371–1377

9   Belhassen L, Kelly RA, Smith TW, Balligand JL (1996) Nitric oxide synthase (NOS3) and contractile responsiveness to adrenergic and cholinergic agonists in the heart. Regulation of NOS3 transcription *in vitro* and *in vivo* by cyclic adenosine monophosphate in rat cardiac myocytes. *J Clin Invest* 97 (8): 1908–1915

10 Singh K, Balligand JL, Fischer TA, Smith TW, Kelly RA (1996) Regulation of cytokine-inducible nitric oxide synthase in cardiac myocytes and microvascular endothelial cells. Role of extracellular signal-regulated kinases 1 and 2 (ERK1/ERK2) and STAT1 alpha. *J Biol Chem* 271 (2): 1111–1117

11 Xuan YT, Tang XL, Banerjee S, Takano H, Li RC, Han H, Qiu Y, Li JJ, Bolli R (1999) Nuclear factor-kappa-B plays an essential role in the late phase of ischemic preconditioning in conscious rabbits. *Circ Res* 84 (9): 1095–1109

12 Macmicking JD, North RJ, LaCourse R, Mudgett JS, Shah SK, Nathan CF (1997) Identification of nitric oxide synthase as a protective locus against tuberculosis. *Proc Natl Acad Sci USA* 94 (10): 5243–5248

13 Wheeler MA, Smith SD, Garcia-Cardena G, Nathan CF, Weiss RM, Sessa WC (1997). Bacterial infection induces nitric oxide synthase in human neutrophils. *J Clin Invest* 99 (1): 110–116

14 Haywood GA, Tsao PS, von der Leyen HE, Mann MJ, Keeling PJ, Trindade PT, Lewis NP, Byrne CD, Rickenbacher PR, Bishopric NH et al (1996) Expression of inducible nitric oxide synthase in human heart failure. *Circulation* 93 (6): 1087–1094

15 Habib FM, Springall DR, Davies GJ, Oakley CM, Yacoub MH, Polak JM (1996)

Tumour necrosis factor and inducible nitric oxide synthase in dilated cardiomyopathy. *Lancet* 347 (9009): 1151–1155

16   Thoenes M, Forstermann U, Tracey WR, Bleese NM, Nussler AK, Scholz H, Stein B (1996) Expression of inducible nitric oxide synthase in failing and non-failing human heart. *J Mol Cell Cardiol* 28 (1): 165–169

17   Wildhirt SM, Dudek RR, Suzuki H, Bing RJ (1995) Involvement of inducible nitric oxide synthase in the inflammatory process of myocardial infarction. *Int J Cardiol* 50 (3): 253–261

18   Ishiyama S, Hiroe M, Nishikawa T, Abe S, Shimojo T, Ito H, Ozasa S, Yamakawa K, Matsuzaki M, Mohammed MU (1997) Nitric oxide contributes to the progression of myocardial damage in experimental autoimmune myocarditis in rats. *Circulation* 95 (2): 489–496

19   MacGowan GA, Mann DL, Kormos RL, Feldman AM, Murali S (1997) Circulating interleukin-6 in severe heart failure. *Am J Cardiol* 79 (8): 1128–1131

20   Torre-Amione G, Kapadia S, Benedict C, Oral H, Young JB, Mann DL (1996) Proinflammatory cytokine levels in patients with depressed left ventricular ejection fraction: A report from the studies of left ventricular dysfunction (SOLVD). *J Am Coll Cardiol* 27: 1201–1206

21   Torre-Amione G, Kapadia S, Lee J, Durand J-B, Bies RD, Young JB, Mann DL (1996) Tumor necrosis factor-α and tumor necrosis factor receptors in the failing human heart. *Circulation* 93: 704–711

22   Cohn JN, Levine TB, Olivari MT, Garberg V, Lura D, Francis GS, Simon AB, Rector T (1984) Plasma norepinephrine as a guide to prognosis in patients with chronic congestive heart failure. *N Engl J Med* 311: 819–823

23   Balligand JL, Ungureanu-Longrois D, Simmons WW, Pimental D, Malinski TA, Kapturczak M, Taha Z, Lowenstein CJ, Davidoff AJ, Kelly RA (1994) Cytokine-inducible nitric oxide synthase (iNOS) expression in cardiac myocytes. Characterization and regulation of iNOS expression and detection of iNOS activity in single cardiac myocytes *in vitro*. *J Biol Chem* 269 (44): 27580–27588

24   Oddis CV, Simmons RL, Hattler BG, Finkel MS (1994) Chronotropic effects of cytokines and the nitric oxide synthase inhibitor, L-NMMA, on cardiac myocytes. *Biochem Biophys Res Comm* 205: 992–997

25   Heymes C, Vanderheyden M, Bronzwaer JG, Shah AM, Paulus WJ (1999) Endomyocardial nitric oxide synthase and left ventricular preload reserve in dilated cardiomyopathy. *Circulation* 99 (23): 3009–3016

26   Gulick T, Pieper SJ, Murphy MA, Lange LG, Schreiner GF (1991) A new method for assessment of cultured cardiac myocyte contractility detects immune factor-mediated inhibition of beta-adrenergic responses. *Circulation* 84 (1): 313–321

27   Balligand JL, Ungureanu D, Kelly RA, Kobzik L, Pimental D, Michel T, Smith TW (1993) Abnormal contractile function due to induction of nitric oxide synthesis in rat cardiac myocytes follows exposure to activated macrophage-conditioned medium. *J Clin Invest* 91 (5): 2314–2319

28 Balligand JL, Ungureanu-Longrois D, Simmons WW, Kobzik L, Lowenstein CJ, Lamas S, Kelly RA, Smith TW, Michel T (1995) Induction of NO synthase in rat cardiac microvascular endothelial cells by IL-1 beta and IFN-gamma. *Am J Physiol* 268 (3 Pt 2): H1293–303

29 Keaney JF, Jr., Hare JM, Balligand JL, Loscalzo J, Smith TW, Colucci WS (1996) Inhibition of nitric oxide synthase augments myocardial contractile responses to beta-adrenergic stimulation. *Am J Physiol* 271 (6 Pt 2): H2646–652

30 Hare JM, Loh E, Creager MA, Colucci WS (1995) Nitric oxide inhibits the positive inotropic response to beta-adrenergic stimulation in humans with left ventricular dysfunction. *Circulation* 92 (8): 2198–2203

31 Hare JM, Givertz MM, Creager MA, Colucci WS (1998) Increased sensitivity to nitric oxide synthase inhibition in patients with heart failure. Potentiation of β-adrenergic inotropic responsiveness. *Circulation* 97: 161–166

32 Drexler H, Kastner S, Strobel A, Studer R, Brodde OE, Hasenfuss G (1998) Expression, activity and functional significance of inducible nitric oxide synthase in the failing human heart. *J Am Coll Cardiol* 32 (4): 955–963

33 Packer M, Colucci WS, Sackner-Bernstein JD, Liang C, Goldscher DA, Freeman I et al (1996) Double-blind, placebo-controlled study of the effects of carvedilol in patients with moderate to severe heart failure. The PRECISE trial. Prospective randomized evaluation of carvedilol on symptoms and exercise. *Circulation* 94 (11): 2793–2799

34 Colucci WS, Packer M, Bristow MR, Gilbert EM, Cohn JN, Fowler MB, Krueger SK, Hershberger R, Uretsky BF, Bowers JA (1996) Carvedilol inhibits clinical progression in patients with mild symptoms of heart failure. US carvedilol heart failure study group. *Circulation* 94 (11): 2800–2806

35 Gealekman O, Abassi Z, Rubinstein I, Winaver J, Binah O (2002) Role of myocardial inducible nitric oxide synthase in contractile dysfunction and beta-adrenergic hyporesponsiveness in rats with experimental volume-overload heart failure. *Circulation* 105 (2): 236–243

36 Gauthier C, Leblais V, Kobzik L, Trochu JN, Khandoudi N, Bril A, Balligand JL, Le Marec H (1998) The negative inotropic effect of beta3-adrenoceptor stimulation is mediated by activation of a nitric oxide synthase pathway in human ventricle. *J Clin Invest* 102 (7): 1377–1384

37 Balligand JL, Kelly RA, Marsden PA, Smith TW, Michel T (1993) Control of cardiac muscle cell function by an endogenous nitric oxide signaling system. *Proc Natl Acad Sci USA* 90 (1): 347–351

38 Han X, Kobzik L, Balligand J-L, Kelly RA, Smith TW (1996) Nitric oxide synthase (NOS3)-mediated cholinergic modulation of Ca^{2+} current in adult rabbit atrioventricular nodal cells. *Circ Res* 78: 998–1008

39 Hare JM, Keaney JF Jr, Balligand JL, Loscalzo J, Smith TW, Colucci WS (1995) Role of nitric oxide in parasympathetic modulation of beta-adrenergic myocardial contractility in normal dogs. *J Clin Invest* 95 (1): 360–366

40 Finkel MS, Oddis CV, Jacob TD, Watkins SC, Hattler BG, Simmons RL (1992) Nega-

tive intropic effects of cytokines on the heart mediated by nitric oxide. *Science* 257: 387–389

41 Brady AJ, Warren JB, Poole-Wilson PA, Williams TJ, Harding SE (1993) Nitric oxide attenuates cardiac myocyte contraction. *Am J Physiol* 265: H176–H186

42 Pagani FD, Baker LS, Hsi C, Knox M, Fink MP, Visner MS (1992) Left ventricular systolic and diastolic dysfunction after infusion of tumor necrosis factor-alpha in conscious dogs. *J Clin Invest* 90 (2): 389–398

43 Oddis CV, Finkel MS (1995) Cytokine-stimulated nitric oxide production inhibits mitochondrial activity in cardiac myocytes. *Biochem Biophys Res Comm* 213 (3): 1002–1009

44 Campbell DL, Stamler JS, Strauss HC (1996) Redox modulation of L-type calcium channels in ferret ventricular myocytes. Dual mechanism regulation by nitric oxide and S-nitrosothiols. *J Gen Physiol* 108 (4): 277–293

45 Xu L, Eu JP, Meissner G, Stamler JS (1998) Activation of the cardiac calcium release channel (Ryanodine receptor) by poly-S-nitrosylation [In Process Citation]. *Science* 279 (5348): 234–237

46 Funakoshi H, Kubota T, Kawamura N, Machida Y, Feldman AM, Tsutsui H, Shimokawa H, Takeshita A (2002) Disruption of inducible nitric oxide synthase improves beta-adrenergic inotropic responsiveness but not the survival of mice with cytokine-induced cardiomyopathy. *Circ Res* 90 (9): 959–965

47 Malik AB, Geha AS (1975) Role of adrenergic mechanisms in the development of cardiac hypertrophy. *Proc Soc Exp Biol Med* 150 (3): 796–800

48 Kudej RK, Iwase M, Uechi M, Vatner DE, Oka N, Ishikawa Y, Shannon RP, Bishop SP, Vatner SF (1997) Effects of chronic beta-adrenergic receptor stimulation in mice [In Process Citation]. *J Mol Cell Cardiol* 29 (10): 2735–2746

49 Stein B, Bartel S, Kirchhefer U, Kokott S, Krause EG, Neumann J, Schmitz W, Scholz H (1996) Relation between contractile function and regulatory cardiac proteins in hypertrophied hearts. *Am J Physiol* 270 (6 Pt 2): H2021–2028

50 Communal C, Singh K, Pimentel DR, Colucci WS (1998) Norepinephrine stimulates apoptosis in adult rat ventricular myocytes by activation of the β-adrenergic pathway. *Circulation* 98: 1329–1334

51 Calderone A, Thaik CM, Takahashi N, Chang DLF, Colucci WS (1998) Nitric oxide, atrial natriuretic peptide, and cGMP inhibit the growth-promoting effects of norepinephrine in cardiac myocytes and fibroblasts. *J Clin Invest* 101: 812–818

52 Nisoli E, Clementi E, Paolucci C, Cozzi V, Tonello C, Sciorati C, Bracale R, Valerio A, Francolini M, Moncada S et al (2003) Mitochondrial biogenesis in mammals: The role of endogenous nitric oxide. *Science* 299 (5608): 896–899

53 Thaik CM, Calderone A, Takahashi N, Colucci WS (1995) Interleukin-1β modulates the growth and phenotype of neonatal rat cardiac myocytes. *J Clin Invest* 96: 1093–1099

54 Cheng W, Li B, Kajstura J, Li P, Wolin MS, Sonnenblick EH, Hintze TH, Olivetti G, Anversa P (1995) Stretch-induced programmed myocyte cell death. *J Clin Invest* 96: 2247–2259

55 Mannick JB, Miao XQ, Stamler JS (1997) Nitric oxide inhibits fas-induced apoptosis. *J Biol Chem* 272 (39): 24125–24128

56 Pinsky DJ, Cai B, Yang X, Rodriguez C, Sciacca RR, Cannon PJ (1995) The lethal effects of cytokine-induced nitric oxide on cardiac myocytes are blocked by nitric oxide synthase antagonism or transforming growth factor β. *J Clin Invest* 95: 677–685

57 Ing DJ, Zang J, Dzau VJ, Webster KA, Bishopric NH (1999) Modulation of cytokine-induced cardiac myocyte apoptosis by nitric oxide, Bak, and Bcl-x. *Circ Res* 84 (1): 21–33

58 Li HL, Suzuki J, Bayna E, Zhang FM, Dalle ME, Clark A, Engler RL, Lew WY (2002) Lipopolysaccharide induces apoptosis in adult rat ventricular myocytes *via* cardiac AT(1) receptors. *Am J Physiol Heart Circ Physiol* 283 (2): H461–H467

59 Arstall MA, Sawyer DB, Fukazawa R, Kelly RA (1999) Cytokine-mediated apoptosis in cardiac myocytes: The role of inducible nitric oxide synthase induction and peroxynitrite generation. *Circ Res* 85 (9): 829–840

60 Olivetti G, Abbi R, Quaini F, Kajstura J, Cheng W, Nitahara JA, Quaini E, Di Loreto C, Beltrami CA, Krajewski S et al (1997) Apoptosis in the failing human heart. *N Engl J Med* 336 (16): 1131–1141

61 Radi R, Beckman JS, Bush KM, Freeman BA (1991) Peroxynitrite oxidation of sulfhydryls. The cytotoxic potential of superoxide and nitric oxide. *J Biol Chem* 266 (7): 4244–4250

62 Ischiropoulos H, Zhu L, Chen J, Tsai M, Martin JC, Smith CD, Beckman JS (1992) Peroxynitrite-mediated tyrosine nitration catalyzed by superoxide dismutase. *Arch Biochem Biophys* 298 (2): 431–437

63 Beckman JS, Koppenol WH (1996) Nitric oxide, superoxide, and peroxynitrite: The good, the bad, and ugly. *Am J Physiol* 271 (5 Pt 1): C1424–437

64 Xia Y, Zweier JL (1997). Superoxide and peroxynitrite generation from inducible nitric oxide synthase in macrophages. *Proc Natl Acad Sci USA* 94 (13): 6954–6958

65 Dhalla AK, Singal PK (1994) Antioxidant changes in hypertrophied and failing guinea pig hearts. *Am J Physiol* 266: H1280–H1285

66 Hill MF, Singal PK (1997) Right and left myocardial antioxidant responses during heart failure subsequent to myocardial infarction. *Circulation* 96 (7): 2414–2420

67 Sam F, Sawyer DB, Xie Z, Chang DL, Ngoy S, Brenner DA, Siwik DA, Singh K, Apstein CS, Colucci WS (2001) Mice lacking inducible nitric oxide synthase have improved left ventricular contractile function and reduced apoptotic cell death late after myocardial infarction. *Circ Res* 89 (4): 351–356

68 Mungrue IN, Gros R, You X, Pirani A, Azad A, Csont T, Schulz R, Butany J, Stewart DJ, Husain M (2002) Cardiomyocyte over-expression of iNOS in mice results in peroxynitrite generation, heart block, and sudden death. *J Clin Invest* 109 (6): 735–743

69 Heger J, Godecke A, Flogel U, Merx MW, Molojavyi A, Kuhn-Velten WN, Schrader J (2002) Cardiac-specific over-expression of inducible nitric oxide synthase does not result in severe cardiac dysfunction. *Circ Res* 90 (1): 93–99

70 Scherrer-Crosbie M, Ullrich R, Bloch KD, Nakajima H, Nasseri B, Aretz HT, Lindsey

ML, Vancon AC, Huang PL, Lee RT et al (2001) Endothelial nitric oxide synthase limits left ventricular remodeling after myocardial infarction in mice. *Circulation* 104 (11): 1286–1291

71   Bachmaier K, Neu N, Pummerer C, Duncan GS, Mak TW, Matsuyama T, Penninger JM (1997) iNOS expression and nitrotyrosine formation in the myocardium in response to inflammation is controlled by the interferon regulatory transcription factor 1. *Circulation* 96 (2): 585–591

72   Kalra DK, Zhu X, Ramchandani MK, Lawrie G, Reardon MJ, Lee-Jackson D, Winters WL, Sivasubramanian N, Mann DL, Zoghbi WA (2002) Increased myocardial gene expression of tumor necrosis factor-alpha and nitric oxide synthase-2: A potential mechanism for depressed myocardial function in hibernating myocardium in humans. *Circulation* 105 (13): 1537–1540

Identification and role of inflammatory oxygen free radicals in cardiac ischemia and reperfusion injury

Catherine Vergely, Gaëlle Clermont, Sandrine Lecour, Antoine Bril and Luc Rochette

Laboratoire de Physiopathologie et Pharmacologie Cardiovasculaires Expérimentales, Institut Fédératif de Recherche n° 100, Facultés de Médecine et de Pharmacie, Université de Bourgogne, 7 Bd Jeanne d'Arc, BP 87900, 21079 Dijon cedex, France

Introduction

Prolonged myocardial ischemia results in a variety of severe cellular, metabolic and ultra-structural damages. It is therefore generally accepted that reperfusion is an absolute prerequisite for the survival of ischemic tissue. However, reperfusion may precipitate arrhythmias, cause myocardial stunning and accelerate necrotic process. Oxygen free radicals have been suggested as possible mediators of reperfusion-induced injury and there is circumstantial evidence that supports this hypothesis. Indirect evidence in support of this concept derives from studies in which antioxidant enzymes, enzyme inhibitors, free radical scavengers and iron chelators are able to protect against reperfusion injury in a number of experimental studies. *In vivo*, polymorphonuclear leukocytes (PMNs) have been hypothesized to induce and to amplify the process of reperfusion injury in post-ischemic myocardium. With *in vivo* models, there are many different cellular and humoral factors making it difficult to determine the importance of specific components in the pathogenesis of myocardial injury. Both ischemia and reperfusion promote the expression of pro-inflammatory gene products and bioactive agents. Furthermore, ischemia induces a pro-inflammatory state that increases tissue vulnerability towards further injury during reperfusion.

The aim of the present chapter is to review the involvement of inflammatory Reactive Oxygen Species (ROS) in the pathophysiology of ischemia and in reperfusion damages. After a brief description of the biochemistry of reactive oxygen species and the methods used for their determination, experimental and clinical evidence for their role in cardiac ischemia and reperfusion injury will be summarized.

Biological chemistry of reactive oxygen species (ROS)

A free radical is defined as any atomic or molecular species that contains one or more unpaired electrons in one of its molecular orbitals. Although some free radi-

Inflammation and Cardiac Diseases, edited by Giora Z. Feuerstein, Peter Libby and Douglas L. Mann

cals are not reactive oxygen species, some reactive oxygen species (ROS) do not qualify as free radicals. Indeed hydrogen peroxide is a very reactive species derived from oxygen but its chemical structure is not a free radical. In contrast, molecular O_2 may be qualified as a free radical because it has two unpaired electrons with parallel spin [1, 2]. The cellular production of oxygen free radicals is a complex system in which both enzymatic and non-enzymatic pathways are involved.

Any aerobic organisms can generate and degrade oxygen free radicals (OFR). OFR include a number of chemically reactive molecules derived from oxygen. The superoxide anion $O_2^{\cdot-}$ created from molecular oxygen by addition of an electron is a typical free radical, in spite of being not very reactive. Physiologically, the production of superoxide anion takes place spontaneously in area of the inner mitochondrial membrane as a part of the respiratory chain. Two molecules of superoxide react together to produce hydrogen peroxide (H_2O_2) and molecular oxygen via a reaction known as dismutation which is accelerated by superoxide dismutases (SOD). The resulting product, H_2O_2, is not a free radical itself as indicated previously, but its role as an intermediate and a signaling molecule is widely recognized.

In a reaction catalyzed by various metal ions (Fe^{2+} or Cu^+) hydroxyl radical ($^{\cdot}OH$) is formed from H_2O_2 and is very reactive with other biomolecules. Amongst other free radicals, nitric oxide ($^{\cdot}NO$) is synthesized enzymatically from L-arginine by NO synthases. NO, which has the ability to cross cell membranes, functions as an intracellular second messenger stimulating guanylate cyclase thereby relaxing smooth muscles in blood vessels. NO is not a locally-acting messenger and its spatial distribution in tissue is large. Membrane-bound proteins are especially important targets for NO and nitrosylation of proteins is known to regulate enzymatic activity [3].

Most of the damages induced by $O_2^{\cdot-}$ and H_2O_2 in $vivo$ are thought to be due to their conversion into $^{\cdot}OH$. Hydroxyl radical is very reactive and it can combine with almost every cellular molecules. Therefore, all the components present in a cell can be considered as $^{\cdot}OH$ scavenger. It has been argued that an antioxidant acting to interfere with damage induced by $^{\cdot}OH$ will also act by binding the transition metal, Fe^{2+} or Cu^+. The action of $^{\cdot}OH$ upon biological compounds (lipids, proteins, DNA) induces the formation of carbon-centered radicals that can then react with O_2 to give peroxyl radicals ($RO_2^{\cdot}$). Similarly, the reaction of $^{\cdot}OH$ with thiols can also produce thiyl radicals ($RS^{\cdot}$). Peroxyl radicals are the major chain-propagating species involved in the process of lipid peroxidation of biological membranes. These reactions lead to the generation of lipid hydroperoxides (LOOH) and to alkoxyl radicals ($RO^{\cdot}$) in the presence of traces of iron [4].

The generation of ROS at the mitochondria level accounts for 1 or 2% of total O_2 consumption under reducing conditions but the intra-mitochondrial concentrations of superoxide are maintained at very low steady-state levels as a result of the high concentrations of SOD present in mitochondria. However, there is evidence that tumor necrosis factor (TNF)-α and interleukin (IL-1) induce apoptosis via mitochondria-derived ROS. It has been recently suggested that membrane-associated oxidases are an important source of ROS. The most extensively characterized membrane oxidases is the phagocytic NADPH oxidase present not only in phagocytic cells but also in non phagocytic cells such as cardiac myocytes and smooth muscle cells [5]. This enzyme catalyzes the one-electron reduction of O_2 to $O_2^{\cdot-}$ with NADPH being the electron donor through the cytochrome b_{558}, a heterodimeric complex of gp91^{phox} and p22^{phox} protein subunits. By analogy with the neutrophil enzyme, the vascular oxidase is thought to span the membrane utilizing intracellular NADH or NADPH. It has been estimated that vascular enzymes are responsible for one third of the production of $O_2^{\cdot-}$-production induced by neutrophils. Furthermore, these vascular enzymes appear to have a moderate constitutive activity. On the other hand, it has been clearly demonstrated that the NADPH oxidase activity is increased by angiotensin II and there is a broad body of evidence that AT_1-angiotensin receptor activation leads to a production of OFR in the vessel wall and that AT_1 receptors are linked to the activation of NADH/NADPH oxidase. Endogenous ROS stimulated by the activation of AT_1 receptors play critical roles as intracellular signaling molecules and low concentrations of intracellular ROS have been demonstrated to activate various members of the MAPK family. Several mechanisms have been proposed for the ROS-induced activation of MAPK, including receptor clustering, protein tyrosine phosphatase inhibition and protein kinase activation. In addition, ROS may directly regulate the activity of transcription factors. As an example, it is known that the transcription factor NF-κB which is a key mediator of the inflammatory response, is activated in response to various stimuli including cytokines and oxidative stress and that the addition of antioxidant compounds or the up-regulation of cellular antioxidant systems can prevent cytokine-induced NF-κB activation. Nitric oxide (NO) is also a redox signaling molecule that can modulate the activity of several transcription factors. In addition, the expression of the endothelial NO synthase (eNOS) is regulated by NF-κB initiating possible feedback loops. NF-κB inhibition by NO probably involves inhibition of IκB degradation.

The biological relevance of each of the three inorganic species – iron, oxygen and nitric oxide (NO) – is crucial. Transition metal ions, in particular iron, are important mediators of oxidative damage. Iron transport and storage proteins like ferritin, transferrin and haemosiderin, efficiently control iron reactivity. It has been proposed that a small "chelatable" ion pool exists in the cytosol which is bound to low molecular weight chelators such as nucleotides, citrate and amino acids [6]. In order to be available to the cell, iron has to be released from proteins, giving rise to a "pool" of "free" iron within the cell. It has been suggested that loosely non-haem iron may initiate free radical generation processes. Therefore, the iron metabolism has to be tightly regulated and, in cells, this regulation is co-ordinated by ferritin and transferring receptors. However, there are many controversies about the role of ferritin in oxidative stress since, under oxidative stress conditions, the intracellular pool of "free" iron is increased. Furthermore, an increase in intracellular ferritin level following exposure of cells to iron has been reported. The mechanisms leading to this enhanced ferritin expression may be considered as being compensatory pathways aimed at counterbalancing the inhibitory effects of oxidants on ferritin synthesis. As a consequence, the use of iron chelators to suppress oxidative damage may prove useful in the therapy of reperfusion injury in heart and in other tissues [7, 8].

While there is general agreement that free radicals are involved in reperfusion injury, their cellular origin *in vivo* remains uncertain. Using cultured endothelial cells, several laboratories have demonstrated that reoxygenation results in production of OFR [9, 10]. The *in vitro* models of anoxia-reoxygenation demonstrated that endothelial cells were not only potential sources of free radicals but also sites of oxidative injury [11]. More generally, superoxide can be produced from xanthine oxidase, arachidonic acid and the mitochondrial enzymes in both endothelial and vascular smooth muscle cells. In fact, it has been demonstrated that in endothelial and vascular smooth muscle cells the most significant system generating oxygen free radicals is the NAD(P)H-dependent oxidase and that the activity of this oxidase is increased by angiotensin II. Indeed, one of the most important attributes of the cardiovascular oxidases is their responsiveness to hormones, haemodynamic forces and local metabolic changes including the uncoupling of NOS III [12].

Under physiological conditions, equilibrium exists between the mechanisms generating and scavenging reactive oxygen species and every organism has antioxidant systems protecting them against the actions of these radicals. An antioxidant is a molecule which, at low concentration, reacts with a free radical and is relatively stable either in a radical or a non-radical form [13]. The protective systems decreasing the negative influence of ROS can be divided into two classes that are the preventive antioxidants and chain breaking antioxidants respectively. Preventive antioxidants intercept oxidizing species before a cellular damage can be observed. Because of the reactivity of the hydroxyl radical, it is obvious that there are no true antioxidants for ˙OH but compounds that scavenge ˙OH only delay or postpone its action. Actually, these agents suppress oxidation processes only slightly compared to true antioxidants. In contrast to preventive antioxidants, chain breaking antioxidants slow or stop the oxidative processes after their initiation, by intercepting the chain-carrying radicals. Typical examples of chain breaking antioxidants are donor antioxidant such as vitamins including tocopherol, ascorbate [14] or sacrificial antioxidant such as nitric oxide (˙NO). In fact ˙NO could play a dual antioxidant effect for cells localized near the endothelium as ˙NO is acting preventively since ˙NO co-ordinates with heme-iron, and also reacting toward oxiradicals as chain-breaking reagent (ROO˙ + ˙NO → ROONO).

Finally, there is evidence showing that hydroxyl radicals are produced during a Ca^{2+} paradox as a transient calcium overload is associated with a burst of free radical production and interacts with this sudden production of free radicals to induce cellular injury. It is well established that an increase in cytosolic Ca^{2+} occurs during a period of ischemia and is increased further upon reperfusion. The mechanisms responsible for this calcium overload at reperfusion are multiple but generally involve the activation of the Na^+/Ca^{2+} exchange. There is evidence that OFR and calcium are involved in the cellular alterations leading to reperfusion injury such as arrhythmias and various compounds that reduce free radicals levels also reduce the incidence of reperfusion arrhythmias [15–17].

Identification and quantification of free radicals: Electron paramagnetic resonance spectroscopy (EPR)

EPR is considered the least ambiguous method for the detection of free radicals and when the free radical has a long lifetime such as ascorbyl free radicals, a direct EPR spectroscopy can be used to identify this species. Unfortunately, it is not always possible to quantify free radicals directly because their concentration may be below the detection limit. On the other hand, oxygen-centered radicals are of particular interest because they are implicated in many *in vivo* reactions. However, their short lifetimes make many of these radical difficult to detect even by direct EPR. The use of modified techniques such as the spin trapping provides a mean to overcome these issues.

Briefly, the spin-trapping technique makes use of a diamagnetic compound called the spin trap, which reacts with a free radical, the spin, giving rise to a relatively stable product called spin-adduct. Many spin trap compounds have been developed but those which find a use in studies on free radicals in biological systems are, with only few exceptions, nitroso and nitrone derivatives. One of the most innovative achievements of spin trapping is the ability to detect superoxide and hydroxyl radical formation in living cells and tissues. Indeed, depending on the radical under investigation, various spin traps may be used. For oxygen, carbon and sulphur radicals, nitrone spin-traps such as the water soluble 5,5-dimethyl-1-pyrroline-N-oxide (DMPO) or the lipid soluble α-phenyl N-tert-butyl nitrone (PBN) are the most commonly used. For NO, iron or sulphur cluster-containing spin traps have been developed which, depending on their hydro- or lipo-solubility, can diffuse across the cell membranes.

Experimental approaches of the role of ROS in cardiac ischemia and reperfusion

Ascorbyl free radicals (AFR)

The myocardium contains many antioxidants including water soluble compounds such as ascorbic acid and glutathione, and lipid soluble antioxidants such as α-tocopherol and ubiquinones. Due to its low redox potential, ascorbate anion (AH-

) is able to give up one single electron to any free radical occurring in a biological system or to generated oxidized biological radical scavengers such as vitamin E. This oxidative process leads to the formation of AFR. Given its relatively long half-life compared to other free radicals such as superoxide anion, hydroxyl, peroxyl and alkoxyl radicals, AFR can be detected by EPR in aqueous solutions at room temperature. Interestingly, because AFR is one of the rare radical species that can be directly observed in biological systems, AFR liberation has been proposed as a marker of oxidative stress both *in vitro* and *in vivo* in studies in which the functional recovery of hearts subjected to ischemia and reperfusion was investigated. The relationship between the severity of myocardial ischemia, the intensity of ascorbyl free radical release and the post-ischemic recovery during reperfusion was investigated in isolated perfused rat hearts submitted to global ischemia, either total (zero-flow ischemia) or low flow (residual flow of 5%) maintained for either 20 or 60 minutes [18]. Coronary effluents were collected at different times during the protocol and were analyzed with EPR spectroscopy. AFR EPR doublet (g = 2.0054, $a_H = 0.188$ MT) was not detected in coronary effluents collected during the control perfusion periods but, during low-flow ischemia, a weak AFR release was noted. Moreover, a sudden and massive AFR liberation was observed at the time of reperfusion. This AFR release was weaker after low-flow ischemia than after zero-flow ischemia and was enhanced when the duration of ischemia increased from 20 to 60 minutes. The large liberation of AFR noticed after global total ischemia was associated with a greater depression in myocardial contractile function and a lower recovery in coronary flow. This study demonstrates that AFR production at the time of reperfusion depends on both duration and severity of the ischemia, and is related to free radical injury [18]. According to previously described ascorbate/AFR properties, it can be suggested that AFR liberation in coronary effluents could represent a marker of oxidative stress during myocardial ischemia and/or reperfusion. This AFR release could be considered as an indication of the severity of the ischemic episode, and could be related to the functional impairment during reperfusion.

A similar conclusion was obtained *in vivo* using an open-chest canine model of myocardial ischemia-reperfusion [19]. In this study AFR release increased reproducibly after an occlusion-reperfusion sequence and the magnitude of AFR rise during reperfusion depended on the duration of coronary occlusion. The greater rise of AFR was accompanied by persistent dyskinesis, indicating myocardial stunning. In other studies Buettner and Jurkiewicz [20] demonstrated that the steady-state AFR EPR signal intensity can serve as an indicator of the degree of free radical oxidative processes taking place in biological systems, when the variables (pH, catalytic metal concentration and ascorbate levels) are controlled. Furthermore, it has been reported that the measurements by EPR of AFR in plasma could be a reliable marker indicating the occurrence of an oxidative stress in patients undergoing aortic cross-clamping ischemia [21].

Primary and secondary radical species

Many studies have provided evidence for a free radical burst starting from the initial minutes of reperfusion using EPR spectroscopy associated with spin trapping. In conditions where cellular antioxidative defenses are overwhelmed, primary radical species may induce radical chains reactions leading to the appearance of secondary radical species. The spin trapping agent 5,5-dimethyl-1-pyrroline-N-oxide (DMPO) was used to investigate oxy-radical production in post-ischemic rat hearts previously exposed to myocardial ischemia. A hydroxyl spin adduct (DMPO-OH) was identified in coronary effluent during the initial seconds of reperfusion. The intensity of the EPR signal in post-ischemic period increased as ischemic duration was prolonged, and a direct relationship between free radical generation and subsequent impaired contractile function has been observed [22]. Superoxide dismutase inhibited the formation of DMPO-OH, suggesting that superoxide anion was initially generated [23]. Zweier et al. performed experiments using hearts in which adventitial iron was removed and the results suggested that, in the absence of iron, $O_2^{\cdot-}$ would be primarily destroyed by the relatively slow reaction of spontaneous dismutation to form H_2O_2. These experiments suggest that the potency of SOD at scavenging free radicals in reperfused myocardium can be modulated by the presence of iron.

Nitrone spin traps, such as DMPO and DEPMPO are very water soluble whereas other spin traps such as PBN and its analogs, are mainly lipid soluble. It is therefore most likely that DMPO is more efficient at trapping free radicals in the extracellular area, while PBN reacts with intracellular free radicals. We therefore investigated the significance of the secondary free radical release during non ischemic perfusion and post-ischemic reperfusion and evaluated the cardiovascular effects of the spin trap used [24]. For that purpose, isolated perfused rat hearts underwent 0, 20, 30 or 60 minutes of a total ischemia, followed by 30 minutes of reperfusion in the absence or presence of PBN (α-phenyl-N-tert-butylnitrone, 3 mM). Functional parameters were recorded and samples of coronary effluents were collected and analyzed using EPR to identify and quantify the amount of spin adducts produced. During non-ischemic perfusion, there was undetectable level of free radical release. In contrast, a large and long-lasting (30 minutes) release of spin adducts was detected from the onset of reperfusion. The free radical species were identified as alkyl and alkoxyl radicals with amounts reaching 40 times the pre-ischemic values. Interestingly, PBN showed a cardioprotective effect, allowing a significant reduction of rhythm disturbances and a better post-ischemic recovery of hearts submitted to 20 minutes of ischemia. However, when the duration of ischemia was increased further, the protective effects of PBN disappeared and toxic effects became more important. These results therefore confirmed the antioxidant and protective properties of a spin trap agent such as PBN but showed the limitation in the used of such compounds. Moreover, we demonstrated that the persistent post-ischemic dysfunction was associated with a sustained production and release of free radical species.

Another observation from our studies [25] is that the spin adduct release rate during reperfusion is not modified by the treatment with the active enantiomers of arginine or NAME. Therefore, the positive or negative modulation of NOS activity does not seem to influence the level of post-ischemic oxidative stress. Several authors have provided evidence that uncoupled electron transfer can occur in NOS, leading to the production of superoxide. In physiological conditions, cells probably maintain sufficient levels of L-arginine for NOS to catalyze NO synthesis, because L-arginine is found in mammalian cells at concentrations by far exceeding the K_M values of these enzymes. However, in conditions such as ischemia and reperfusion, where a leak in amino acids is observed, the availability of L-arginine and tetrahydrobiopterin could be impaired and would participate in NOS-induced generation of $O_2^{\cdot-}$. These results indicate that, in isolated rat heart, cardiac ˙NO synthases might not be major components implicated in the oxidative burst that follows a global myocardial ischemia.

Nitric oxide

˙NO is a gaseous free radical that possesses a broad array of biological functions. Although there is a large number of techniques used to detect ˙NO in cell suspensions and isolated tissue preparations, EPR spectroscopy is considered the best technique available. EPR methods require the stabilization of ˙NO using endogenous and exogenous spin traps. Spin trapping in combination with EPR can characterize ˙NO in real time and at their loci of production. The most frequently used iron chelates for the *in vivo* spin trapping of ˙NO are iron-N-methyl-D-glucamine dithiocarbamate [Fe(MGD)$_2$] [26] and iron-diethyl dithiocarbamate [Fe(DETC)$_2$].

MGD is able to diffuse into the tissue and to selectively bind NO in biological systems after complexing with reduced iron Fe(II). The [NO-Fe(MGD)$_2$] complex formed gives rise to a typical triplet EPR spectrum and is a relatively stable product [27]. Several studies applied this spin-trapping technique to quantify myocardial NO levels in the isolated rat heart model directly. Using the ferrous iron complex of [Fe(MGD)$_2$] a specific and water-soluble NO spin trap, it has been shown that myocardial NO levels were markedly increased after 30 minutes of global ischemia and that the intensity of NO formation was directly proportional with the duration of ischemia [27].

There has been considerable controversy regarding whether reperfusion results in increased or decreased ˙NO formation in the heart. It has been hypothesized that if ˙NO is increased upon reperfusion it might react with $O_2^{\cdot-}$ resulting in the formation of the potent cytotoxic oxidant ONOO˙ [28].

During the past years, the effect of myocardial ischemia on ˙NO production, *in vivo*, has been controversial. In recent studies, direct quantification of ˙NO was investigated using a rat model of myocardial ischemia *in vivo* [29]. In these experiments, the characteristic triplet spectrum of the $[NO\text{-}Fe(MGD)_2]$ complex appeared in the infracted area eight hours after left coronary artery occlusion and an increase in the NO adduct was measured as a function of the duration of ischemia. This increase was specifically observed in the ischemic area since no ESR triplet was observed in the non-ischemic area of the heart. The presence of the $[Fe(MGD)_2]$ spin trap in the ischemic area could be due to a reduced blood flow.

In these experiments, the origin of NO produced specifically in the ischemic area was investigated. NO might be synthetized from L-arginine by NOS activation but as reported by Zweier et al. [27], NO could also be generated in the ischemic heart by direct reduction of nitrite into NO under the acid and highly reduced conditions that occur during ischemia. A treatment of the animals with the inducible NOS inhibitor, aminoguanidine, prevented the formation of the $[NO\text{-}Fe(MGD)_2]$ complex suggesting that the generation of NO detected in the ischemic area mostly derived from the activation inducible NOS.

Ischemia-reperfusion injury and neutrophils in clinical approaches

Multiple aspects of inflammation have been demonstrated to be involved in reperfusion injury. Accumulating evidence has indicated that myocardial ischemia elicits an acute inflammatory response that is greatly increased by reperfusion. Several mechanisms have been proposed for reperfusion injury, including generations of OFR and calcium overload. Among the consequences of the inflammatory process, superoxide, hydrogen peroxide and hydroxyl radicals that are all products of the membrane-bound NADPH oxidase enzyme have been identified. Polymorphonuclear leukocytes (PMNs) are integrated into the acute inflammatory response to tissue injury and possess the capacity to produce OFR. Most stimuli that induce superoxide generation by PMNs also cause the release of myeloperoxidase from azurophil granules. Myeloperoxidase, which is one of the major constituents of neutrophil granules, is able to produce highly reactive toxic products such as hypochloric acid. Hypochloric acid is considered to be primarily responsible for the OFR-dependent cytotoxicity of PMNs.

There is a large body of research on the incidence of ischemia-reperfusion on leukocyte activation, chemotaxis, leukocyte-endothelial cell adhesion and transmigration. Activated leukocytes interact with the vascular endothelium *via* a series of distinct steps. The first step is initiated by ischemia and reperfusion-induced increases in endothelial P-selectin surface expression which interacts with its leukocyte counterreceptor, P-selectin glycoprotein 1. This low affinity interaction between leukocyte β_2 integrins such as CD11a/CD18 with endothelial intercellular adhesion molecule 1 (ICAM-1) results in leukocyte adherence and cessation of lateral movement. Then the leucocyte transmigration into interstitial compartment is facilitated by an adhesion molecule [30].

In experimental models, PMN accumulation is accelerated by reperfusion and occurs preferentially in the sub-endocardial area. In addition, regional plugging of the microvasculature by PMNs is likely to be enhanced by various microvascular alterations. In dogs, the depletion of circulating neutrophils has been reported to protect against the fall in coronary flow during reperfusion of ischemic myocardium [31]. Furthermore several reports have indicated that PMN depletion reduced myocardial infarct size when administered before [32] or at the times of reperfusion [33]. Currently many investigators are proposing leukocytes as the source of free radicals in the reperfused heart, however, it should be noted that free-radical mediated injury has been shown to occur in many leukocyte free systems. Therefore, it could be suggested that reactive oxygen species from several sources contribute to the post-ischemic myocardial injury.

In clinical practice, a sequence ischemia-reperfusion is associated with thrombolytic therapy, aortic cross-clamping, cardiopulmonary bypass or organ transplantation. The development of thrombolytic therapy that causes lysis of platelet thrombi allows the restoration of blood flow to the affected area of tissue within hours of the ischemic insult. In patients undergoing cardiopulmonary bypass (CPB) procedures, it is well known that some cases of organ dysfunction involving kidneys, lungs, liver, central nervous system and cardiovascular system are observed. The pathogenesis of the development of postoperative organ dysfunction is multifactorial. First, it is believed that the organ dysfunction is triggered at least in part by a systemic inflammatory response to CPB, induced by the exposure of blood elements to non-physiological surfaces. Second, there is evidence suggesting that ROS may play a significant role in the pathogenesis of these phenomena. However, the origin and the exact mechanism of ROS production in the setting of cardiac surgery remain nuclear. Recently, we investigated the time course and the origin of ROS release in patients undergoing open heart surgery [34]. For this purpose, peripheral and coronary sinus time-collected samples were taken during coronary artery bypass grafting and the oxidative stress was examined by both direct and indirect approaches. Direct detection of alkyl and alkoxyl radicals was assessed by EPR associated with the spin-trapping technique using α-phenyl-N-tert-butylnitrone (PBN). Before cross-clamping, a small amount of PBN-alkyl-alkoxyl adducts was detected both in coronary sinus and in peripheral blood samples at similar concentrations. During cross claming, the spin adduct concentrations steadily increased in the peripheral blood and during the reperfusion period, spin adduct concentrations remained elevated in the peripheral blood. In the coronary sinus, the spin adduct production seemed to be more pronounced at the beginning of reoxygenation since a peak occurred three minutes after removing the clamp. In addition, a correlation existed between the spin adduct production during CPB and the cross clamping duration as well as between the spin adduct production and the postoperative CPK MB concentrations. The fact that, after 30 minutes of cross clamping, a significant decrease in the plasma antioxidant status was observed in both peripheral and coronary sinus samples which persists during the entire reperfusion period provides confirmation that an oxidative stress is activated in such surgical procedures. Indeed, these findings suggest that a myocardial radical activation seems to occur within the first three minutes of reperfusion in the coronary sinus. However, this study also established that no significant difference existed between peripheral and coronary sinus samples. Therefore, it seems reasonable to hypothesize that the myocardial ROS release could have been masked by the high systemic radical activation preceding the myocardial blood transit.

An alternative hypothesis could be that the surgical procedure itself is responsible for the release of ROS in the peripheral circulation. To test this hypothesis, the investigation of a second group of patients showed that no difference occurred in ROS concentration between samples collected before anesthesia, just before CPB, i.e., after the anesthesia procedure, and the pre-CPB surgery, which includes the sternothomy collection of internal mammary artery or saphenous vein grafts. Therefore, anesthesia and surgical trauma are not likely to be responsible for the peripheral oxidative stress observed [34]. Other components that could participate in the peripheral free radical production include the poor perfusion of peripheral tissues or the high oxygen tension level used during CPB. It could be concluded from these studies that an overall inflammation and activated neutrophils could be a prominent source of ROS. However several technical issues, such as the use of mannitol before myocardial reperfusion, that are related to the clinical setting could have minimized the ROS release from the myocardium and need to be further investigated. Furthermore, the production of primary ROS within myocardium during reperfusion could induce specific intracellular effects that cannot be evidenced in plasma using traditional spin-trapping technique. Finally, the positive correlation showed between the rate of PBN adducts produced during CPB and the duration of aortic cross clamping might be attributable to the cross-clamping but also the duration of CPB itself. Actually, the production of PBN adducts systemic for a majority, could be the result of the enlarged duration of the CPB procedure. A correlation was also found between the PBN adduct production and the concentration of creatine phosphokinase in muscle band of patients one hour after the end of intervention. ROS circulating in the extracorporeal circuit and passing through heart during the reperfusion period could increase the myocardial damage related to ischemia-reperfusion. The presence of alkyl-alkoxyl radicals in blood from patients undergoing CPB could result from the action of primary ROS such as hydroxyl or superoxide on cellular and plasma components. These secondary radical species then participate in radical chain reactions, in particular lipid peroxydation, and can induce deleterious effect within tissues. The increased PBN adduct concentrations support the evidence that a free radical aggression occurs during CPB [34]. In addition, our results show that peripheral alkyl-alkoxyl radical release exists from the onset (during the cross-clamping period) to the end of the CPB procedure independently, at least to some extent, of reperfusion of the ischemic myocardium.

Taken together, these results suggest that the peripheral oxidative stress observed during CPB leads in large part to neutrophil activation [35]. Indeed, it is known that the CPB procedure is associated with a major inflammatory response [35] potentially responsible for an activation of neutrophils that represents a prominent source of systemic primary oxygen free radical production. The synergistic action of free radicals, activation and infiltration of neutrophils in reperfused tissues has been well recognized to enhance myocardial damages during any ischemic episode. Moreover, the high oxygen tension used during CPB, concomitant with neutrophil activation could also lead to oxidative stress [37, 38] and could be critical in preventing injuries during ischemic insults. Therefore, several investigators suggested that future strategies of myocardial protection should not be limited to interventions targeting the heart itself, but should take into account the systemic response as shown during CPB procedures [37, 39]. These concepts should be particularly relevant for high-risk patients, who are more prone to multiple organ injuries.

Conclusion

Reperfusion of the ischemic myocardium is necessary for tissue salvage, but it has to be recognized that this procedure is itself associated with cellular injuries. Experimental evidence has indicated that myocardial reperfusion can promote potentially cardiotoxic inflammatory reactions and PMNs are among the cellular mediators implicated in myocardial reperfusion injury because PMNs are an important source of OFRs. In addition to direct activation of PMNs during reperfusion period, complement activation indirectly increases neutrophil recruitment and infiltration into the myocardial risk region. Therefore, the development of pharmacologic interventions aimed at modulating the responses of the organism to the "oxygen paradox" associated with reperfusion represents a clinical hope.

References

1   Halliwell B, Gutteridge JMC (1989) The chemistry of oxygen radicals and other oxygen-derived species. In: *Free radicals in biology and medicine* (2nd edition), Clarendon Press, Oxford, 22–81

2   Halliwell B, Gutteridge JMC (1989) A consideration of atomic structure and bounding. In: *Free radicals in biology and medicine* (2nd edition), Clarendon Press, Oxford, 509–524

3   Moncada S, Palmer RM, Higgs EA (1989) Biosynthesis of nitric oxide from L-arginine. A pathway for the regulation of cell function and communication. *Biochem Pharmacol* 38: 1709–1715

4   Fridovich I (1998) Oxygen toxicity: A radical explanation. *J Exp Biol* 201 (Pt 8): 1203–1209

5   Griendling KK, Sorescu D, Ushio-Fukai M (2000) NAD(P)H oxidase: Role in cardio-vascular biology and disease. *Circ Res* 86(5): 494–501

6   Rothman RJ, Serroni A, Farber JL (1992) Cellular pool of transient ferric iron, cheletable by deferoxamine and distinct from ferritin, that is involved in oxidative cell injury. *Mol Pharmacol* 42: 703–710

7   Hasinoff BB, Hellmann K, Herman EH, Ferrans VJ (1998) Chemical, biological and clinical aspects of dexrazoxane and other bisdioxopiperazines. *Curr Med Chem* 5 (1): 1–28

8   Menasché P, Antebi H, Alcindor LG, Teiger E, Perez G, Giudicelli Y, Nordmann R, Piwnica A (1990) Iron chelation by deferoxamine inhibits lipid peroxidation during cardiopulmonary bypass in humans. *Circulation* 82 (5 Suppl): IV390–396

9   Arroyo CM, Carmichael AJ, Bouscarel B, Liang JH, Weglicki WB (1990) Endothelial cells as a source of oxygen-free radicals. An ESR study. *Free Radic Res Commun* 9 (3–6): 287–296

10   Zweier JL (1988) Measurement of superoxide-derived free radicals in the reperfused heart. Evidence for a free radical mechanism of reperfusion injury. *J Biol Chem* 263 (3): 1353–1357

11   Kramer JH, Dickens BF, Misik V, Weglicki WB (1995) Phospholipid hydroperoxides are precursors of lipid alkoxyl radicals produced from anoxia/reoxygenated endothelial cells. *J Mol Cell Cardiol* 27 (1): 371–381

12   Mollnau H, Wendt M, Szocs K, Lassegue B, Schulz E, Oelze M, Li H, Bodenschatz M, August M, Kleschyov AL et al (2002) Effects of angiotensin II infusion on the expression and function of NAD(P)H oxidase and components of nitric oxide/cGMP signalling. *Circ Res* 90 (4): E58–65

13   Halliwell B, Gutteridge JMC (1989) Protection against oxidants in biological systems. In: *Free radicals in biology and medicine* (2nd edition), Clarendon Press, Oxford, 86–179

14   Buettner GR (1993) The pecking order of free radicals and antioxidants: Lipid peroxidation, alpha-tocopherol, and ascorbate. *Arch Biochem Biophys* 300(2): 535–43

15   Abadie C, Ben Baouali A, Maupoil V, Rochette L (1993) An alpha-tocopherol analogue with antioxidant activity improves myocardial function during ischemia reperfusion in isolated working rat hearts. *Free Radic Biol Med* 15: 209–215

16   Bolli R (1991) Oxygen-derived free radicals and myocardial reperfusion injury: An overview. *Cardiovasc Drugs Ther* 5 (Suppl 2): 249–268

17   Shattock MJ, Matsuura H, Hearse DJ (1991) Functional and electrophysiological effects of oxidant stress on isolated ventricular muscle: A role for oscillatory calcium release from sarcoplasmic reticulum in arrythmogenesis? *Cardiovasc Res* 25: 645–651

18   Vergely C, Maupoil V, Benderitter M, Rochette L (1998) Influence of the severity of myocardial ischemia on the intensity of ascorbyl free radical release and on postichemic recovery during reperfusion. *Free Radic Biol Med* 24(3): 470–479

19 Sharma MK, Buettner GR, Spencer KT, Kerber RE (1994) Ascorbyl free radical as a real-time marker of free radical generation in briefly ischemic and reperfused hearts. An electron paramagnetic resonance study. *Circ Res* 74 (4): 650–658

20 Buettner GR, Jurkiewicz BA (1993) Ascorbate free radical as a marker of oxidative stress: An EPR study. *Free Radic Biol Med* 14 (1): 49–55

21 Pietri S, Seguin JR, d'Arbigny PD, Culcasi M (1994) Ascorbyl free radical: A noninvasive marker of oxidative stress in human open-heart surgery. *Free Radic Biol Med* 16 (4): 523–528

22 Zweier JL, Kuppusamy P, Lutty GA (1988) Measurement of endothelial cell free radical generation: Evidence for a central mechanism of free radical injury in postischemic tissues. *Proc Natl Acad Sci USA* 85 (11): 4046–4050

23 Arroyo CM, Kramer JH, Dickens BF, Weglicki WB (1987) Identification of free radicals in myocardial ischemia/reperfusion by spin trapping with nitrone DMPO. *FEBS Lett* 221 (1): 101–104

24 Vergely C, Tabard A, Maupoil V, Rochette L (2001) Isolated perfused rat hearts release secondary free radicals during ischemia reperfusion injury: Cardiovascular effects of the spin trap alpha-phenyl N-tert-butylnitrone. *Free Radic Res* 35 (5): 475–489

25 Vergely C, Perrin-Sarrado C; Clermont G, Rochette L (2002) Postischemic recovery and oxidative stress are independent of nitric-oxide synthases modulation in isolated rat heart. *J Pharmacol Exp Ther* 303 (1): 149–157

26 Lecour S, Maupoil V, Siri O, Tabard A, Rochette L (1999) Electron spin resonance detection of nitric oxide generation in major organs from LPS-treated rats. *J Cardiovasc Pharmacol* 33 (1): 78–85

27 Zweier JL, Wang P, Kuppusamy P (1995) Direct measurement of nitric oxide generation in the ischemic heart using electron paramagnetic resonance spectroscopy. *J Biol Chem* 270 (1): 304–307

28 Wang P, Zweier J (1996) Measurement of nitric oxide and peroxynitrite generation in the postischemic heart. *J Biol Chem* 271 (46): 29223–29230

29 Lecour S, Maupoil V, Zeller M, Laubriet A, Briot F, Rochette L (2001) Levels of nitric oxide in the heart after experimental myocardial ischemia. *J Cardiovasc Pharmacol* 37: 55–63

30 Williams FM (1996) Neutrophils and myocardial reperfusion injury. *Pharmacol Ther* 72 (1): 1–12

31 Engler RL, Dahlgren MD, Morris DD, Peterson MA, Schmid-Schonbein GW (1986) Role of leukocytes in response to acute myocardial ischemia and reflow in dogs. *Am J Physiol* 251 (2 Pt 2): H314–H323

32 Simpson PJ, Fantone JC, Mickelson JK, Gallagher KP, Lucchesi BR (1988) Identification of a time window for therapy to reduce experimental canine myocardial injury: Suppression of neutrophil activation during 72 hours of reperfusion. *Circ Res* 63 (6): 1070–1079

33 Litt MR, Jeremy RW, Weismann HF, Winkelstein JA, Becker LC (1989) Neutrophil depletion limited to reperfusion reduces myocardial infarct size after 90 minutes of

ischemia. Evidence for neutrophil-mediated reperfusion injury. *Circulation* 80 (6): 1816–1827

34 Clermont G, Vergely C, Jazayeri S, Lahet JJ, Goudeau JJ, Lecour S, David M, Rochette L, Girard C (2002) Systemic free radical activation is a major event involved in myocardial oxidative stress related to cardiopulmonary bypass. *Anesthesiology* 96: 80–87

35 Belligan G (2000) Leukocytes: Friend or foe. *Intensive Care Med* 26 (Suppl 1): S111–S118

36 Wan S, Leclerc JL, Vincent JL (1997) Inflammatory response to cardiopulmonary bypass: Mechanisms involved and possible therapeutic strategies. *Chest* 112 (3): 676–692

37 Ihnken K, Winkler A, Schlensak C, Sarai K, Neidhart G, Unkelbach U, Mulsch A and Sewell A (1998) Normoxic cardiopulmonary bypass reduces oxidative myocardial damage and nitric oxide during cardiac operations in the adult. *J Thorac Cardiovasc Surg* 116(2): 327–334

38 Knight PR, Holm BA (2000) The three components of hyperoxia. *Anesthesiolgy* 93 (1): 3–5

39 Menasché P (1995). The inflammatory response to cardiopulmonary bypass and its impact on postoperative myocardial function. *Curr Opin Cardiol* 10 (6): 597–604

40 Zweier JL, Wang P, Samouilou A, Kuppusamy P (1995) Enzyme-independent formation of nitric oxide in biological tissues. *Nat Med* 8: 804–809

The immune and complement system
and cardiac diseases

Immune-mediated myocarditis and interleukin-10

Kenichi Watanabe[1], Makoto Kodama[2] and Yoshifusa Aizawa[2]

[1]Department of Clinical Pharmacology, Niigata University of Pharmacy and Applied Life Sciences, Kamisin-ei-cho, Niigata 950-2081; [2]First Department of Medicine, Niigata University School of Medicine, Niigata, Japan

Human myocarditis

Introduction

Myocarditis has been described during and following a wide variety of viral, rickettsial, bacterial and protozoal diseases etc. Infectious agents cause myocardial damage by various mechanisms:

1. invasion of the myocardium
2. production of a myocardial toxin, e.g., diphtheria, and
3. immunologically-mediated myocardial damage [1–4].

Evidence for immune-mediated mechanism is the demonstration of a marked increase in major histocompatibility complex antigen expression in the biopsy specimens from patients with myocarditis.

Viral myocarditis

There are approximately two dozen viruses that may be associated with clinical evidence of myocarditis [1–5]. The myocarditis characteristically develops after a lag period of several weeks following the initial systemic infection, suggesting the involvement of an immunological mechanism. Although infection with Coxsackie virus B is more common, both Coxsackie A and B viruses produce myocarditis. Although most infections are probably benign, self-limited, and sub-clinical, Coxsackie myocarditis appears to be particularly virulent in neonates. Rarely, Coxsackie myocarditis is fatal in adults. Most patients recover completely within weeks.

Inflammation and Cardiac Diseases, edited by Giora Z. Feuerstein, Peter Libby and Douglas L. Mann
© 2003 Birkhäuser Verlag Basel/Switzerland

Giant cell myocarditis

Giant cell myocarditis is a rare disease of unknown etiology characterized by the presence of multinucleated giant cells in the myocardium. It has been occasionally called acute isolated myocarditis, or granulomatous myocarditis, this condition is typically a rapidly fatal disease, often in young to middle-aged adults [5, 6]. Although little evidence aside from the histological findings supports this view, it has been suggested that the cause is an autoimmune reaction. Multinucleated giant cells are found particularly at the margins of the areas of myocardial necrosis; and the giant cells appear to be of macrophage, rather than myocyte origin. The onset is typically rapid, with dyspnea, chest pain, orthopnea and hypotension. Overt congestive heart failure and sudden death may occur. Therapy is invariably unsuccessful, although corticosteroids and immunosuppressive agents have been used.

Experimental autoimmune myocarditis

Introduction

There are two major clinical problems in the field of myocarditis. Firstly, patients with severe-type myocarditis die during the active phase from refractory heart failure, ventricular arrhythmia or cardiogenic shock because there is no specific therapy for acute myocarditis. The next problem is that some patients who have been able to survive the active phase develop dilated cardiomyopathy in the chronic phase. It is well known that Coxsackie B viruses are detected in the myocardium in a significant proportion of patients with myocarditis and in patients with dilated cardiomyopathy.

Human myocarditis can be classified into lymphocytic myocarditis and giant cell myocarditis according to the histopathologic findings. Giant cell myocarditis was believed to be a rare and fatal disease of unknown etiology. However, a recent report indicates that it is more prevalent in human myocarditis than previously recognized [5, 6]. In that report, the left ventricular function of patients with lymphocytic myocarditis improved during long-term follow-up. On the other hand, a progressive decline in the left ventricular systolic function was observed in patients with giant cell myocarditis. This observation implies that giant cell myocarditis is more likely to progress into dilated cardiomyopathy than lymphocytic myocarditis.

It is well understood that myocarditis is a kind of organ-destructive autoimmune disease mediated by T-cell immunity. We have focused on the antigenicity of cardiac myosin in clinical and experimental studies. Experimental autoimmune myocarditis, the clinical and pathological features of which are quite different from those of viral infection, was provoked in Lewis rats by immunization with cardiac myosin fragments.

Cardiac myosin for experimental autoimmune myocarditis

The development of organ-specific autoimmune disease varies with antigens and animal strains. Various experimental models of autoimmune myocarditis were reported during the last half century [7–10]. Heart-specific antigens, such as cardiac myosin, membranous protein, and sarcoplasmic reticulum protein, which were purified from heart tissue, were challenged in inbred strains of animals. From these studies, a model of myocarditis was established by immunizing rats with cardiac myosin. This rat model has several unique characteristics such as the prevalence of myocarditis having 100%, resemblance to human fulminant myocarditis, and the appearance of multinucleated giant cells in the lesions.

Cardiac myosin is composed of two heavy chains and four light chains. The myosin is a large peptide consisting of more than 4,000 amino acids. Three major myocarditogenic epitopes have been identified. Using an antigen-reactive proliferation assay of hybridoma cells, which are derived from lymphocytes of a murine model, the myocarditogenic epitope is localized on residues 334-352 of the murine cardiac myosin α-chain. In the rat model, residues 1,539–1,555 of the rat cardiac myosin α-chain would be the myocarditogenic epitope of experimental autoimmune myocarditis. Direct sub-fragment analysis revealed that several myocarditogenic epitopes actually existed in cardiac myosin. The most effective epitope was identified as a 96 amino acid residues from 1,070 to 1,165 by enzymatic digestion analysis using porcine cardiac myosin β-chain [7–11].

Experimental autoimmune myocarditis

Cardiac myosin, which is prepared from the ventricular muscle of pig hearts, is dissolved in a solution of potassium chloride 0.3 mol/l, and phosphate-buffered sodium chloride 0.2 mol/l, at a concentration of 10 mg/ml [8, 9, 12]. The antigen solution is mixed with an equal volume of complete Freund's adjuvant supplemented with mycobacterium tuberculosis at a concentration of 11 mg/ml. Lewis rats are injected with 0.2 ml of the antigen-adjuvant emulsion into their footpads. The morbidity of experimental autoimmune myocarditis is 100% in rats immunized using this protocol [8, 12]. The myosin-immunized rats become ill and immobile at day 14, and then their activity gradually recovers beginning in the fourth week. About 25% of the myosin-immunized rats die from day 16 to day 28 (the phase of acute myocarditis). All hearts from these rats are enlarged and their surface color changes to a whitish-yellow (Figs. 1 and 2b). There is massive effusion in the pericardium. Histologically, immense cell infiltrates, giant cells and broad myocardial necrosis were seen in all the ventricular walls, as shown in Figure 1.

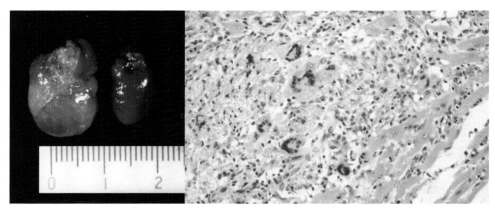

Figure 1
Heart and histologic findings of a rat with experimental autoimmune myocarditis.
Left panel: Massive pericardial effusion and enlargement of the heart are evident in a rat with experimental autoimmune myocarditis. Heart weights of rats with normal (right) and myocarditis (left) are 0.98 g and 1.77 g, respectively. Right panel: Multinucleated giant cells are observed in the lesion (hematoxylin-eosin staining).

About 15% of the rats died between day 28 and day 84. All the hearts from these rats showed extensive myocardial fibrosis and massive pericardial effusion such as dilated cardiomyopathy (the phase of chronic and dilated cardiomyopathy, Fig. 2d).

Interleukin-10

Introduction

Cytokines play important roles in the pathogenesis of myocarditis. Cardiac myosin-specific T-cells are activated by antigen presentation from resident dendritic cells after entering the myocardium [1, 7, 13]. The activated T-cells secrete various cytokines and chemokines, which recruit and activate inflammatory cells in the myocardium. T-helper Type 2 (Th2)-associated cytokine interleukin (IL)-10 has a variety of immunomodulatory properties involving the inhibition of T-helper Type 1 (Th1) cells, macrophages, and pro-inflammatory cytokines [13–15]. IL-10 inhibits the inflammatory response by inhibiting the activation of nuclear factor-κB [16]. Recent reports have suggested that the profound immunosuppressive effects of IL-10 may be effective against transplanted organ rejection, immune complex diseases, and sepsis. Clinical trials of IL-10 have been carried out in patients with these disorders [17, 18].

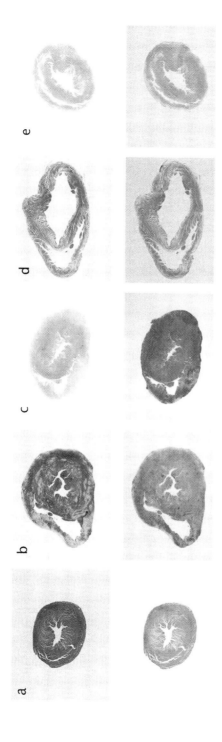

Figure 2
Effects of murine IL-10 on myocardial infiltration and heart size (acute and chronic phases).
Figures show representative data for each group. Upper panel, Azan-Mallory staining; lower panel, hematoxylin-eosin staining: a, Group-N (normal rat); b, Group-V (acute phase on day 21); c, Group-IL-10 (acute phase on day 21); d, Group-V (chronic phase on day 56); e, Group-IL-10 (chronic phase on day 56); Scale bar is 10 mm.

Cytokines generally have a very short circulating half-life *in vivo*. For example, the circulating half-life of IL-10 is < 20 minutes. Therefore, repeated administration has been necessary to observe the effects of cytokines *in vivo*. However, the repeated administration of cytokines results in their fluctuation from extremely high peak levels to basal levels in the serum, which may cause untoward systemic effects.

IL-10 in experimental autoimmune myocarditis

Figure 3 shows the myocardial cytokine expression in this model. IL-2 and IL-12 mRNA appear in the heart at the onset of the disease.

Subsequently, mRNA of IL-1β, interferon-γ (IFN-γ) and tumor necrosis factor-α (TNF-α) increase. These cytokines are released from day 14 to day 19 after immunization. In addition to these, myocardial-inducible nitric oxide synthase (iNOS) is released around day 25. In the recovery phase, IL-10 appears in the heart (from day 25 to day 36). These cytokines are key-players in the pathogenesis of this model [7–18].

Rats with myocarditis that survive the acute phase developed post-myocarditis dilated cardiomyopathy after one month or more. Macroscopically, the hearts of the rats are enlarged and diffusely discolored (Fig. 2d). Transforming growth factor-β (TGF-β), collagen and fibronectin mRNA appear in the heart from day 14 to day 45 after immunization. Collagen and other extracellular matrix components play a role in protecting the left ventricle from extreme expansion after myocardial damage, but they may also interfere with the left ventricular diastolic function and metabolism of the residual myocardial fibers. Management of adequate replacement fibrosis may be a therapeutic strategy for post-myocarditis dilated cardiomyopathy [7, 19].

Gene transfer by electroporation

Introduction

Cardiovascular gene therapy in human subjects

Since 1994, the year in which the first cardiovascular gene therapy trial was initiated, cardiovascular applications have increased from 3% to 17% of all gene therapy trials. Clinical trials of cardiovascular gene therapy, whether using viral (53%), plasmid DNA (39%) or DNA-liposome (8%) vectors, have thus far disclosed no evidence indicative of inflammatory or other complications, including death, directly attributable to the vector used. Indeed, despite the fact that the initial cardiovascular gene therapy trials targeted patients with end-stage vascular disease, including critical limb ischemia and refractory myocardial ischemia, the mortality rate for

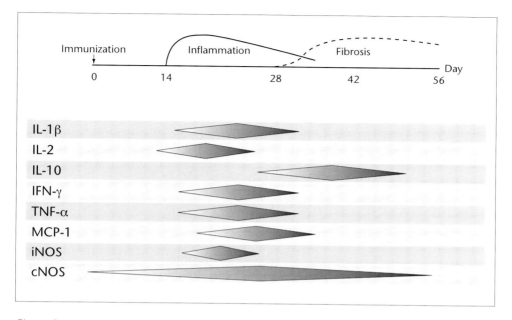

Figure 3
Messenger RNA expression of inflammatory molecules in the rat heart with experimental autoimmune myocarditis.
Interleukin (IL)-2 mRNA appears in the heart at the onset of the disease. Subsequently, mRNA expressions of IL-1β, IFN-γ and tumor necrosis factor-α (TNF-α) increase. In the recovery phase, IL-10 appears in the heart [7].

patients enrolled in cardiovascular gene therapy clinical trials reported to date compares favorably with the mortality rate for similar groups of patients in contemporary controlled studies of medical or interventional therapies. The most common cause of morbidity reported after cardiovascular gene transfer is lower extremity edema. Concerns regarding the potential for angiogenic cytokines to promote the progression of atherosclerosis are not supported by angiographic follow-up of patients with coronary or peripheral vascular disease. The levels and duration of gene expression investigated for therapeutic angiogenesis transfer have not been associated with hemangioma formation [20, 21].

Gene therapy of cytokine
Various cytokines have been cloned and their functions *in vivo* have been intensively explored in many laboratories. Their functions can be analyzed by the adminis-

tration of recombinant proteins. However, the half-life of these cytokines is generally so short that high doses and repeated administration are needed in order to obtain an effective concentration of the cytokines *in vivo*.

Recent progress in molecular biotechnology makes it possible to introduce exogenous genes into animal tissues and achieve efficient expression of the transferred gene. Adenovirus, retrovirus, adeno-associated virus and others are widely used as carriers to introduce exogenous genes into animal cells. While these vectors can efficiently transfer exogenous genes into the target cells, it is still possible that the protein encoded by viral genes could induce immunological responses that might be inappropriately attributed to cytokine function. On the other hand, direct injection of plasmid DNA into the skeletal muscle has several advantages over transfer using viral vectors [22–27].

Electroporation

Electroporation has been widely used to introduce DNA into various types of cells *in vitro*. Gene transfer by electroporation *in vivo* (DNA injection followed by application of electric fields) has been effective for introducing DNA into mouse skin, chick embryos, rat liver, and murine melanoma [22–27]. Gene transfer into the muscle by electroporation *in vivo* is more efficient and the therapeutic effect of IL-10 on autoimmune myocarditis can be analyzed.

Intramuscular DNA injection by electroporation

Plasmid pCAGGS-IL-10 is constructed by inserting murine IL-10 cDNA into the unique EcoRI site between the CAG promoter and a 3'-flanking sequence of the rabbit β-globin gene of the pCAGGS expression vector (Fig. 4) [22, 25].

Fifty micro liters with 200 μg of closed circular plasmid DNA at 4 μg/μl in saline are injected four times (total murine IL-10 is 800 μg/rat) into the bilateral tibialis anterior muscles using a disposable insulin syringe with a 27-gauge needle. A pair of electrode needles is inserted into the muscle to a depth of 5 mm to encompass the DNA injection sites, and electric pulses are delivered using an electric pulse generator connected to a switch box, and monitored using a graphic pulse analyzer [22, 25].

Time-course of IL-10 levels in the blood after a single administration of IL-10 in normal rat

The levels of serum murine IL-10 on days 2 (126 ± 14 pg/ml), 4 (308 ± 16 pg/ml), 6 (320 ± 23 pg/ml), 8 (192 ± 34 pg/ml), 10 (82 ± 9 pg/ml) and 14 (35 ± 8 pg/ml) are sig-

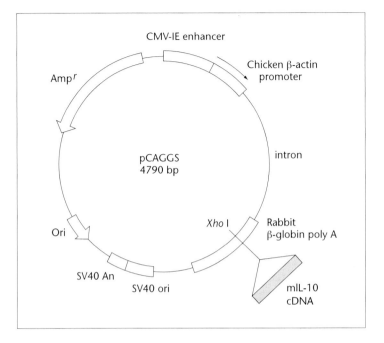

Figure 4
Structure of the murine IL-10 expression plasmid.
Plasmid pCAGGS-IL-10 is constructed by inserting murine (m) IL-10 cDNA into the unique EcoRI site between the CAG promoter and a 3'-flanking sequence of the rabbit β-globin gene of the pCAGGS expression vector.

nificantly higher than that on day 0 (not detected). The level of murine IL-10 peaks on day 6 (Fig. 5).

These murine IL-10 levels are over 50 pg/ml until day 10, and are greater than the peak value of serum rat IL-10 during the natural course of progression of myocarditis in this model (42 ± 4 pg/ml on day 27).

Preventive effects of IL-10 plasmid administration (Group-IL10) in myocarditis

Rats in the myosin-immunized group (Group-V) become ill and immobile on day 14. Twelve of 30 rats in Group-V died between days 19 and 21, and all the hearts from these rats show extensive myocarditis and massive pericardial effusion. The 21-day and 56-day survival rates in Group-IL10 are higher ($30/30 = 100\%$ and $30/30 = 100\%$) than those in Group-V ($18/30 = 60\%$ and $15/30 = 50\%$).

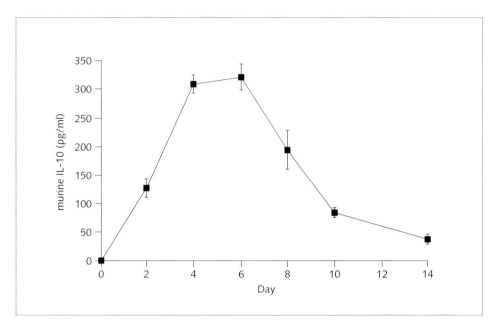

Figure 5
Time course of the serum concentration of murine IL-10 after transfer to normal rats by in vivo electroporation.
The levels of serum murine IL-10 on days 2, 4, 6, 8, 10 and 14 are significantly higher than that on day 0. These murine IL-10 levels are over 50 pg / ml until day 10, and are greater than the peak value of serum rat IL-10 (42 ± 4 pg / ml on day 27) during the natural course of progression of myocarditis in this model.

Central venous pressure and left ventricular end-diastolic pressure are higher, and mean blood pressure, left ventricular pressure and ± dP/dt are lower in Group-V than in normal rats (Group-N). These parameters improve in Group-IL10 (Fig. 6). Although massive pericardial effusion is observed in most of the surviving rats in Group-V on day 21, there is little effusion in Group-IL10. Figure 2 shows representative photographs of thin sections stained with hematoxylin-eosin and Azan-Mallory.

The normal hearts do not show any inflammation, but those in Group-V rats show massive inflammation (stained light blue, which indicates inflammation) in the acute phase (Fig. 2b). The area of myocarditis in Group-IL-10 is smaller than that in Group-V (Fig. 2c). In the chronic phase, a dilated left ventricle and myocardial fibrosis (stained light blue, which indicates fibrosis) are observed in Group-V (Fig. 2d). These findings provide some insight into the effectiveness of IL-10 treatment against not only myocarditis but also post-myocarditis dilated cardiomyopathy.

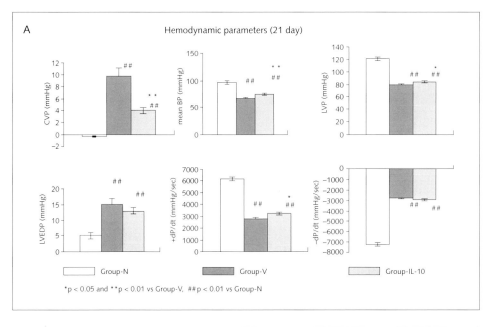

A   Hemodynamic parameters (21 day)

Group-N   Group-V   Group-IL-10

*p < 0.05 and **p < 0.01 vs Group-V, ##p < 0.01 vs Group-N

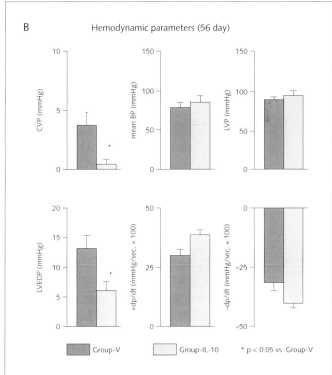

B   Hemodynamic parameters (56 day)

Group-V   Group-IL-10   * p < 0.05 vs. Group-V

Figure 6
Effects of IL-10 on hemodynamic parameters (A is acute phase, and B is chronic phase). Administration of mIL-10 improves central venous pressure (CVP), mean blood pressure (mean BP), peak left ventricular pressure (LVP), left ventricular end-diastolic pressure (LVEDP) and + dP/dt [22].

Conclusion

The model of myocarditis by immunizing rats with cardiac myosin resembles human fulminant myocarditis. IL-10 has a variety of immunomodulatory properties. Among the non-viral techniques for *in vivo* gene transfer, the direct injection of plasmid DNA into the muscle is simple, inexpensive and safe. IL-10 treatment for myocarditis increases the survival rate, attenuates myocardial lesions and decreases the left ventricular end-diastolic pressure. These findings provide evidence that gene transfer into the muscle by electroporation *in vivo* is efficient, and IL-10 may be used for the treatment of autoimmune myocarditis.

Acknowledgments
This research was supported by grants from "Niigata Yujin Memorial Grant", "The Ministry of Education, Science, Sports and Culture of Japan" and "the Promotion and Mutual Aid Corporation for Private Schools of Japan".

References

1   Matsumori A (2002) Cytokines in experimental myocarditis. In: Cooper LT Jr (ed): *Myocarditis*. Humana Press, USA, 109–134

2   Wynne J, Braunwald E (2001) The cardiomyopathies and myocarditides. In: Braunwald E (eds): *Heart diseases*, Saunders Co., USA, 1783–1797

3   Peters NS, Pool-Wilson PA (1991) Myocarditis-continuing clinical and pathologic confusion. *Am Heart J* 121: 942–948

4   Reyes MP, Lerner AM (1985) Coksakievirus myocarditis – with special reference to acute and chronic effects. *Prog Cardiovasc Dis* 27: 373–381

5   Dec GW, Palacios IF, Fallon JT, Aretz HT, Mills J, Lee DCS, Johnson RA (1985) Acute myocarditis in the spectrum of acute dilated cardiomyopathies: clinical features, histologic correlates, and clinical outcome. *N Eng J Med* 312: 885–890

6   Davidoff R, Palacios I, Southern J, Fallon JT, Newell J, Dec GW (1991) Giant cell *versus* lymphocytic myocarditis: a comparison of their clinical features and long-term outcomes. *Circulation* 83: 953–961

7   Kodama M, Okura Y, Aizawa Y, Izumi T (2002) Animal models of autoimmune myocarditis. In: Cooper LT Jr (eds): *Myocarditis*. Humana Press, USA. 197–214

8   Kodama M, Hanawa H, Saeki M, Hosono H, Inomata T, Suzuki K, Shibata A (1994) Rat dilated cardiomyopathy after autoimmune giant cell myocarditis. *Circ Res* 75: 278–284

9   Kodama M, Matsumoto Y, Fujiwara Y Masani F, Izumi T, Shibata A (1991) A novel experimental model of giant cell myocarditis induced in rats by immunization with cardiac myosin fraction. *Clin Immunol Immunopathol* 57: 250–262

10 Wagmann KW, Zhao W, Griffin AC, Hickey WF (1994) Identification of myocardito-genic peptides derived from cardiac myosin capable of inducing experimental allergic myocarditis in the Lewis rat. *J Immunol* 153: 892–900

11 Inomata T, Hanawa H, Miyanishi T, Yajima E, Nakayama S, Maita T, Kodama M, Izumi T, Shibata A, Abo T (1995) Localization of porcine cardiac myosin epitopes that induce experimental autoimmune myocarditis. *Circ Res* 76:726–733

12 Watanabe K, Ohta Y, Nakazawa M, Higuchi H, Hasegawa G, Naito M, Fuse K, Ito M, Hirono S, Tanabe N et al (2000) Low dose carvedilol inhibits progression of heart failure in rats with dilated cardiomyopathy. *Br J Pharmacol* 130: 1489–1495

13 Okura Y, Yamamoto T, Goto S, Inomata T, Hirono S, Hanawa H, Feng L, Wilson CB, Kihara I, Izumi T et al (1997) Characterization of cytokine and iNOS mRNA expression *in situ* during the course of experimental autoimmune myocarditis in rats. *J Mol Cell Cardiol* 29: 491–502

14 Liblau RS, Singer SM, McDevitt HO (1995) Th1 and Th2 CD4+ T cell in the patho-genesis of organ-specific autoimmune diseases. *Immunol Today* 16: 34–38

15 Fiorentino DF, Bond MW Mosmann TR, Ward PA (1989) Two types of mouse T helper cell, IV: Th2 clones secrete a factor that inhibits cytokine production by Th1 clones. *J Exp Med* 170: 2081–2095

16 Lentsch AB, Shanley TP, Sarma V, Ward PA (1997) *In vivo* suppression of NF-kappa-B and preservation of I kappa-B alpha by interleukin-10 and interleukin-13. *J Clin Invest* 100: 2443–2448

17 Shanley TP, Schmal H, Friedl HP, Jones ML, Ward PA (1995) Regulatory effects of intrinsic IL-10 in IgG immune complex-induced lung injury. *J Immunol* 154: 3454–3460

18 Nishio R, Matsumori A, Shioi T, Ishida H, Sasayama S (1999) Treatment of experi-mental viral myocarditis with interleukin-10. *Circulation* 1102–1108

19 Ma M, Watanabe K, Wahed MII, Inoue M, Sekiguchi T, Kouda T, Ohta Y, Nakazawa M, Yoshida Y, Yamamoto T et al (2001) Inhibition of progression of heart failure and expression of TGF-β mRNA in rats with heart failure by the ACE inhibitor quinapril. *J Cardiovascul Pharmacol* 38: S51–S54

20 Isner JM, Vale PR, Symes JF, Losordo DW (2001) Assessment of risks associated with cardiovascular gene therapy in human subjects. *Circ Res* 89: 389–400

21 Baumgartner I, Rauh G, Pieczek A, Wuensch D, Magner M, Kearney M, Schainfeld R, Isner JM (2000) Lower-extremity edema associated with gene transfer of naked DNA vascular endothelial growth factor. *Ann Intern Med* 132: 880–884

22 Watanabe K, Nakazawa M, Fuse K, Hanawa H, Kodama M, Aizawa Y, Ohnuki T, Gejyo F, Maruyama H, Miyazaki J (2001) Protection against autoimmune myocarditis by gene transfer of interleukin-10 by electroporation. *Circulation* 104: 1098–1100

23 Heller R, Jaroszeski M, Atkin A, Moradpour D, Gilbert R, Wands J, Nicolau C (1996) *In vivo* electroinjection and expression in rat liver. *FEBS Lett* 389: 225–228

24 Rols MP, Delteil C, Golzio M, Dumond P, Cros S, Teissie J (1998) *In vivo* electrically mediated protein and gene transfer in murine melanoma. *Nat Biotechnol* 16: 168–171

25   Aihara H, Miyazaki J (1998) Gene transfer into muscle by electroporation *in vivo*. *Nat Biotechnol* 16: 867–870

26   Maruyama H, Sugawa M, Moriguchi Y, Imazeki I, Ishikawa Y, Ataka K, Hasegawa S, Ito Y, Higuchi N, Kazama JJ et al (2000) Continuous erythropoietin delivery by muscle-targeted gene transfer using *in vivo* electroporation. *Hum Gene Ther* 11: 429–437

27   Adachi O, Nakano A, Sato O, Kawamoto S, Tahara H, Toyoda N, Yamato E, Matsumori A, Tabayashi K, Miyazaki J (2002) Gene transfer of Fc-fusion cytokine by *in vivo* electroporation. *Gene Ther* 9: 577–583

Immunomodulation in heart failure: experimental models

Shigetake Sasayama

Hamamatsu Rosai Hospital, 25 Shogen-cho, Hamamatsu, Shizuoka 430-8525, Japan

Introduction

Heart failure is a syndrome rather than a disease. The syndrome still remains an obscure clinical entity and even its definition is disputed. Traditionally, congestive heart failure (CHF) has been viewed as a pathophysiologic state in which the heart is unable to function properly as a pump to deliver adequate blood to the peripheral organ systems and the therapeutic endpoint was directed towards hemodynamic improvement. When cardiac output is reduced as a consequence of ventricular dysfunction, several neurohormonal mechanisms including sympathetic nervous system and renin-angiotensin-aldosterone systems are activated in an attempt to preserve circulatory homeostasis. This activation, however, turns out to be detrimental and constitutes the centerpiece of pathogenesis of CHF. Thus, neurohormonal events have provided an important target for pharmacological interventions. More recently, it has become apparent that direct myocyte injury and dysfunction can be caused by cell-mediated immune responses [1, 2]. There is a growing body of evidence that a major subset of heart disease may be expressed by non-lethal alterations of myocyte function induced by immune cells and their cytokines [3–10]. Therefore, in addition to inhibition of neurohormonal factors, immunomodulating or anticytokine therapy has now been considered to pave a new way in the management of heart failure [11–14].

Role of cytokines in pathogenesis of heart failure

A number of clinical studies have demonstrated that patients with CHF express excessive levels of cytokines in plasma [3–8]. Most cytokines act as local autocrine or paracrine mediators and do not act in endocrine fashion. Therefore, systemic elevation of cytokines by spill-over of the locally-expressed excess molecules into the circulation produces a series of pathologic reactions. A continuous infusion of cytokine in rat provoked a time-dependent depression in left ventricular (LV) func-

Inflammation and Cardiac Diseases, edited by Giora Z. Feuerstein, Peter Libby and Douglas L. Mann
© 2003 Birkhäuser Verlag Basel/Switzerland

tion and structure [15]. Transgenic mice with cardiac-specific over-expression of cytokine developed dilated cardiomyopathy (DCM) with increased mortality [16]. Injection of recombinant cytokine in murine models of myocarditis also increased mortality of the animals [17]. Elevated circulating levels of cytokines are actually noted in patients with heart failure, correlating with the severity [18–21]. But the net biological effect of cytokines seems to be determined primarily by the body compartment in which they are produced, and not by the ambient serum level [16, 22, 23].

Pro-inflammatory cytokines modulate cardiovascular functions by a variety of mechanisms. When cardiac myocytes were cultured in the presence of culture supernatants from activated immune cells, beta-adrenergic agonist-mediated increases in cultured cardiac myocyte contractility and intracellular cAMP accumulation were inhibited [24]. Suppressive activity was attributed to the macrophage-derived cytokine interleukin (IL)-1 and tumor necrosis factor (TNF) that altered β-receptor or guanine nucleotide binding protein function by the uncoupling of agonist-occupied receptors from adenyl cyclase. In primary cultures of adult rat ventricular myocytes, IL-1β and interferon (IFN)-γ individually increased inducible nitric oxide synthase (iNOS) mRNA abundance. Cytokine-pretreated myocytes exhibited a depressed contractile response to isoproterenol in the presence of L-arginine. This altered contractile function of cardiac myocytes was considered to be due to induction of myocyte iNOS [25]. In the canine model of myocardial ischemia, IL-1β induced sustained myocardial dysfunction. Thereby, nitric oxide (NO) produced by iNOS and the resultant formation of peroxynitrite were shown to be involved in the pathogenesis of this cytokine-induced sustained myocardial dysfunction *in vivo* [26]. TNF-α, IL-6, and IL-2 were shown to inhibit contractility of isolated hamster papillary muscles in a concentration-dependent manner. On the basis of effects of the NOS inhibitor N-monomethyl-L-arginine (L-NMMA), these negative inotropic effects of cytokines were suggested to be mediated by enhanced NO production by a constitutive myocardial NOS [27]. In both the ventricles and the isolated adult cardiac myocyte, TNF-α exerted a concentration- and time-dependent negative inotropic effect which was associated with decreased levels of peak intracellular calcium during the systolic contraction [28] and a rapid increase in the hydrolysis of [14] sphingomyelin in cell free extracts together with an increase in ceramide mass [29]. Thus, the negative inotropic effect of TNF-α observed here was considered to be the direct result of alterations in intracellular calcium homeostasis or by activation of the neutral sphingomyelinase pathway. The sphingolinoid signaling cascade was shown to be involved in cardiac cell death, therefore inhibitory effect of myocardial contraction by TNF-α was also suggested to be related to cardiomyocyte apoptosis [30]. More recently, in transgenic mice with cardiac-specific over-expression of TNF-α, only a low level of apoptosis was demonstrated in cardiac myocytes and most of the cells undergoing apoptosis were shown to be non-myocytes. Thereby, cardiac expression of transcripts encoding both pro-and anti-apoptotic proteins were enhanced. Therefore, it was suggested that TNF-α does not sufficiently induce apoptosis in cardiac myocytes *in vivo* and apoptosis of myocyte itself was not considered to significantly contribute to the pathogenesis of congestive heart failure [31].

Myocarditis and dilated cardiomyopathy (DCM)

Since the original report by Levine et al. [3], a number of clinical studies have demonstrated that patients with CHF express excessive levels of TNF-α in plasma [4, 6, 8, 10]. Positive TNF-α immunoreactivity was also noted in myocardial tissues of patients with heart failure [32–34], suggesting that the heart is capable of synthesizing TNF-α. On the other hand, similar temporal changes in T cell infiltration and expression of cytokines in the myocardium suggest that infiltrating cells rather than resident heart cells may be responsible for expression of cytokines [34–37]. Currently, an intensive interest has been generated to define the role of TNF-α in the progression of heart failure. TNF-α has been recognized as a common mediator of the immune system and its biologic activities overlap with other cytokines. TNF-α genes are located close to the MHC genes, which genetically control TNF-α production. DCM has been shown to be associated with human lymphocyte Class II antigen expression [38], expression of which is increased by TNF-α infusion [39]. The circulating levels of TNF-α in heart failure patients showed direct correlation with severity of heart failure in terms of New York Heart Association (NYHA) functional class [40]. However, exact mechanism responsible for cytokine production in heart failure still remains unclear.

DCM has been considered as an end result of preceding myocarditis. Then we assessed a causal relationship between DCM and myocarditis in murine models [37, 41]. When myocarditis was induced in mice with inoculation with encephalomyocarditis (EMC) virus, DCM became apparent within 7–10 days after infection ensued. Over the following three-month period, heart weight increased with further dilation of the LV cavity. Thereby, myocardial hypertrophy and interstitial fibrosis preceded in the absence of the acute inflammatory process and heart assumed the characteristic pattern of DCM [37, 41]. By this time, most of the culturable virus had been eliminated. However, the viral genome was still detectable in the myocardial tissue by the polymerase chain reaction gene amplification technique [37]. In this model, pro-inflammatory cytokines, IL-1β and TNF-α were induced rapidly within three days after infection. Immunoregulatory cytokines, IFN-γ and IL-2 mRNAs started to be detected from 3–7 days after inoculation. Gene expression of these cytokines continued for three months after virus inoculation particularly in the absence of inflammatory process. IL-1β which was expressed relatively in large amount, positively correlated with ventricular mass and with the extent of fibrosis. In patients undergoing cardiac transplantation for DCM, IL-1β mRNA was shown to be elevated in coronary arteries and in myocardium, suggesting that IL-1β may play a part in the pathogenesis of heart failure [42]. The fundamental process involved in the viral infection leading to DCM is the initial activation of protective immune responses followed by an immune-mediated destructive response against the heart in the later stage [43–45]. In the murine model of myocarditis and heart failure, administration of recombinant human IL-2 in the acute stage increased survival rate with less intense pathologic changes of myocardium, whereas the same amount of IL-2 exacerbated the severity of the disease and reduced survival rate in the later stage [45]. Thus, the same cytokine may modulate different stages and disease types in different ways and the net effects of the host response may ultimately depend on a balance between the beneficial and injurious effects of cytokines [9].

The role of cytokines in pressure overload hypertrophy

Cardiac hypertrophy is an important risk factor for the development of heart failure. In the Framingham Heart Study, the echocardiograph determined left ventricular mass was shown to be associated with all outcome events [46]. The importance of cardiac hypertrophy in the response to overload was already noted in the 19th century. Austin Flint postulated that protection of cardiac dilatation by hypertrophy has a limit as the muscle of the heart cannot increase indefinitely [47]. William Osler also described three phases in the hypertrophic response of the heart to acute mechanical overload and a role for maladaptive hypertrophy in causing heart failure [48]. In the middle of the 1960s, experimental evidence was provided by Meerson [49] to support these earlier hypotheses. He defined the sequence of events during the development of hypertrophy as three distinctive stages: The initial stage of myocardial damage and impairment of contractile function; the second stage of stable hyperfunction in which normal myocardial function is restored; and the third stage of a gradual deterioration of myocardial function, leading to overt heart failure.

We had postulated that hypertrophy initially provides important compensatory mechanisms permitting to normalize chamber wall stress and to restore relatively normal pumping ability [50, 51]. However, this physiological hypertrophy may progress to pathological hypertrophy, ultimately leading to heart failure if the overload is sufficiently intense and sustained [52]. We proposed that cytokine may also participate in this pathologic transition.

We developed a well-characterized model that displays compensated pressure-overload hypertrophy and congestive heart failure [53]. When Dahl salt sensitive rats (DS) were fed a high-salt diet, they developed rapidly characteristic LV hypertrophy associated with a substantial rise in blood pressure. Thereby, systolic myocardial function was completely normal. In subsequent weeks all of these rats developed severe dilation. These changes are in striking contrast to those observed

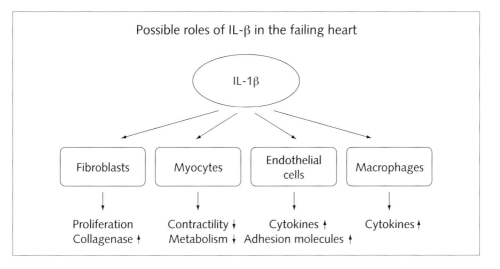

Figure 1

IL-1β exerts various biological effects on heart. IL-1β activates fibroblasts which might significantly affect the remodeling process. IL-1β decreases cardiac contractility and induces sustained myocardial dysfunction. IL-1β possibly activates cytotoxic T cells, which might cause direct myocyte injury and induce cell adhesion molecules regulating persistent inflammatory cell traffic within the myocardium. IL-1β also recruits macrophages that again induce the expression of multiple cytokines.

in corresponding Dahl salt-resistant rats (DR), which are derived from the same colony and genetically indistinguishable except for a polymorphism in the renin gene [54]. The latter rats did not develop systemic hypertension with the same diet and showed normal age-related growth of the heart.

In this model, we observed the increased expression of IL-1β in the hypertrophied heart which was further increased with the development of CHF [55]. Immunohistochemical studies revealed that IL-1β protein localized in the endothelial cells of the arterioles and the infiltrating macrophages in the hypertrophied myocardium (Fig. 1).

The amount of IL-1β mRNA correlated with the ventricular mass. The expression of myocyte chemotactic and activating factor/monocyte chemo-attractant protein-1 (MCAF/MCP-1), a potent chemotactic factor for macrophages was also increased together with an increased number of macrophages in the interstitium. In fact, it has been suggested that activated monocytes and macrophages recruited and activated by chemokines are important cellular sources for the increased levels of circulating pro-inflammatory cytokines [56].

Elevated circulating levels of C-C chemokines have been demonstrated in patients with CHF [57] as well as in those with acute myocardial infarction [58]. *In vitro* studies on isolated peripheral blood suggested that a platelet-myocyte interaction may contribute to the enhanced chemokine levels in CHF, and serum from CHF patients enhanced oxygen radical generation in myocyte. This effect was inhibited by neutralizing antibodies against MCP-1, reflecting increased monocyte activity [57].

Mechanism of expressions of cytokines by mechanical overload

In order to assess the mechanism by which mechanical stress is converted into the gene expression of cytokines, endothelial cells isolated from human umbilical veins were cultured on flexible silicone membranes. When cyclic mechanical stress was applied to the cell by deforming the culture plate by computer-controlled vacuum, the levels of MCAF/MCP-1 in the culture medium was significantly elevated [59]. Northern blot analysis indicated that mRNA levels of MCAF/MCP-1 were up-regulated by cyclic stretch as a function of intensity. Oscillatory shear stress in cultured human endothelium up-regulates adhesion molecules associated with enhanced monocyte adherence [60]. The pattern of adhesion molecule induction with oscillatory flow stress was similar to that seen after cytokine stimulation, being associated with the recruitment of macrophages. When focal adhesion was formed by integrin receptor engagement and clustering, the integrins linked to intracellular cytoskeletal complexes and bundles of actin filaments [58]. Both integrins and the actin cytoskeleton have been considered as mechanochemical transducers which convert mechanical force into gene induction of chemokines [61]. In the human endothelial cells with cyclic stretch, the actin cytoskeleton disruption abolished the stretch induced gene expression of chemokines [62]. Analysis with specific enzyme inhibitors indicated that phospholipase C, protein kinase C and tyrosine kinase were also involved in this chemokine induction [59]. Taken together, it can be postulated that mechanical stretch induces gene expression of chemotactic factors for macrophages (Fig. 2). Recruited macrophages are the main source of production of cytokines, notably IL-1β. Although there is no one cytokine that is acting alone in the development of heart failure but many cytokines are acting in concert within the framework of entire cytokine network, IL-1β has been thought to play a key role in the pathogenesis of heart failure [63].

Endothelin signaling pathway in the process of hypertrophy

Stretch activates multiple second messenger systems and directly induces proto-oncogene expression and protein synthesis. Mechanical stretch also stimulates the

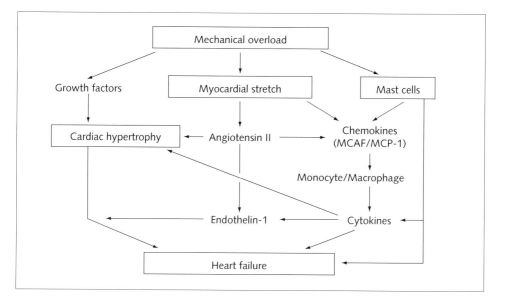

Figure 2

Pathophysiological diagram to explain the main determinants of cardiac hypertrophy and the later development of heart failure.

autocrine release of angiotensin (Ang) II from the early stage which synergistically activates intracellular protein kinase cascades and induces various growth actor genes [64, 65] (Fig. 2). In the rat model of pressure overloaded hypertrophy, the local renin-angiotensin system was significantly up-regulated at the stage of compensated hypertrophy at 11 weeks [66]. In an *in vitro* stretch model of load-induced cardiac hypertrophy, Ang II was shown to play a key role in the hypertrophic process in terms of protein synthesis and expression of the immediate early gene critical for cell proliferation. Both of these responses were inhibited by Ang II receptor antagonist [64, 65], or specific angiotensin converting enzyme (ACE) inhibition [67, 68]. Our observation in the compensated hypertrophy of DS rat offered additional support to the hypothesis that locally produced Ang II may act as an endogenous growth factor for the myocardium. Activation of the renin-angiotensin system remained at the similar level in the failing stage. The mRNA levels of angiotensinogen and ACE were similarly elevated in both compensated and failing stages of hypertrophy. However, the extent of increase was greater in ACE mRNA. Therefore, the local Ang production appeared to be critically regulated at the converting enzyme level [66].

Circulating [69, 70] and myocardial [71, 72] concentrations of endothelin-1 (ET-1) are elevated in patients with CHF and endothelin receptor antagonists improve overall LV function [73–77] as well as long-term survival [78, 79] in chronic heart failure. ET-1 is a potent vasoconstrictor peptide produced in the myocardium and exerts various pathophysiological roles in the cardiovascular system including effects on cardiac myocyte growth and phenotype [80]. ET-1 expression is induced in cultured neonatal cardiac myocytes by β1-adrenergic stimulation associated with the accelerated conversion of big ET-1 to bioactive mature ET-1 mediated by up-regulation of endothelin converting enzyme-1 (ECE-1) [81]. In DS rats, plasma and myocardial ET-1 in both right and left ventricles remained the same as in the age-matched control DR rats at the compensated hypertrophy but were markedly augmented after overt heart failure ensued [82]. The lack of increases of serum and myocardial ET-1 was also observed in the compensated hypertrophy of SHR [83, 84]. In the failing heart, ET-1 was demonstrated immunohistochemically to be localized in cardiac myocytes and LV ET-1 concentrations showed a significant correlation with ventricular function and LV systolic wall stress [82]. The increase in ET-1 peptide levels in the failing stage was associated with a concomitant increase in the mRNA levels of preproET-1 and ECE-1 [66]. Though the magnitude of increase in the pre-proET-1 mRNA was much higher than in the ECE mRNA suggesting a critical regulation of ET-1 synthesis at the precursor level, the local production of ET-1 is also mediated by accelerated conversion of big ET-1 by an increased ECE-1 transcript during the development of heart failure (Fig. 2).

ET-1 receptor blocker substantially attenuated the progression of LV dysfunction and significantly improved mortality rate [66, 82]. These effects were not considered to be related to the reduction of afterload, because lowering of blood pressure to the same extent by α1-receptor agonist failed to improve hemodynamic measures and survival of the animals [82]. Therefore, the accelerated expression of ET-1 appeared to directly cause systolic dysfunction during transition from hypertrophy to heart failure. It has been shown that ET-1 may exert a depressant effect on myocyte through inhibitory G-coupled protein (Gi) pathway [85, 86], a depletion of cyclic AMP in cardiac myocyte [87], a decrease in sarcoplasmic Ca^{2+} ATPase [88] or direct toxic effect [89]. Treatment with the ET-1 receptor antagonist, bosentan, and ACE inhibitor, temocapril, started from the compensated stage equally improved survival of the animals. Thereby, ACE inhibitor blunted the development of hypertrophy, but ET receptor blocker ameliorated LV dysfunction while the effect of ACE inhibitor to be more related to an improvement of hypertrophy and remodeling, while the combined use of ACE inhibitor and ET-1 receptor blocker further potentiate the inhibitory effects of transition from compensated hypertrophy to heart failure [66].

Role of mast cells in maladaptive hypertrophy

Mast cells are multifunctional cells that contain various mediators such as histamine, proteases and leukotriene as well as cytokines [90–93]. They are found in almost all major organs of the body and are involved in many types of inflammation and repair process. Patella et al. [94] demonstrated that mast cell density is higher in failing human hearts than in normal control hearts. Panizo et al. [95] also showed that the number of ventricular mast cells was augmented in SHR as compared with WKY rats and there was a direct correlation between the number of mast cells and the degree of collagen volume fraction. After treatment with ACE inhibitor, quinapril, the mast cell count was decreased. Therefore, mast cells are considered to play a role in the remodeling process and progression of heart failure. In order to assess effects of mast cells on cardiac structure and function, Mast cell granules (MCGs) were prepared from the rat peritoneal lavage. Cardiomyocytes and non-myocytes were isolated from neonatal rats and were incubated separately with mast cell granules for 24 hours. MCG caused death of cardiomyocytes by apoptosis in a concentration-dependent manner. When non-myocardial cells were cultured with MCGs, proliferation of the cells was promoted. Thus, mast cells are considered to accelerate the progression of heart failure by producing systolic dysfunction with loss of cardiomyocyte by apoptosis and diastolic dysfunction with proliferation of fibroblasts [96].

On the basis of these data, we hypothesized that myocardial mast cells may play a role in cytokine mediated inflammatory response and tissue repairing process and transition from compensated hypertrophy to heart failure. Then, we assessed a critical role of mast cells during the development of heart failure using w/c-kit mutant mice in which mast cells are nearly absent [97]. Mast cell deficient mice and their normal male litter-mates were exposed to 15 weeks of pressure overload by banding of the abdominal aorta. Thereby, ventricular mass increased by more than 50% in wild type but this increase remained by less than 10% in the mutant group. Fractional shortening determined by trans-thoracic echocardiography decreased gradually after eight weeks of banding in the wild type, while it remained unchanged in the mutant mice. Histological studies revealed a prominent increase in perivascular fibrosis only in wild type mice, whereas in the mutant mice, the extent of fibrosis was nearly the same as that in the sham-operated mice. In addition there was a trend toward a lesser amount of interstitial fibrosis in mutant mice compared with wild type. TUNEL assay also revealed more apoptotic cardiac myocytes in wild type mice than in the mutant mice, although the difference did not reach the statistical significance. All of these data support the view that mast cells contribute substantially to the transition toward heart failure (Fig. 2).

Then, we examined effects of a mast cell stabilizer, tranilast, [98, 99] on the progression of heart failure in pressure overload hypertrophy. Pressure overload was again produced in nine-week-old male C57BL/6 mice by banding of the abdominal aorta. Four weeks after surgery, the animals were randomized to treatment with tranilast for 11 weeks or with the vehicle for the same period of time. At 15 weeks, the systolic blood pressure remained the same in the two groups but the magnitude of cardiac hypertrophy, systolic dysfunction and left ventricular chamber dilation were significantly less in the tranilast treated group. All of these observations suggest that mast cells play a significant role in the pathophysiologic manifestations of heart failure in pressure-overload hypertrophy [97].

An increase in muscle length evokes not only a change in cardiac performance but also a multigene response.

Summary

An increase in muscle length evokes multigene growth signals as well as an increase in its ability to do work as a function of the length-tension relationship. These signals include up-regulation of cytokines. Cytokines accelerate the growth of myocyte and left ventricular remodeling and are responsible for non-lethal down-modulation of cardiac function.

The treatment of heart failure may be directed to blunt this maladapting signaling. The redundancy of the signaling pathways that control these processes, however, makes it difficult to completely inhibit these and other maladaptive response by a single measure. In view of existing knowledge on the biological effect of cytokines, we have proposed anticytokine therapy will provide a new direction for the management of heart failure [13, 14, 100–102]. The cytokine-mediated systemic response may initially be beneficial but when sustained becomes deleterious. Mast cells also evoke a healing response as well as attacking invaders before they accelerate the development of heart failure (Fig. 2). Therefore, the same therapeutic approach could act differently depending upon the disease state of the individual patient.

We can anticipate that therapy will move into cells to target and inactivate the redundant systems responsible for maladaptive signaling in patients with heart failure.

References

1   Lange LG, Schreiner GF (1992) Immune cytokines and cardiac disease. *Trends Cardiovasc Med* 2: 145–151

2   Barry WH (1994) Mechanisms of immune-mediated myocyte injury. *Circulation* 89: 2421–2432

3   Levine B, Kalman J, Mayer L, Fillit HM, Packer M (1990) Elevated circulating levels of tumor necrosis factor in severe chronic heart failure. *N Eng J Med* 323: 236–241

4   Matsumori A, Yamada T, Suzuki H, Matoba Y, Sasayama S (1994) Increased circulating cytokines in patients with myocarditis and cardiomyopathy. *Br Heart J* 72: 561–566

5   Plents G, Song ZF, Tjan TDT, Koenig C, Baba HA, Erren M, Flesch M, Wichter T, Scheld HH, Deng MC (2001) Activation of the cardiac interleukin-6 system in advanced

heart failure. *Eur J Heart Fail* 3: 415–421

6   Blum A, Miller H (2001) Pathophysiological role of cytokines in congestive heart failure. *Annu Rev Med* 52: 15–27

7   Yamaoka-Tojo M, Tojo T, Inomata T, Machida Y, Osada K, Izumi T (2002) Circulating levels of interleukin 18 reflect etiologies of heart failure: Th1/Th2 cytokine imbalance exaggerates the pathophysiology of advanced heart failure. *J Card Fail* 8: 21–27

8   Adamopoulos S, Parissis JT, Kremastinos DT (2001) A glossary of circulating cytokines in chronic heart failure. *Eur J Heart Fail* 3: 517–526

9   Sasayama S, Matsumori A, Kihara Y (1999) New insights into the pathophysiological role for cytokines in heart failure. *Cardiovasc Res* 42: 557–564

10   Bradham WS, Moe G, Wendt KA, Scott AA, Konig A, Romanova M, Naik G, Spinale FG (2002) TNF-alpha and myocardial matrix metalloproteinases in heart failure; relationship to LV remodeling. *Am J Physiol (Heart Circ Physiol)* 282: H1288–H1295

11   Sasayama S, Matsumori A (1996) Vesnarinone: a potential cytokine inhibitor. *J Card Fail* 2: 251–258

12   Bozkurt B, Torre-Amione G, Warren MS, Whitmore J, Soran OZ, Feldman AM, Mann DL (2001) Results of targeted anti-tumor necrosis factor therapy with etanercept (ENBREL) in patients with advanced heart failure. *Circulation* 103: 1044–1047

13   Deswal A, Misra A, Bozkurt B (2001) The role of anti-cytokine therapy in the failing heart. *Heart Fail Rev* 6: 143–151

14   Damas JK, Gullestad L, Aukrust P (2001) Cytokines as new treatment targets in chronic heart failure. *Curr Control Trials Cardiovasc Med* 2: 271–277

15   Bozkurt B, Kribbs SB, Clubb FJ, Michael LH, Didenko VV, Hornsby PJ, Seta Y, Oral H, Spinale FG, Mann DL (1998) Pathophysiologically relevant concentrations of tumor necrosis factor-alpha promote progressive left ventricular dysfunction and remodeling in rats. *Circulation* 97: 1382–1391

16   Kubota T, McTiernan CF, Frye CS, Slawson SE, Lemster HB, Koretsky AP, Demetris AJ, Feldman AM (1997) Dilated cardiomyopathy in transgenic mice with cardiac-specific overexpression of tumor necrosis factor-alpha. *Circ Res* 81: 627–635

17   Yamada T, Matsumori A, Sasayama S (1994) Therapeutic effect of anti-tumor necrosis factor-alpha antibody on the murine model of viral myocarditis induced by encephalomyocarditis virus. *Circulation* 89: 846–851

18   Ferrari R, Bachetti T, Confortini R, Opasich C, Febo O, Corti A, Cassani G, Visioli O (1995) Tumor necrosis factor soluble receptors in patients with various degrees of congestive failure. *Circulation* 92: 1479–1486

19   Torre-Amione G, Kapasida S, Benedict CR, Oral H, Young JB, Mann DL (1996) Pro-inflammatory cytokine levels in patients with depressed left ventricular ejection fraction: A report from the studies of left ventricular dysfunction (SOLVD). *J Am Coll Cardiol* 27: 1201–1206

20   Testa M, Yeh M, Lee P, Fanelli R, Loperfido F, Berman JW, LeJemtel TH (1996) Circulating levels of cytokines and their endogenous modulators in patients with mild to

severe congestive heart failure due to coronary artery disease or hypertension. *J Am Coll Cardiol* 28: 964–971

21 MacGowan GA, Mann DL, Kormas RL, Feldman AM, Murali S (1997) Circulating interleukin-6 in severe heart failure. *Am J Cardiol* 79: 1128–1131

22 Bryant D, Becker L, Richardson J, Shelton J, Franco F, Peshock R, Thompson M, Gioroir B (1998) Cardiac function in transgenic mice with myocardial expression of tumor necrosis factor-alpha. *Circulation* 97: 1375–1381

23 Kapadia SR, Oral H, Lee J, Nakano M, Taffet GE, Mann DL (1997) Hemodynamic relation of tumor necrosis factor-alpha gene and protein expression in adult feline myocardium. *Circ Res* 81: 187–195

24 Gulick T, Chung MK, Pieper SJ, Lange LG, Schreiner GF (1989) Interleukin-1 and tumor necrosis factor inhibit cardiac myocyte β-adrenergic responsiveness. *Proc Natl Acad Sci USA* 86: 6753–6757

25 Balligand JL, Ungureanu-Longrois D, Simmons WW, Pimental D, Malinsky TA, Kapturczak M, Taha Z, Lowenstein CJ, Davidoff AJ, Kelly RA et al (1994) Cytokine-inducible nitric oxide synthase (iNOS) expression in cardiac myocytes: Characterization and regulation of iNOS expression and detection of iNOS activity in single cardiac myocytes *in vitro. J Biol Chem* 269: 27580–27588

26 Oyama J, Shimokawa H, Momii H, Cheng X, Fukuyama N, Arai Y, Egashira K, Nakazawa H, Takeshita A (1998) Role of nitric oxide and peroxynitrite in the cytokine-induced sustained myocardial dysfunction in dogs *in vivo. J Clin Invest* 101: 2207–2214

27 Finkel MS, Oddis CV, Jacob TD, Watkins SC, Hattler BG, Simmons RL (1992) Negative inotropic effects of cytokines on the heart mediated by nitric oxide. *Science* 257: 387–389

28 Yokoyama T, Vaca L, Rossen RD, Durante W, Hazarika P, Mann DL (1993) Cellular basis for the negative inotropic effects of tumor necrosis factor-α in the adult mammalian heart. *J Clin Invest* 92: 2303–2312

29 Oral H, Mann DL (1997) Sphigosine mediates the immediate negative inotropic effects of tumor necrosis factor-α in the adult mammalian cardiac myocyte. *J Biol Chem* 272: 4836–4842

30 Known KA, Page MT, Nguyen C, Zechner D, Gutierrez V, Comstock KL, Glembotski CC, Quintana PJE, Sabbadini RA (1996) Tumor necrosis factor alpha-induced apoptosis in cardiac myocytes. Involvement of the sphingolipid signaling cascade in cardiac cell death. *J Clin Invest* 98: 2854–2865

31 Kubota T, Miyagishima M, Frye CS, Alber SM, Bounoutas GS, Kadokami T, Watkins SC, McTiernan CF, Feldman AM (2001) Over-expression of tumor necrosis factor-alpha activates both anti- and pro-apoptotic pathways in the myocardium. *J Mol Cell Cardiol* 33: 1331–1344

32 Doyama K, Fujiwara H, Fukumoto M, Tanaka M, Fujiwara Y, Oda T, Inada T, Ohtani S, Hasegawa K, Fujiwara T et al (1996) Tumor necrosis factor is expressed in cardiac tissues of patients with heart failure. *Int J Cardiol* 54: 217–225

33 Torre-Amione G, Kapadia S, Lee J, Durand J-B, Bies RD, Young JB, Mann DL (1996)

Tumor necrosis factor-alpha and tumor necrosis factor receptors in the failing human heart. *Circulation* 93: 704–711

34   Retter AS, Fishman WH (2001) The role of tumor necrosis factor in cardiac disease. *Heart Dis* 3: 319–325

35   Kalra D, Sivasubramanian N, Mann DL (2002) Angiotensin II induces tumor necrosis factor biosynthesis in the adult mammalian heart through a protein kinase C-dependent pathway. *Circulation* 105: 2198–2205

36   Kalra D, Zhu X, Ramchandani MK, Lawrie G, Reardon MJ, Lee-Jackson D, Winters WL, Sivasubramanian N, Mann DL, Zoghbi WA (2002) Increased myocardial gene expression of tumor necrosis factor-alpha and nitric oxide synthase-2: A potential mechanism for depressed myocardial function in hibernating myocardium in humans. *Circulation* 105: 1517–1519

37   Shioi T, Matsumori A, Sasayama S (1996) Persistent expression of cytokine in the chronic stage of viral myocarditis in mice. *Circulation* 94: 2930–2937

38   Carlquist JF, Menlove RL, Murray MB, O'Connell JB, Anderson JL (1991) HLA class II (DR and DQ) antigen associations in idiopathic dilated cardiomyopathy: Validation study and meta-analysis of published HLA association studies. *Circulation* 83: 515–522

39   Freund YR, Dedrick RL, Jones PP (1990) cis-Acting sequences required for Class II gene regulation by interferon gamma and tumor necrosis factor alpha in a murine macrophage cell line. *J Exp Med* 171: 1283–1299

40   Seta Y, Shan K, Bozkurt B, Oral H, Mann DL (1996) Basic mechanism in heart failure: the cytokine hypothesis. *J Card Fail* 2: 243–249

41   Matsumori A (1993) Animal models: Pathological findings and therapeutic considerations. In: Banatvala JE (ed): *Viral infections of the heart*. Edward Arnold, London, 110–137

42   Francis SE, Holden H, Holt CM, Duff GW (1998) Interleukin-1 in myocardium and coronary arteries of patients with dilated cardiomyopathy. *J Mol Cell Cardiol* 30: 215–223

43   Lodge PA, Herzum M, Olszewski J, Huber SA (1987) Coxsackie virus B-3 myocarditis: Acute and chronic forms of the disease caused by different immunopathogenic mechanisms. *Am J Pathol* 128: 455–463

44   Yokoyama T, Nakano M, Bednarczyk JL, McIntyre BW, Entman M, Mann DL (1997) Tumor necrosis factor-alpha provokes a hypertrophic growth response in adult cardiac myocytes. *Circulation* 95: 1247–1252

45   Kishimoto C, Kuroki Y, Hiraoke Y, Ochiai H, Kurokawa M, Sasayama S (1994) Cytokine and murine Coxsackie virus B3 myocarditis: Interleukin-2 suppressed myocarditis in the acute stage but enhanced the condition in the subsequent stage. *Circulation* 89: 2836–2842

46   Levy D, Garrison RJ, Savage DD, Kannel WB, Castelli WP (1990) Prognostic implications of echocardiographically determined left ventricular mass in the Framingham Heart Study. *N Engl J Med* 322: 1561–1566

47   Flint A (1870) *A practical treatise on the diagnosis, pathology, and treatment of diseases of the heart* (2nd ed). HC Lea, Philadelphia, 33

48   Osler W (1982) *The principles and practice of medicine.* Appleton & Co, New York, 632

49   Meerson FZ (1963) The myocardium in hyperfunction, hypertrophy and heart failure. *Circ Res* 25 (Suppl): 1–163

50   Sasayama S, Ross J Jr, Franklin D, Blooor CM, Bishop S, Dilley R (1976) Adaptations of the left ventricle to chronic pressure overload. *Circ Res* 38: 172–178

51   Sasayama S, Franklin D, Ross J Jr. (1997) Hyperfunction with normal inotropic state of the hypertrophied left ventricle. *Am J Physiol* 232: H418–H425

52   Takahashi M, Sasayama S, Kawai C, Kotoura H (1980) Contractile performance of the hypertrophied ventricle in patients with systemic hypertension. *Circulation* 62: 116–126

53   Inoko M, Kihara Y, Morii I, Fujiwara H, Sasayama S (1994) Transition from compensatory hypertrophy to dilated, failing left ventricules in Dahl salt-sensitive rats. *Am J Physiol* 267: H2471–H2482

54   Rapp TP, Wang SM, Dene H (1989) A genetic polymorphism in the renin gene of Dahl rats co-segregates with blood pressure. *Science* 243: 542–544

55   Shioi T, Matsumori A, Kihara Y, Inoko M, Ono K, Iwanaga Y, Yamada T, Iwasaki A, Matsushima K, Sasayama S (1997) Increased expression of interleukin-1β and myocyte chemotactic and activating factor/monocyte chemoattractant protein-1 in the hypertrophied and failing heart with pressure overload. *Circ Res* 81: 664–672

56   Arai KI, Lee F, Miyajima A, Miyatake S, Arai N, Yokota T (1990) Cytokines: coordinators of immune and inflammatory responses. *Annu Rev Biochem* 59: 783–836

57   Aukrust P, Ueland T, Mueller F, Andreassen AK, Nordoy I, Aas H, Kjekshus J, Simonsen S, Froland SS, Gullestad L (1998) Elevated circulating levels of C-C chemokines in patients with congestive heart failure. *Circulation* 97: 1136–1143

58   Matsumori A, Furukawa Y, Hashimoto T, Yoshida A, Ono K, Shioi T, Okada M, Iwasaki A, Nishio R, Matsushima K et al (1997) Plasma levels of the monocyte chemotactic and activating factor/monocyte chemo-attractant protein-1 in patients with acute myocardial infarction. *J Mol Cell Cardiol* 29: 419–423

59   Okada M, Matsumori A, Ono K, Furukawa Y, Shioi T, Iwasaki A, Matsushima K, Sasayama S (1998) Cyclic stretch up-regulates production of interleukin-8 and monocyte chemotactic and activating factor/monocyte chemo-attractant protein-1 in human endothelial cells. *Arterioscler Thromb Vasc Biol* 18: 894–901

60   Chappell DC, Varner SE, Nerem RM, Medford RM, Alexander RW (1998) Oscillatory shear stress stimulates adhesion molecule expression in cultured human endothelium. *Circ Res* 82: 532–539

61   Vandenburgh HH (1992) Mechanical forces and their second messengers in stimulating cell growth *in vitro*. *Am J Physiol* 262: R350–R355

62   Clark EA, Brugge JS (1995) Integrins and signal transduction pathways: the road taken. *Science* 268: 233–239

63   Long CS (2001) The role of interleukin-1 in the failing heart. *Heart Fail Rev* 6: 81–94

64 Sadoshima J, Xu Y, Slayter HS, Izumo S (1993) Autocrine release of angiotensin II mediates stretch-induced hypertrophy of cardiac myocytes *in vitro*. Cell 75: 977–984

65 Yamazaki T, Komuro I, Kudoh S, Zou Y, Shiojima I, Mizuno T, Takano H, Hiroi Y, Ueki K, Tobe K et al (1994) Angiotensin II partly mediates mechanical stress-induced cardiac hypertrophy. *Circ Res* 77: 258–265

66 Iwanaga Y, Kihara Y, Inagaki K, Onozawa Y, Yoneda T, Kataoka K, Sasayama S (2001) differential effects of angiotensin II *versus* endothelin-1 inhibitions in hypertrophic left ventricular myocardium during transition to heart failure. *Circulation* 104: 606–612

67 Shunkert H, Jackson B, Tang SS, Hirsch AT, Apstein CS, Lorell BH (1990) Distribution and functional significance of cardiac ACE in hypertrophied rat hearts. *Circulation* 86: 1913–1920

68 Feldman A, Weinberg EO, Ray P, Lorell BH (1993) Selective changes in gene expression during compensated hypertrophy and the transition to cardiac decompensation in rats with chronic aortic banding. *Circ Res* 73: 184–192

69 Haynes WG, Webb DJ (1993) The endothelin family of peptides: Local hormones with diverse roles in health and disease? *Clin Sci* 84: 485–500

70 Cody RJ, Hass GJ, Binkley PF, Capers Q, Kelley R (1992) Plasma endothelin correlates with extent of pulmonary hypertension in patients with chronic congestive heart failure. *Circulation* 85: 504–507

71 Ry SD, Andreassi MG, Clerico A, Biagini A, Giannessi D (2001) Endothelin-1, endothelin-1 receptors and cardiac natriuretic peptides in failing human heart. *Life Sci* 68: 2715–2730

72 Kakinuma Y, Miyauchi T, Yuki K, Murakoshi N, Goto K, Yamaguchi I (2001) Novel molecular mechanism of increased myocardial endothelin-1 expression in the failing heart involving the transcriptional factor hypoxia-inducible factor-1α induced for impaired myocardial energy metabolism. *Circulation* 103: 2387–2394

73 Shimoyama H, Sabbah NH, Borzak S, Tanimura M, Shevlyagin S, Scicli G, Goldstein S (1996) Short-term hemodynamic effects of endothelin receptor blockade in dogs with chronic heart failure. *Circulation* 94: 779–784

74 Kiowski W, Sutsch G, Hunziker P, Muller P, Kim J, Oechslin E, Schmitt R, Jones R, Bertel O (1995) Evidence for endothelin-1 mediated vasoconstriction in severe chronic heart failure. *Lancet* 346: 732–736

75 Torre-Amione G, Young JB, Durand J, Bozkurt B, Mann DL, Kobrin I, Pratt CM (2001) Hemodynamic effects of tezosentan, an intravenous dual endothelin receptor antagonist, in patients with Class III to IV congestive heart failure. *Circulation* 103: 973–980

76 Berger R, Stanek B, Hulsmann M, Frey B, Heher S, Pacher R, Neunteufl T (2001) Effects of endothelin A receptor blockade on endothelial function in patients with chronic heart failure. *Circulation* 103: 981–986

77 Schalcher C, Cotter G, Reisin L, Bertel O, Kobrin I, Guyene TT, Kiowski W (2001) The dual endothelin receptor antagonist tezosentan acutely improves hemodynamic parameters in patients with advanced heart failure. *Am Heart J* 142: 340–349

78 Sakai S, Miyauchi T, Kobayashi M, Goto K, Sugishita Y (1996) Inhibition of myocar-

dial endothelin pathway improves long-term survival in heart failure. *Nature* 384: 353–355

79   Spieker LE, Noll G, Ruschitzka FT, Luscher TF (2001) Endothelin receptor antagonists in congestive heart failure: a new therapeutic principle for the future? *J Am Coll Cardiol* 37: 1493–1505

80   Miyauchi T, Masaki T (1999) Pathophysiology of endothelin in the cardiovascular system. *Annu Rev Physiol* 61: 391–415

81   Kaburagi S, Hasegawa K, Morimoto T, Araki M, Sawamura T, Masaki T, Sasayama S (1999) The role of endothelin-converting enzyme-1 in the development of α1-adrenergic- stimulated hypertrophy in cultured neonatal rat cardiac myocytes. *Circulation* 99: 292–298

82   Iwanaga Y, Kihara Y, Hasegawa K, Inagaki K, Yoneda T, Kaburagi S, Araki M, Sasayama S (1998) Cardiac endothelin –1 plays a critical role in the functional deterioration of left ventricles during the transition from compensatory hypertrophy to congestive heart failure in salt-sensitive hypertensive rats. *Circulation* 98: 2065–2073

83   Li JS, Schiffrin L (1995) Effect of chronic treatment of adult spontaneously hypertensive rats with an endothelin receptor antagonist. *Hypertension* 25: 495–500

84   Hiroe M, Hirata Y, Fujita N, Umezawa S, Ito H, Tsujino M, Koike A, Nogami A, Takamoto T, Marumo F (1991) Plasma endothelin-1 levels in idiopathic dilated cardiomyopathy. *Am Heart J* 68: 1114–1115

85   Inoko M, Kihara Y, Sasayama S (1995) Neurohumoral factors during transition from left ventricular hypertrophy to failure in Dahl salt-sensitive rats. *Biochem Biophys Res Commun* 206: 814–820

86   Ono K, Tsujimoto G, Sakamoto A, Eto K, Masaki T, Ozaki Y, Satake M (1994) Endothelin-A receptor mediates cardiac inhibition by regulating calcium and potassium currents. *Nature* 370: 301–304

87   Jones LG (1996) Inhibition of cyclic AMP accumulation by endothelin is pertussis toxin sensitive and calcium independent in isolated adult feline cardiac myocytes. *Life Sci* 58: 115–123

88   Hartong R, Villarreal FJ, Giordano F, Hilal Dandan R, McDonough PM, Dillmann WH (1996) Phorbol myristate acetate-induced hypertrophy of neonatal rat cardiac myocytes is associated with decreased sarcoplasmic reticulum Ca^{2+} ATPase gene expression and calcium reuptake. *J Mol Cell Cardiol* 28: 2467–2477

89   Prasad MR (1991) Endothelin stimulates degradation of phospholipids in isolated rat hearts. *Biochem Biophys Res Commun* 174: 952–957

90   Church MK, Levi-Schaffer F (1997) The human mast cell. *J Allergy Clin Immunol* 99: 155–160

91   Welle M (1997) Development, significance, and heterogeneity of mast cells with particular regard to the mast cell-specific proteases chymase and tryptase. *J Leukoc Biol* 61: 233–245

92   Marone G, de Crescenzo G, Adt M, Patella V, Arbustini E, Genovese A (1995) Immuno-

logical characterization and functional importance of human heart mast cells. *Immunopharmacology* 31: 1–18

93 Galli SJ, Wershil BK (1995) Mouse mast cell cytokine production: role in cutaneous inflammatory and immunological responses. *Exp Dermatol* 4: 240–249

94 Patella V, Marino I, Arbustini E, Lampater-Schummert B, Verga L, Adt M, Marone G (1998) Stem cell factor in mast cells and increased mast cell density in idiopathic and ischemic cardiomyopathy. *Circulation* 97: 971–978

95 Panizo A, Mindan FJ, Galindo MF, Cenarruzabeitia E, Hernandez M, Diez J (1995) Are mast cells involved in hypertensive heart disease? *J Hypertens* 8: 815–822

96 Hara M, Matsumori A, Ono K, Kido H, Hwang M-W, Miyamoto T, Iwasaki A, Okada M, Nakatani K, Sasayama S (1999) Mast cells cause apoptosis of cardiomyocytes and proliferation of other intramyocardial cells *in vitro*. *Circulation* 100: 1443–1449

97 Hara M, Ono K, Hwang M-W, Iwasaki A, Okada M, Nakatani K, Sasayama S, Matsumori A (2002) Evidence for a role of mast cells in the evolution to congestive heart failure. *J Exp Med* 195: 375–381

98 Zampini P, Riviera AP, Tridente G (1983) *In vitro* inhibition of histamine release from mouse mast cells and human basophils by an anthranilic acid derivative. *Int J Immunopharmacol* 5: 431–435

99 Hara K, Komatsu H, Tsutsumi N, Ujiie A, Ikeda S, Kobayashi T, Kudo I, Inoue K (1994) Suppressive effects of the anti-allergic drugs, tranilast and azelastine, on the lysophosphatidylserine-dependent activation of rat mast cells. Biol Pharm Bull 17: 1121–1123

100 Sasayama S (1995) Immune modulation of cardiac function: A new frontier. *J Card Fail* 1: 331–335

101 Shioi T, Matsumori A, Kakio T, Kihara Y, Sasayama S (2001) Proinflammatory cytokine inhibitor prolongs the survival of rats with heart failure induced by pressure overload. *Jpn Circ J* 65: 584–585

102 McMurray J, Pfeffer MA (2002) New therapeutic options in congestive heart failure. Part II. *Circulation* 105: 2223–2228

The role of complement in myocardial inflammation and reperfusion injury

Elaine J. Tanhehco[1] and Benedict R. Lucchesi[2]

[1]Henry Ford Hospital, 2799 West Grand Boulevard, 4047 E&R, Detroit, MI 48202, USA;
[2]University of Michigan Medical School, Department of Pharmacology, 1150 W. Medical Center Drive, 1301C Medical Science Research Building III, Ann Arbor, MI 48109-0632, USA

Introduction

The complement system represents a major physiologic defense mechanism, which in addition has the potential for initiating tissue damage at the initial site of injury, in many cases, being directed towards the vascular endothelium. A major question concerns the role of the complement system as a direct mediator of tissue injury, as well as its ability to promote the inflammatory response associated with myocardial ischemia and/or reperfusion. As a major component of the innate immune system, complement is able to discriminate self from non-self and to bring about the removal of pathogens and non-self antigens by inducing signaling mechanisms that initiate pro-inflammatory, opsonic, phagocytic, and cytolytic actions.

Reperfusion of the ischemic myocardium results in irreversible tissue injury and cell necrosis, leading to decreased cardiac function and alterations in electrophysiological properties. While early reperfusion of the heart is essential in preventing further tissue damage due to ischemia, reintroduction of blood flow can expedite the death of vulnerable, but still viable, myocardial tissue by initiating a series of events involving both intra- and extracellular mechanisms. Extensive efforts have focused on the role of cytotoxic reactive oxygen species, complement activation, neutrophil adhesion, and the interactions between complement and neutrophils during myocardial reperfusion injury [1]. Without reperfusion, myocardial cell death evolves slowly over the course of hours. In contrast, reperfusion after an ischemic insult of sufficient duration initiates an inflammatory response, involving complement activation, followed by the recruitment and accumulation of neutrophils into the reperfused myocardium. Modulation of the inflammatory response, therefore, constitutes a potential pharmacological target to protect the heart from reperfusion injury [2]. The present discussion will be approached from the position that ischemia/reperfusion injury is a multifactorial process in which the duration of perfusion deprivation sets the stage for events that will serve to perpetuate the demolition of tissue during the subsequent period of reperfusion. Recognition of the initiating factor(s) involved in myocardial reperfusion injury should aid in development

Inflammation and Cardiac Diseases, edited by Giora Z. Feuerstein, Peter Libby and Douglas L. Mann
© 2003 Birkhäuser Verlag Basel/Switzerland

of interventions to selectively or collectively attenuate the sequence of events that mediate extension of tissue injury beyond that caused by the ischemic insult. The reader is referred to recent publications that present a detailed discussion of the role of the complement system and inflammatory conditions [3–6].

The complement system

The complement system (Fig. 1) consists of more than 30 serum or cellular components including activating proteins, receptors, and positive and negative regulators that form an independent immune system. The functions of the complement related proteins include, opsonization of target sites, modulating chemotaxis, lysis of microorganisms, neutralization of viruses, control of vascular permeability, removal of immune complexes and control of the immune response.

The classical complement pathway

The classical pathway can be activated when preformed antibody binds to antigen, forming an antigen-antibody complex. This activation proceeds when C1 complex (C1q, C1r, and C1s) attaches to the Fc portion of an IgM or IgG antibody. C1s is formed, which, in conjunction with C4, will merge to bring about the formation of C4b. In this proteolytic process, C4a is dissociated from the parent C4 and can serve as a weak anaphylatoxin in comparison to the C3a and C5a chemotactic factors. C4b merges with plasma C2 to form the C4b2a classical pathway C3 convertase. C4b2a subsequently cleaves C3 (present in human plasma at a concentration of 1.2 mg/ml) *via* the amplification cascade. Once the amplification pathway is initiated, C3 can rejoin with C4b2a (the classical pathway C3 convertase) to form C4b2aC3b, through the loss of its C3a product. This multifaceted complex (C4b2aC3b) can cleave plasma C5 (85 µg/ml) to generate C5a, another anaphylatoxin, and C5b.

C5a is the most potent anaphylatoxin arising from direct complement activation and directly alters vasculature tone and permeability in addition to facilitating the recruitment of neutrophils to the zone of inflammation. C5b is the first component of the terminal pathway that ultimately functions to form the membrane attack complex (MAC). C5b loosely associates with biological membranes and has binding sites for C6 and C7. The resulting trimolecular complex, C5b-7, can associate with the cell membrane, possibly through phospholipid binding sites within the C7 protein. After C5b-7 attachment, plasma C8 and C9 associate with the complex. C9 enhances the lytic capacity of the membrane attack complex, a process independent of an enzymatic mechanism. The MAC that inserts into the target cell is lethal *via* formation of a lesion (hole) in the membrane, thereby rendering the cell incapable of maintaining its intracellular water and electrolyte composition.

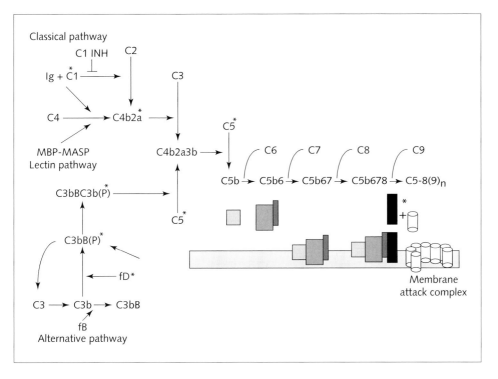

Figure. 1
Schematic diagram of the classical, alternative, and lectin pathways of complement activation. Although the separate pathways are activated under different conditions, each converge at complement component C3. Full activation of the complement system yields the lytic moiety C5b-9 (MAC). The cleavage products C4a, C3a, and C5a are also biologically active. Sites indicated by an asterisk (*) represent targets for therapeutic intervention. C1 Inhibitor (C1 INH); mannan-binding lectin (MBL); MBL associated serine protease (MASP); Factor D (f D); Factor B (f B).

Activation of the alternative complement pathway

As plasma C3 (1.2 mg/ml) circulates throughout the vasculature, spontaneous activation of the protein occurs at very low levels. The removal of C3a induces a conformational change in the protein that leads to the exposure of an internal thioester that is protected in native C3. The C3 thioester is able to form covalently linked complexes with any nucleophile. The ability to bind to any molecule with a hydroxyl or amino group implies that activated C3b could potentially deposit on the surface of any biological cell (host or foreign). Along the surface of normal vascular endothelial cells, regulatory molecules, known as "regulators of complement activation" (RCA), are present and serve to control the extent of alternative pathway activation and the potential for complement mediated tissue injury. The loss of endogenous regulator moieties, either through tissue injury or the presence of discordant foreign surfaces, permits alternative pathway activation to occur, resulting in tissue injury and/or death. C3b that is not inactivated by either the RCA or ester hydrolysis, complexes with Factor B at the target site. Factor D, a plasma serine protease, proteolytically cleaves the resultant C3bB complex. In the process, the Ba and Bb fragments are formed. C3bBb can then function as a "C3 convertase" in a situation analogous to the previous description of the classical pathway convertase. If the RCA cannot dissociate the alternative pathway C3 convertase, a C5 convertase can form, ultimately leading to the assembly of the cytolytic membrane attack complex.

The initiation of the alternative pathway of complement activation consists of binding of C3b or C3 (H20) to Factor B (Fig. 1). The serum concentration of the serine protease, Factor D, determines the extent to which the alternative pathway may be activated. The enzyme normally is found in low concentrations in the circulation. Factor D catalyzes the cleavage of bound Factor B, producing Ba and Bb. Bb then binds to C3b, forming the alternative pathway C3 convertase, C3bBb. Once stabilized by properdin, surface bound C3bBb can participate in an amplification loop that promotes further complement activation by generating additional amounts of C3b.

The relatively low plasma concentration of Factor D limits the cascade of reactions comprising the alternative pathway, thereby making the enzyme an ideal target for regulation of the alternative pathway. The importance of Factor D is reflected in that nine times the physiological concentration is necessary for it to become non-limiting. Depletion of Factor D from human serum prevents lysis of rabbit erythrocytes. Likewise, monoclonal antibodies against Factor D prevent rabbit erythrocyte hemolysis by human serum as well as inhibit the cleavage of C3 to C3b by cobra venom factor. Thus, the inactivation of Factor D with the use of a specific anti-Factor D antibody may be an effective means of modulating human complement-mediated tissue damage [7]. Monoclonal antibody to Factor D inhibited the alternative complement activation and the production of Bb, C3a, sC5b-9, and C5a. Up-regulation of CD11b on neutrophils and CD62P on platelets was significantly inhibited by monoclonal antibody 166-32. This is consistent with the inhibition of the release of neutrophil-specific myeloperoxidase and elastase and platelet thrombospondin. The antibody suppressed the production of pro-inflammatory cytokine, interleukin 8 [8]. The monoclonal anti-Factor D antibody, MAb 166-32, inhibited hemolysis of rabbit erythrocytes by human complement as well as prevented degradation of myocardial function in human plasma perfused rabbit hearts. Decreased amounts of the Bb fragment in the lymphatic effluent of MAb 166-32 treated hearts support the hypothesis that the antibody neutralizes the catalytic activity of Factor

D, in turn arresting activation of the alternative complement pathway. Activation of the human complement system by rabbit tissue occurs mainly *via* the alternative pathway. Irreversible injury of rabbit myocardium challenged with human plasma is predominantly due to formation of the membrane attack complex on the coronary vasculature. The latter observation is consistent with the understanding that the perfused vascular bed, and primarily the endothelium, represents the primary target of host immunity in hyper-acute rejection. The rabbit isolated heart, perfused in the presence of human plasma, serves as a paradigm for xenotransplantation with full appreciation for the fact that complement activation in the process of organ rejection represents only one, albeit, an important component of the rejection phenomenon. As a structural and functional interface, the endothelium is the site at which inflammatory cells move from the bloodstream through the vessel wall into the parenchyma. The endothelium interacts with the complement system, the coagulation and inflammatory cascades, circulating leukocytes, the immune system, the smooth muscle in the vessel wall, and the surrounding matrix and cardiomyocytes. A better understanding of its many roles may lead to expansion of our therapeutic possibilities and better outcomes overall [9].

Activation of the lectin pathway

The lectin pathway is mediated by mannan-binding lectin (also known as mannan-binding protein, or MBP). The mannan-binding protein binds mannose and N-acetyl glucosamine residues found in many microbial carbohydrates but not usually found in the carbohydrates of humans. The MBP has a structure similar to that of C1q – a multimeric molecule with globular binding regions and a collagenous stalk associated with a protease termed MBL associated serine protease (MASP). The latter is homologous with C1r and C1s in the classical complement pathway. The MBL-MASP complex activates C4 in a manner similar to that involving C1.

To summarize, activation of the lectin pathway begins when mannan-binding protein (MBP) binds to the mannose groups of microbial carbohydrates. Two more lectin pathway proteins called MASP1 and MASP2 (equivalent to C1r and C1s of the classical pathway) now bind to the MBP (Fig. 1). This forms an enzyme similar to C1 of the classical complement pathway that is able to cleave C4 and C2 to form C4bC2a, the C3 convertase capable of enzymatically splitting hundreds of molecules of C3 into C3a and C3b.

The regulators of complement activation (RCA)

The reactants resulting from activation of the alternative pathway do not discriminate between host and foreign cells. Therefore, regulatory mechanisms are present to prevent complement activation and host tissue damage under normal conditions. A number of regulatory proteins, both soluble and membrane-bound, have been identified.

Four membrane-associated proteins found on endothelial cells and most peripheral blood cells function as regulators of the complement cascade:

1. Decay accelerating factor (DAF, CD55);
2. Complement receptor Type 1 (CR1; CD35);
3. Membrane cofactor protein (MCP; CD46); and
4. Homologous restriction factor (HRF), also known as C8 binding protein.

DAF and CR1 regulate complement activation by preventing association (or affecting dissociation) of C3b with factor Bb, and/or C4b with C2a; the result is inactivation of the convertases. MCP possesses cofactor activity in the factor I-mediated degradation of C3b to iC3b, as well as in the degradation of C4b. DAF and MCP, together, control activation of the complement cascade at the critical level of the C3 convertases. Protection against the lytic action of the MAC may occur by regulating activation of the earlier portions of the cascade at the level of the convertases. In addition, there are two inhibitors of the membrane attack complex, homologous restriction factor, and CD59, which, by binding to C8, prevent the unfolding of the first C9 molecule needed for membrane insertion. CD59 also prevents binding of subsequent C9 molecules and their polymerization into the MAC transmembrane ring structure. DAF, HRF and CD59 are bound to the cell membrane through glycosyl phosphatidylinositol anchors.

The so-called regulators of complement activation offer a mechanism for preventing the excessive generation of activated complement products, thus confining the event near the site of injury in an effort to protect normal tissues from complement-mediated "bystander" cell lysis. The membrane associated regulators of complement activation include complement receptor 1 (CR1), decay accelerating factor (DAF, CD55) and membrane cofactor protein (MCP, CD56) are expressed by nearly all cell types, including endothelium, epithelial cells, fibroblasts and leukocytes. Plasma associated regulators of complement activation include Factor H (alternative pathway inhibitor) and C4b-binding protein (C4bp). The latter, in concert with factor I, splits C4b molecules. In addition, C4bp interferes with C2a association with C4b and promotes C4b2a dissociation into C4b and C2a. CD59, an 18-to-20 kDa glycoprotein present on many hematopoietic and non-hematopoietic cells is involved in the binding to C8 and preventing insertion of C9 to complete formation of the MAC. The expression and isolation of soluble forms of the membrane and plasma-associated regulators of complement activation has resulted in their use in experimental models of complement mediated tissue injury.

Pharmacologic inhibition of the complement cascade is typified by the ability of the soluble form of complement receptor 1 (sCR1) to decrease infarct size in the rat

[10]. Soluble CR1 is formed through the removal of the membrane spanning and cytoplasmic regions of the protein, thereby resulting in a soluble form of the molecule. CR1 inhibits both the alternative and classical pathways of complement. In addition to its involvement in the processing and clearance of immune complexes with C3b or C4b on their surface, CR1 acts as a cofactor for the proteolysis of C3b and C4b by Factor I. In rats subjected to coronary occlusion/reperfusion, the soluble form of human CR1 reduced infarct size; neutrophil infiltration and assembly of cell associated MAC [10]. *In vitro* and *in vivo* studies [11] have demonstrated the inhibition of complement activation using human recombinant soluble decay accelerating factor (DAF; CD55). DAF accelerates the inactivation of the C3 and C5 convertases, a mechanism of action resembling that of endogenous CR1. Zalman et al. [12] isolated a soluble form of homologous restriction factor (HRF, C8-binding protein), which binds C8 and C9 and regulates the assembly of the MAC. However, a potential disadvantage of complement inhibition during the latter portions of the cascade, which does not prevent activation of C3 or production of the anaphylatoxins, is problematic. The recent description of CAB-2, a molecule that comprises portions of the human complement regulatory proteins MCP and DAF, is another example of how complement mediated tissue responses may be modulated [13]. The complement regulatory proteins are most effective at controlling the activation of homologous complement, and the complement of closely related species, but they are much less effective regulators of complement from more divergent species [14, 15]. The availability of other recombinant inhibitors of the complement system is anticipated with enthusiasm.

The lack of sufficient human organs available for transplantation has increased interest in xenotransplantation with the anticipation that the pig will serve as a source of organs. The pig is considered an attractive species because of its availability in large numbers and many anatomical and physiological similarities to humans. Discordant xenotransplantation is accompanied by complement activation, hyper-acute rejection, and graft loss in minutes to hours. Because the major barriers in hyper-acute rejection include natural antibody, complement activation, and blood coagulation, many ways to inhibit these pathways have been developed. Hyper-acute rejection, but not subsequent irreversible accelerated acute rejection, can be overcome in discordant cardiac xenografts by various means of complement inhibition; including use of donor organs expressing species specific transgenic regulators of complement activation, treatment with inhibitors of C5b-9 such as antibodies to C5 and C8 or C6 and inhibitors of C3 and C5 convertases.

Soluble CR1 is one approach under consideration and has been reported to prolong xenograft survival [16]. Complement inhibition alone using a recombinant sCR1 prevented hyper-acute rejection but not subsequent irreversible accelerated acute rejection of discordant pig-to-cynomolgus monkey cardiac xenografts, which occurs within one week. To inhibit accelerated acute rejection, which is associated with a rise in serum xenoreactive antibody and a cellular infiltrate, triple therapy with standard immunosuppressive agents (cyclosporine, cyclophosphamide, and steroids was combined with continuous complement inhibition using sCR1. Monkeys that received sCR1 plus immunosuppressive triple therapy showed minimal evidence of rejection when euthanized on days 21 and 32 in comparison to controls.

Complement inhibition by C1-inhibitor has been shown to reduce myocardial ischemia-reperfusion injury in animal models. In a recent study, de Zwaan et al. [17] examined the effects of intravenous C1-inhibitor, after reperfusion therapy, in patients with acute myocardial infarction. The authors concluded that continuous 48-hour treatment with C1-inhibitor provided safe and effective inhibition of complement activation after reperfused acute myocardial infarction and may reduce myocardial injury.

In vitro expression of human regulators of complement activation, such as hDAF or MCP on the surface of pig cells has been shown to protect them from lysis by human complement [18–20]. Hearts from hDAF transgenic pigs are not hyperacutely rejected when transplanted heterotopically into the abdomen of cynomolgus monkeys and prolonged survival can be obtained when combined with immunosuppression [21]. Shiraishi et al. [22] investigated the use of an adenovirus-mediated gene transfer of triple human complement regulating proteins in xenogeneic pig liver perfusion. The livers were harvested 24 hours after gene transfer and then were reperfused ex vivo with fresh human blood for two hours. In immunohistochemical staining, each complement regulating protein showed a distribution similar to that of the LacZ expression. The complement deposition on the porcine liver (C3, membrane attack component (MAC)) decreased significantly in the treated organs as compared to the controls. Thus, the adenovirus-mediated multiple gene transfer of human complement regulating proteins effectively suppressed the complement activation in xenogenetic pig liver perfusion.

The effect of ischemia on the regulatory proteins of the complement system exerts an important influence on the degree to which the complement cascade contributes to reperfusion injury. The ischemic insult may lead to altered function of membrane bound regulatory proteins (regulators of complement activation). During ischemia, phospholipases may be activated thereby cleaving the glycolipid anchor, which maintains the regulators of complement activation on the cell surface. Phospholipase C, with specific activity against phosphatidyl inositol functions in myocardial metabolism and is activated in response to myocardial ischemia. There is suggestive evidence that the loss of expression of CD59 occurs in association with MAC deposition in infarcted myocardial tissue. In post-ischemic liver, CD59 deposits were noted in the endothelium of ischemic and non-ischemic tissues thus refuting the hypothesis of loss of the glycolipid anchored complement regulator as a mechanism for uncontrolled complement activation in ischemia and reperfusion. However, in areas of tissue necrosis, deposits of C9 were found suggesting the presence of the MAC.

Role of complement activation in myocardial ischemia/reperfusion injury

Activation of the complement system in the setting of myocardial ischemic injury represents an integrated mechanism through which the ischemic tissue undergoes cellular injury and, ultimately, necrosis. It is firmly established that consumption of classical complement components by heart subcellular membranes *in vitro* and *in vivo* occurs in the acutely infarcted myocardium. The deposition of C1q, an early component of the classical pathway activation occurs in experimental models of myocardial ischemia and reperfusion injury [23]. Ischemia-induced complement activation, as evidenced by the deposition of complement components, is not apparent immediately in with brief episodes of ischemia [24, 25]. This would suggest that ischemic insults of limited duration, in contrast to longer intervals of ischemia, might not invoke irreversible injury associated with the complement cascade. Evidence of limited complement deposition begins within 45–60 minutes in the absence of reperfusion and progresses over the course of several hours, but is enhanced markedly within minutes upon reperfusion [25]. Yasojima et al. [26] demonstrated that complement activation in infarcted human myocardium continues long after the initial ischemic insult. A sublytic-assembly of complement proteins (C5b-C7) on targeted cells in an ischemic region may participate in transmembrane events manifest as alterations in cardiac function and/or alterations in membrane electrophysiology. The localization of complement components was examined using sections of rat [27] and baboon [28] myocardium obtained after regional myocardial ischemia. Localization of complement proteins in most infarcted myocardial fibers and vessels coincided with sequestration of polymorphonuclear leukocytes [23]. However, neither deposition of complement proteins nor leukocytes was observed in myocardial tissue that was not subjected to an ischemic insult.

An antibody directed against the neoantigen of the human C5b-9 complex was used to identify MAC deposits in infarcted human myocardial tissue obtained at autopsy. Limited to no detection of the MAC was observed with a monoclonal antibody to complement S-protein, indicating that the terminal complement components were deposited mainly in the form of membrane-damaging C5b-9 complexes [26]. It is hypothesized that initial ischemia may cause alterations in the ability of the cardiac myocytes to regulate complement turnover at the membrane level. The resulting deposition of C5b-9 on the cell membranes could contribute to functional disturbances (signal transduction) and irreversible damage (altered intracellular electrolyte and water balance) of myocardial cells during ischemia and reperfusion. Other studies have shown a significant increase in the deposition of C5b-9, C3bBb, and the degradation products of the anaphylatoxins in the plasma of patients after acute myocardial infarction. The findings support the concept that complement activation is involved during myocardial ischemia and the evolution of an acute myocardial infarction [29-31].

Complement activation and membrane signaling

Activation of the complement cascade does not always result in cell death, but can elicit cellular responses, which serve to repair or further damage the jeopardized tissue. Deposition of sublytic amounts of the MAC stimulates the release of the inflammatory mediators monocyte chemo-attractant protein-1 and IL-8 [32] and augments expression of intercellular adhesion molecule-1 (ICAM-1) and E-selectin [33], which serve to mediate leukocyte recruitment. A non-lethal complement attack also triggers the release of von Willebrand factor, which participates in the coagulation cascade [34], and oxygen radicals, which further tissue injury during reperfusion [35–37]. Ironically, pre-exposure to a sublytic concentration of complement protects cells from subsequent, complement-mediated damage [38, 39].

The terminal complement complexes (TCC), C5b-7, C5b-8, and C5b-9, also initiate cell-signaling pathways that may affect the outcome of an ischemic episode. Pertussis-toxin sensitive G-proteins [40] and PKC activity [41] are influenced by TCC binding to the plasma membrane. In addition, the terminal components increase intracellular calcium, which can potentially activate one or more enzymes (e.g., phospholipase C, adenylate cyclase, protein kinase C, etc.) [42, 43]. The hemolytically inactive form of C5b-9, iC5b-9, up-regulates endothelial leukocyte adhesion molecule-1, ICAM-1 and vascular cell adhesion molecule-1 (VCAM-1) expression and amplifies tissue factor activity in endothelial cells [44]. Thus, complement may adversely impact ischemic cardiac myocytes independently of its direct lethal effects by facilitating deleterious immune mechanisms, including increasing the leukocyte population within the area at risk and promoting free radical-mediated damage.

Tanhehco et al. [45] investigated the effects of sub-lethal complement activation on infarct size in an ex vivo model of ischemia and reperfusion. It was observed that reperfused rabbit isolated hearts exposed to a sublytic concentration of human plasma before the induction of regional ischemia developed significantly smaller infarcts compared with hearts perfused with buffer alone. An anti-C5a antibody, implicating C5a as the protective factor in our paradigm, abrogated the protective effect of limited exposure to human plasma.

Rabbit hearts preconditioned with two cycles of five minutes ischemia followed by 10 minutes of reperfusion (IPC) or with the ATP-sensitive potassium channel opener, diazoxide (10 mg/kg), exhibited significantly smaller infarcts compared with control. These treatments also significantly reduced C1q, C1r, C3, C8, and C9 mRNA in the areas at risk of infarction. The K (ATP) channel blocker 5-hydroxy-decanoate (10 mg/kg) attenuated infarct size reduction elicited by ischemic preconditioning or exposure to diazoxide. There were no significant differences in complement gene expression in the non-risk regions and livers of all groups. Western blot analysis revealed that ischemic preconditioning also reduced membrane attack complex expression in the area at risk of infarction. The data demonstrate that preconditioning significantly decreases reperfusion-induced myocardial complement expression *in vivo* [46] and that a sub-lethal complement mediated event can reduce tissue injury similar to that known to occur with ischemic or pharmacological pre-conditioning.

Free radicals and the complement cascade

Free radical generation during reperfusion of the ischemic myocardium increases C1q, C1r, C3, C8, and C9 mRNA and MAC production by the isolated heart [47]. The antioxidants N-(2-mercaptopropionyl)-glycine (MPG) or the intracellular superoxide dismutase mimetic, SC-52608, inhibit free radical-stimulated complement expression. Damaging oxidants are produced during the inflammatory response, which comprises a major part of many pathological conditions, including ischemia/reperfusion injury. Thus, the local activation of complement by free radicals may occur during oxidative stress and may contribute to the tissue injury associated with this event. Furthermore, the "explosive" production of reactive metabolites of oxygen upon reperfusion coincides with the rapid expression of tissue complement during reintroduction of molecular oxygen to the previously ischemic isolated heart perfused in the total absence of plasma proteins [25] or *in vivo* during regional myocardial ischemia and reoxygenation [24].

The metabolism of xanthine by xanthine-oxidase generates reactive oxygen species, most notably the superoxide anion (O_2^-) and hydrogen peroxide (H_2O_2). Both entities cause cellular damage and propagate the generation of free radicals *via* the Fenton and Haber-Weiss reactions. Exposure to xanthine and xanthine oxidase is an accepted method for evaluating the effects of free radicals on cell structure and function. Perfusion of isolated hearts with the enzyme system results in tissue edema, disorganization of myofilaments and mitochondrial swelling in myocytes. Treatment with xanthine/xanthine oxidase also alters the hemodynamic function of the myocardium, decreasing contractility and coronary flow, as well as inducing mitochondrial dysfunction. The combination of MPG and SC-52608 significantly preserved the hemodynamic function of hearts exposed to xanthine/xanthine oxidase, suggesting that free radicals mediate the decline in function [47].

MPG and SC-52608 primarily scavenge hydroxyl and superoxide anions, respectively. Both are lipid soluble and have been shown to attenuate ischemia/reperfusion injury, presumably through their antioxidant capabilities. Recent data demonstrate that these agents effectively inhibit complement expression stimulated by exposure to free radicals [47].

MPG and SC-52608 significantly inhibited complement mRNA synthesis of C1q, C1r, C3, C8, and C9 compared with xanthine/xanthine oxidase perfused hearts. The antioxidants also attenuated C1r, C3 and C8 mRNA expression below control levels, indicating that perfusion of isolated hearts with buffer alone slightly stimulates complement production. The differential sensitivity to reactive oxygen species of the complement components measured suggests that several distinct mechanisms may govern the transcription of each complement gene. The intracellular signaling events and transcriptional regulators involved in expression of complement genes remain largely unknown [47]. Reactive oxygen species initiate the transcription of a variety of genes, as well as activate the transcription factor NF-κB, which regulates several inflammatory genes [48, 49]. In addition, it has been suggested that NF-κB mediates C3 expression in human epithelial cells [50].

Under physiological conditions, free radicals can originate from a variety of sources. Neutrophils destroy invading and native cells *via* the production of oxidants and their cytotoxic metabolites [1]. Since C3a and C5a are chemo-attractants, increased local complement production may recruit these cell types into the area at risk, and maintain the presence of free radical donating-inflammatory cells throughout the reperfusion period. Yasojima et al. [26] demonstrated that complement activation in infarcted human myocardium continues long after the initial ischemic insult. Mitochondria may also leak oxidants during respiration, while intracellular enzymes, such as xanthine oxidase, generate free radicals during catalysis [1, 51]. Aside from the lipid peroxidation and the intracellular calcium overload associated with oxidative stress, tissue-derived complement may also contribute to the mechanism of free radical induced cytotoxicity.

There is a compelling body of data to indicate that free radicals stimulate complement production in the myocardium. Since free radicals and complement activation participate in a variety of inflammatory processes, these two events may promote one another and advance tissue injury. Furthermore, the burst of free radical production is most intense within the first few moments of reperfusion and is related closely to the expression of mRNA encoding for the tissue production of the complement proteins. It is noteworthy that in the absence of reperfusion, and thus the absence of a free radical burst, that tissue complement expression is minimal or absent. In addition, intracellular free radical scavengers can suppress the expression of complement protein synthesis in response to reperfusion. Thus, the accumulating evidence favors the concept that the tissue derived complement proteins as well as those formed in the liver participate in extending the tissue injury during the period of reperfusion.

Inflammatory response and the role of complement in myocardial ischemia and reperfusion injury

Flynn et al. [52] used a feline model of ischemia/reperfusion injury and demonstrated that intravenous ibuprofen given immediately and two hours after coronary artery ligation decreased myocardial infarct size. In contrast, aspirin did not diminish infarct size when used over a wide dose range; in fact, at some doses it tended to increase infarct size. *In vitro* studies with granulocytes exposed to zymosan, activated plasma demonstrated a similar dichotomy between ibuprofen and aspirin. Ibuprofen inhibited granulocyte aggregation, superoxide production, lysosomal enzyme release, and granulocyte-mediated endothelial cytotoxicity, while aspirin was without effect on these modalities. It is proposed that ibuprofen's beneficial effect in experimental myocardial ischemia is related to its ability to inhibit activated granulocytes and thus to diminish myocardial cell death in experimental infarction. The conclusions are supported by related studies in which ibuprofen inhibited zymosan-induced neutrophil adherence [53]. Recognizing that C5a facilitates the adhesion of polymorphonuclear leukocytes to the vascular endothelium in the inflammatory zone, Simpson and colleagues [54] inhibited the C5a-induced recruitment of neutrophils to the ischemic myocardium in a canine model of regional ischemia using iloprost, a stable analogue of prostacyclin. Furthermore, a monoclonal antibody to C5a, which inhibits neutrophil cytotoxic activity, but does not affect formation of the membrane attack complex or myocardial neutrophil accumulation, decreased infarct size in pigs [55]. The reported observations support the concept of an important role for the alternative complement pathway and C5a in the propagation of myocardial injury during reperfusion. Other investigators [56] demonstrated the presence of neutrophil chemotactic activity in reperfusion canine cardiac lymph after myocardial ischemia and infarction. The ability of post-ischemic cardiac lymph to alter neutrophil function was prevented by rabbit antiserum to canine C5a.

The anaphylatoxins, C3a and C5a, generated subsequent to complement activation during reperfusion not only have potent vasoactive actions on the coronary vasculature, but also serve as potent chemo-attractants and activators for cellular constituents of inflammation (mainly neutrophils). However, C5a is a more potent neutrophil-activating peptide in this regard. Shandelya et al. [57] reported the necessity of complement activation and neutrophils together contributing to contractile dysfunction associated with myocardial ischemia and reperfusion injury in the rat isolated heart and attributed the neutrophil-mediated injury due to C5a generation upon reperfusion of the rat myocardium. In a rabbit model of ischemia and reperfusion injury, Ivey et al. [58] demonstrated that higher concentrations of C5a were associated with earlier stages of reperfusion and was not detectable during the ischemic period. The increase in C5a generation was found to correlate with increases in neutrophil accumulation within the ischemic zone during reperfusion. As C5a concentrations began to decline, interleukin-8 (IL-8) concentrations in myocardial tissue increased, demonstrating a biphasic generation of neutrophil chemotactic factors. *In vivo* studies of myocardial ischemia/reperfusion injury demonstrate that localization of neutrophils in the ischemic myocardium occurs within the initial few hours of reperfusion [59]. The localization of the inflammatory cells corresponds with the appearance of C5a-dependent chemotactic activity in the lymph draining the reperfused region [60].

In addition to direct activation of neutrophils through C5a generation during the reperfusion period, complement activation indirectly increases neutrophil recruitment and infiltration into the myocardial risk region. Formation and deposition of the MAC is noted in reperfused myocardial tissue but not the non-involved region or ischemic region that has not been subjected to reperfusion [25]. Although MAC deposition in lytic titers may ultimately lead to myocyte death, sublytic amounts of MAC deposition may alter protein synthesis in viable cells within the ischemic region. *In vitro* studies with human umbilical endothelial cells (HUVECs) suggest that C5b-9 deposition increases expression of the adhesion molecule responsible for leukocyte rolling [33]. Expression of other neutrophil adhesion molecules is increased in the presence of cytokines. Tissue content of the cytokine, tumor necrosis factor-α (TNF-α) is increased during reperfusion of the previously ischemic myocardium. *In vitro* data suggest that C5b-9 deposition in the presence of TNF-α increases the leukocyte adhesion molecules E-selectin, as well as intracellular adhesion molecule-1 (ICAM-1), which would subsequently increase neutrophil adhesion to the vascular endothelium.

The observations cited above, implicate interactions between the complement system and neutrophil activation in increasing irreversible tissue injury in response to myocardial ischemia. The role of the neutrophil in extending tissue injury beyond that due to the ischemic insult itself is supported by studies in which interventions designed to reduce the number of neutrophils, their adhesion, their function or leukotactic activity, reduce infarct size [59, 61]. It is reasonable to conclude that complement activation results in direct activation of leukocytes through anaphylatoxin generation or increases leukocyte adhesion due to C5a or MAC generation. Therefore, modulation of complement activation represents a potential approach to limiting neutrophil-dependent tissue damage during myocardial ischemia and reperfusion injury.

Direct lytic effects of the membrane attack complex

In vivo studies indicate that the terminal complex, C5b-9, accumulates selectively in the infarcted myocardium, an observation consistent with the concept that the complement system may play a role in the pathogenesis of ischemic myocardial injury [24]. An important aspect of the study revealed that, in the absence of reperfusion, C5b-9 accumulation occurred as a late event when most of the jeopardized myocardium was probably irreversibly injured (necrotic). In the presence of reperfusion, however, the complement system is activated rapidly and could increase the extent of injury upon reperfusion. Although complement activation may facilitate a cytotoxic, neutrophil-mediated inflammatory response, the question arises as to whether or not activation of the complement system, in the absence of circulating blood components, is capable of inducing tissue injury and cell death.

Homeister et al. [62] developed an *in vitro* model to examine the direct effects of complement activation on heart function, myocardial tissue damage, and to determine which complement components mediate tissue injury. Rabbit isolated hearts were perfused with human plasma using a modified Langendorff apparatus. The addition of human plasma (a source of complement) to the perfusate resulted in complement activation as evidenced by the generation of Bb, C3a, C5a, and fluid phase C5b-9 (sC5b-9). Functional changes in cardiac performance became apparent 7–15 minutes after plasma addition and developed fully over the next 20–30 minutes. The plasma-mediated alterations in cardiac function were not elicited when an inhibitor of complement activation (FUT-175) was present or when heat-inactivated plasma was used. The effects of complement activation on myocardial function could not be reproduced by treatment with recombinant human C5a, zymosan-activated plasma, or plasma selectively depleted of C8. Complement activation directly mediated tissue injury in a manner consistent with plasmalemmal disruption as a result of C5b-9 formation. The addition of sCR1, the extracellular domain of the membrane-associated regulator of complement activation, to the perfusion medium prevented deterioration in cardiac function in response to human plasma. Ultrastructural changes were present in tissues perfused with human plasma along with immunohistochemical evidence for presence of the terminal C5b-9 complex. Treatment with sCR1 prevented the ultrastructural changes and the formation of the terminal complex. Thus, complement activation in the absence of blood cellular elements, elicited a direct cytotoxic effect upon the rabbit myocardium. The regulators of complement activation on the endothelial cells of the rabbit heart are incapable of regulating activation of the human complement cascade, thereby allowing for the unopposed activation of the human complement system and membrane-associated assembly of the cytolytic membrane attack complex on the endothelial cells and myocytes of the rabbit heart. The observed protection offered by sCR1 against the cytolytic effects resulting from activation of the human complement system is consistent with *in vivo* studies in which sCR1 reduced infarct size in the heart made regionally ischemic and reperfused [10].

Endogenous tissue formation of complement proteins and the terminal membrane attack complex

It has always been assumed, that the liver is the primary source of the complement proteins. This concept was challenged by a group of investigators [25] who used the reverse transcriptase polymerase chain reaction (RT-PCR) technique to establish that the mRNAs for complement proteins C3 and C9 are expressed in rabbit heart. Rabbit liver, brain, spleen, and kidney were also shown to express C3 and C9 mRNAs. Western blotting established that the mRNAs in heart are translated into the corresponding proteins. It was further established that marked up-regulation of the mRNAs occurred in Langendorff-perfused isolated hearts subjected to ischemia and reperfusion. C3 mRNA was always expressed at higher levels than C9 mRNA, but C9 mRNA showed greater up-regulation under stress. Compared with levels in control hearts subjected to five minutes of normoxic perfusion, hearts subjected to 30 minutes of ischemia followed by one hour of reperfusion had a 4.72-fold increase in C3 mRNA and a 19.5-fold increase in C9 mRNA. By contrast, C3 mRNA in hearts subjected to 3.5 hours of normoxic perfusion showed no change, and those subjected to 3.5 hours of ischemia only a 1.72-fold increase, while C9 mRNA levels increased by 5.17 fold after 3.5 hours of normoxic perfusion and 12.5 fold after 3.5 hours of ischemia. The results demonstrated for the first time that heart tissue is capable of expressing genes and proteins of the complement system, although it is not certain which cell types are responsible. They further demonstrate that ischemia and reperfusion of the heart promotes a rapid up-regulation of the mRNAs encoding the complement proteins C3 and C9, and that these abnormal levels considerably exceed those of normal liver. These observations are consistent with the hypothesis that local production of complement proteins may contribute significantly to the degree of tissue injury to the ischemic myocardium, and that complement expression is augmented during at the time of reperfusion. The concept that reperfusion serves a critical role in mediating complement deposition is demonstrated by the observation that, in the absence of reperfusion, MAC accumulation occurs only as a late event. However, in the presence of reperfusion, the complement activation occurs rapidly, suggesting an important role of reperfusion in mediating the activation of complement. Such results in model systems are consistent with what is known about human myocardial infarction. Deposition of the MAC and other indicators of complement activation have been noted in areas of myocardial injury while the surrounding normal tissue remains relatively free of complement components [26]. Taken together, these results indicate that activation of the complement pathway in the ischemic/reperfused heart leads to deposition of the MAC and subsequent myocardial injury, and that inhibition of the complement cascade limits that injury. These observations support the hypothesis that local production by heart tissue might be a major source of injurious complement components that participate in directly injuring tissue by formation of the MAC as well as orchestrating the site-specific migration of inflammatory cells to the jeopardized region undergoing reperfusion.

There is a compelling body of data demonstrating the rapid accumulation of the terminal complement complex in the ischemic myocardium upon reperfusion as opposed to the delayed appearance of the lytic complex with prolonged ischemia [24, 25, 63]. Reactive oxygen species are formed immediately upon reperfusion and have been demonstrated to participate in the up-regulation of mRNA leading to the expression of complement components and formation of the MAC [47]. It is of significance that reperfusion, and not simulated ischemia, initiates intrinsic apoptosis injury in cardiomyocytes [64]. Thus, cells exposed to one hour simulated ischemia followed by three hours of reperfusion exhibited more cell death and membrane damage than cells exposed to four hours of ischemia without reoxygenation [64, 65]. The latter studies suggest that reperfusion and the immediate formation of oxygen free radicals initiate cytochrome C release within minutes, and apoptosis within hours; events that are associated with a significant increase in cell death and contractile dysfunction. These observations are similar to what is observed with the reperfusion-induced complement activation and raise the possibility that complement activation and assembly of the membrane attack complex may participate in the development of apoptosis.

Pharmacological inhibition of the complement cascade during myocardial ischemic stress

The administration of cobra venom factor (CVF), a protein derived from the Indian king cobra *Naja naja kaouthia*, functions as an uncontrollable C3 convertase (CVFBb) in most mammalian species, resulting in the unregulated consumption of C3, thereby preventing further activation of the complement system and ultimate formation of the MAC. Dogs administered CVF have negligible amounts of circulating C3 before the induction of myocardial ischemia. The complement deficient animals develop smaller myocardial infarcts compared to animals that did not receive CVF [66].

Protectin (CD59), a regulator of complement activation, is an 18-to-20-kDa protein present on many hematopoietic and non-hematopoietic cells that inhibits the formation of the MAC by binding to C8 and C9. Vakeva et al. [67] analyzed the expression of various membrane regulators of complement activation (RCA) in normal and infarcted human myocardium in an effort to address the question of why the strictly controlled complement system reacts against autologous heart tissue subjected to ischemia and reperfusion. CD59 is expressed by normal myocardium. Infarcted cells, however, exhibit a substantial decrease in the expression of this regulator of MAC formation. Ischemia and ischemic injury, therefore, induce a change in the sell surface regulators of complement activation and decrease the ability of the affected cell to prevent assembly of the MAC or to shed the complex from cell membrane. The pharmacological inhibition of the complement cascade during myocardial ischemia and/or infarction has received increased attention in the cardiovascular literature. Soluble complement receptor type 1 (sCR1), a recombinant version of the endogenous membrane-bound regulatory protein CR1 (CD35), reduced infarct size in a rat model of myocardial ischemia and reperfusion injury [10]. sCR1 and CR1 act by preventing the formation of the classical and alternative C3 and C5 convertases, which amplify the formation of the anaphylatoxins and the cytolytic membrane attack complex. In addition, sCR1 decreased post-ischemic myocardial contractile dysfunction and enhanced the recovery of coronary blood flow. It is noted that complement activation occurs in post-ischemic myocardium and is necessary for activation of the neutrophil oxidative burst with the generation of reactive oxygen species. The process of neutrophil adhesion, however, is not affected by sCR1 and may be independent of complement factors.

The relative contributions of the classical and alternative complement pathways in an experimental model of xenograft rejection were examined in the rabbit perfused isolated heart exposed to human plasma [68]. The study made use of a selective inhibitor of the alternative complement pathway, sCR1 (desLHR-A). This truncated version of sCR1 lacks the C4b-binding sites of the long homologous repeat region A. The truncated molecule, while equipotent to sCR1 with regard to inhibition of the alternative pathway, possesses negligible effects upon the classical pathway. The latter lacks the long homologous repeat sequence-A responsible for the majority of C4b binding and prevent alternative pathway mediated hemolysis. Thus, deletion of the C4b-binding site from sCR1 results in a new pharmacologic moiety, sCR1 (desLHR-A) that selectively inhibits the alternative pathway of human complement.

Complement activation is induced by cardiopulmonary bypass, and previous work found that late complement components (C5a, C5b-9) contribute to neutrophil and platelet activation during bypass. Rinder et al. [69] used a simulated extracorporeal model that involves activation of complement (C3a and sC5b-9), platelets (CD62P expression, leukocyte-platelet conjugate formation), and leukocytes (increased CD11b expression and neutrophil elastase), to examine an anti-human C8 monoclonal antibody that inhibits C5b-9 generation for its effects on cellular activation. The results of the study led the authors to conclude that the membrane attack complex, C5b-9, is the major complement determinant of platelet activation during extracorporeal circulation, whereas C5b-9 blockade has little effect on neutrophil activation. These data also suggest a role for platelet activation or C5b-9 (or both) in the loss of monocytes and neutrophils to the extracorporeal circuit.

Pexelizumab (h5G1.1-SC), a short-acting, recombinant complement C5 inhibitor, is being examined in several clinical trials under the acronyms of CARDINAL (Complement and ReDuction of Infarct Size after Angioplasty or Lytics) with two sub-studies COMPLY (COMplement Inhibition in Myocardial Infarction and COMMA (COMplement Inhibition in Myocardial Infarction Treated with PTCA). The endpoints focus on the prevention of complications of cardiovascular surgery, such as complement activation during cardiopulmonary bypass procedures that is accompanied by a systemic inflammatory response leading to substantial clinical morbidity. Activation of complement during cardiopulmonary bypass contributes significantly to this inflammatory process. Fitch et al. [70] examined the capability of pexelizumab to prevent pathological complement activation and tissue injury in patients undergoing cardiopulmonary bypass procedures. The study results suggested that the single-chain antibody specific for human C5 was safe, well tolerated and effectively inhibited complement activation. There was no increase in infection associated with administration of the antibody. Pexelizumab had no effect on infarct size, but did have a dose-dependent effect on mortality reduction. In addition to significantly reducing sC5b-9 formation and leukocyte CD11b expression, C5 inhibition attenuated cognitive deficits, and blood loss. Thus, C5 inhibition may represent an acceptable therapeutic strategy for preventing complement-mediated inflammation and tissue injury. This general approach could be extended to the use of antibodies against C2 to block the classical pathway and to factor D [7] to block the alternative pathway. In this way, inhibition of one of the pathways, or of the membrane attack complex could be achieved independently. The goal would be to achieve specific control of one pathway involved in inducing tissue damage, while leaving intact the other pathways needed to serve vital immunologic functions.

Commonly used therapeutic agents such as the glycosaminoglycan anticoagulant heparin and its inactive derivative N-acetylheparin have been implicated in the inhibition of complement activation both *in vivo* and *in vitro* [68, 71–73]. The ability of glycosaminoglycans to modulate activation of the complement cascade was demonstrated initially by the failure of guinea-pig plasma to hemolyze sheep erythrocytes while in the presence of heparin sulfate [74]. Glycosaminoglycans possessing highly sulfated structural domains are capable of regulating the complement cascade at a variety of steps [75–79].

The observations regarding the cardioprotective effects of heparin or N-acetyl heparin provide support for the concept involving activation of the complement system in ischemia/reperfusion injury. There is sufficient evidence to suggest that the therapeutic uses of heparin may extend beyond its traditional role as an anticoagulant, providing an opportunity to offer therapeutic benefits for a wide range of inflammatory disorders [80]. Saliba and colleagues [81] demonstrated the effects of heparin in large doses on the extent of myocardial necrosis after left anterior descending coronary artery occlusion in the dog. The cytoprotective action of glycosaminoglycans and the lack of dependence upon plasma drug concentrations and anticoagulant/antithrombotic activity provide further support for the role of glycosaminoglycans as modulators of the complement cascade. Studies suggesting that the glycosaminoglycans inhibit complement activation *in vivo* provide a strong motivation for further examination of related compounds using experimental models of tissue injury in which complement is reported to have a deleterious role [73]. Along with the aforementioned reports examining the effects of glycosaminoglycan administration beyond the clinical anticoagulant action, recent data suggest their potential application as modulators of the immune system in the management of inflammatory states involving tissue injury secondary to ischemia and reperfusion. The fact that heparin administration, for purposes of anticoagulation, is routine in the management of patients during coronary artery balloon angioplasty, thrombolytic therapy and cardiopulmonary bypass would suggest that some degree of protection against complement mediated injury has unknowingly been put into practice. The opportunity exists to develop heparin derivatives that lack anticoagulant activity while retaining other biological properties, especially those with the potential to control the inflammatory response.

The extensive clinical use of heparin and related glycosaminoglycans has led to a study of the potential cytoprotective properties of heparin and a non-anticoagulant derivative, N-acetyl-heparin, in experimental models of myocardial injury [68, 71, 72]. N-acetyl heparin has limited ability to interact with antithrombin III thereby rendering it devoid of anticoagulant properties. The comparison with N-acetyl heparin provided a method to assess the relative contribution of heparin's anticoagulant properties in mediating a cytoprotective action. There is compelling evidence to suggest that the therapeutic uses of heparin may extend beyond its traditional role as an anticoagulant, providing an opportunity to offer therapeutic benefits for a wide range of inflammatory diseases.

The putative anti-complementary properties of a low molecular weight heparin (LMWH) derivative with structural modifications that altered the sulfation characteristics present upon the glycosaminoglycan pentasaccharide have been examined in experimental models of myocardial ischemia/reperfusion injury [82]. The degree of glycosaminoglycan sulfation has been associated with complement inhibition. LU 51198, a highly sulfated, low molecular weight heparin derivative, reduced myocardial injury resulting from activation of the human complement system under conditions in which the rabbit heart was perfused in the presence of normal human plasma. The lymphatic fluid effluent from rabbit hearts perfused in the presence of human plasma showed a progressive increase in immunoreactive sC5b-9 indicative of formation of the membrane attack complex. The presence of LU 51198 in the perfusion medium suppressed the formation of sC5b-9 throughout the time the heart was perfused in the presence of human plasma, a result that coincided with protection of the heart from complement-mediated functional alterations when hemodynamic variables were used as the arbiter of myocellular injury.

Glycosaminoglycans such as heparin and N-acetyl heparin accelerate the dissociation of an enzymatically active complex designated as the C3 convertase, C3bBb, by causing the potentiation of an endogenous regulatory molecule associated with this complex. A serum protein, Factor H, controls the formation of the alternative complement pathway C3 and C5 convertases *in vivo*. Heparin augments Factor H activity in the fluid phase and in the presence of C3b attached to an activating surface, thus limiting the subsequent formation and deposition of the terminal cytolytic membrane attack complex. Factor H acts on C3b in three ways: Serving as a cofactor in the Factor I-mediated cleavage of C3b to iC3b; accelerating the spontaneous decay of the alternative pathway C3 convertase; and displacing factor B from the C3-convertase enzyme complex (C3bBb). In addition, glycosaminoglycans such as heparin and its modified derivatives are known to interact with components of the classical complement pathway. The function of the C3 convertase is to cleave serum C3 to C3b, forming a positive amplification feedback pathway for the ultimate purpose of MAC formation. Depending on the extent of the formation and deposition of MAC on the target cell, two outcomes can be expected. If a limited number of cytolytic complexes are formed on the cell surface, myocardial cells may be subjected to reversible alterations in function. In contrast, multiple insertions of the cytolytic complex result in a disruption in the intracellular water and electrolyte composition, thereby leading to irreparable injury of the cell membrane and cell death. Previous investigations have demonstrated the ability of heparin and N-acetyl heparin to inhibit the complement-mediated hemolysis of erythrocytes in a concentration-dependent fashion, an observation that further solidifies a role for the reduction of inflammatory processes *via* glycosaminoglycan administration.

Summary

The direct and indirect involvement of complement in the development of a number of pathologies including ischemia/reperfusion injury and transplant rejection lends credence to the belief that the components of the complement system are potential therapeutic targets. The limited data available to-date indicates that a number of interventions may serve to regulate multiple steps in the complement cascade. Particular attention should be given to heparin and related glycosaminoglycans that are used extensively in clinical practice for the purpose of inhibiting blood coagulation. The glycosaminoglycans, however, provide an opportunity to explore those pathophysiological conditions in which the complement system has an important role.

Despite extensive clinical use, little attention has been given to the potential anti-inflammatory and cytoprotective properties of this class of compounds, the actions of which go beyond serving the purpose of anticoagulation. New therapeutic agents based upon expression of endogenous regulators of complement activation are under development. The future looks encouraging for gaining deeper insight into the importance of the complement system in molecular and cellular biology. The ability to pharmacologically modulate the complement system should provide a better appreciation of how it functions in health and disease with the anticipation of being able to better manage clinical events secondary to inappropriate activation of the complement cascade.

While the long-term effects of inhibition of the inflammatory response remain to be determined, the results derived from previous studies provide convincing arguments for inhibition of inflammation as a therapeutic tool for the reduction of cellular injury. It should be noted that therapeutic strategies designed to inhibit one facet of inflammation might have profound effects on other aspects of the inflammatory response. For example, inhibition of complement would not only eliminate the direct effects of complement activation mediated primarily by the anaphylatoxins and MAC, but also decrease the intensity of the inflammatory response. The protection afforded by inhibiting inflammation would not only benefit the myocardium, but any tissue or organ that has been subjected to a period of ischemia followed by reperfusion. Among the areas of consideration is that which involves the inflammatory response to tissue/organ ischemia that is exacerbated further by reperfusion. The development of pharmacologic interventions to modulate inflammation represents an area of importance and in need of continued research.

Acknowledgements
The Cardiovascular Research Fund, University of Michigan Medical School, Department of Pharmacology supported studies from the senior investigator's laboratory.

References

1   Lucchesi BR (1994) Complement, neutrophils and free radicals: Mediators of reperfusion injury. *Arzneimittel-Forschung* 4: 420–432

2   Homeister JW, Lucchesi BR (1994) Complement activation and inhibition in myocardial ischemia and reperfusion injury. *Annu Rev Pharmacol Toxicol* 34: 17–40

3   Cooper NR (1999) Biology of the complement system. In: Feron DT, Haynes BF, Nathan C (eds): *Inflammation, basic principles and clinical correlates*. Lippincott Williams & Wilkins, Philadelphia, 281–315

4   Wolpart MJ (2001) Complement. *N Engl J Med* 344 (Part I): 1059–1066

5   Wolpart MJ (2001) Complement. *N Engl J Med* 344 (Part II): 1140–1044

6   Kilgore KS, Todd RF, III, Lucchesi BR (1999) Reperfusion injury. In: Feron DT, Haynes BF, Nathan C (eds): *Inflammation, basic principles and clinical correlates*. Lippincott Williams & Wilkins, Philadelphia, 1047–1060

7   Tanhehco EJ, Kilgore KS, Liff DA, Murphy KL, Fung MS, Sun WN, Sun C, Lucchesi BR (1999) The anti-factor D antibody, MAb 166-32, inhibits the alternative pathway of the human complement system. *Transplant Proc* 31: 2168–2171

8   Fung M, Loubser PG, Undar A, Mueller M, Sun C, Sun WN, Vaughn WK, Fraser CD Jr. (2001) Inhibition of complement, neutrophil, and platelet activation by an anti-factor D monoclonal antibody in simulated cardiopulmonary bypass circuits. *J Thorac Cardiovasc Surg* 122: 113–122

9   Stoica SC, Goddard M, Large SR (2002) The endothelium in clinical cardiac transplantation. *Ann Thorac Surg* 73: 1002–1008

10 Weisman HF, Bartow T, Leppo MK, Mash HC Jr, Carson GR, Concino MF, Bayle MP, Roux KH, Weisfeldt ML, Fearon DT et al (1990) Soluble human complement receptor type 1: *In vivo* inhibitor of complement suppressing post-ischemic myocardial inflammation and necrosis. *Science* 249: 146–151

11 Moran P, Beasley H, Gorrell A, Martin E, Gribling P, Fuchs H, Gillett N, Burton LE,

Caras IW (1992) Human recombinant soluble decay accelerating factor inhibits complement activation *in vitro* and *in vivo*. *J Immunol* 149: 1736–1743

12 Zalman LS, Brothers MA, Muller-Eberhard HJ (1989) Isolation of homologous restriction factor from human urine. Immunochemical properties and biologic activity. *J Immunol* 143: 1943–1947

13 Ko J-L, Lobell R, Sardonini C, Alessi MK, Yeh CG (1997) A soluble chimeric complement inhibitory protein that possesses both decay-accelerating and factor I cofactor activities. *J Immunol* 158: 2872–2881

14 Rollins SA, Zhao J, Ninomiya H, Sims PJ (1991) Inhibition of homologous complement by CD59 is mediated by a species-selective recognition conferred through binding to C8 within C5b-8 or C9 within C5b-9. *J Immunol* 146: 2345–2351

15 Ninomiya H, Sims PJ (1992) The human complement regulatory proteins CD59 binds to the a-chain of C8 and to the "b" domain of C9. *J Biol Chem* 267: 13675–13680

16 Davis EA, Pruitt SK, Greene PS, Ibrahim S, Lam TT, Levin JL, Baldwin WM, Sanfilippo F, Baldwin WM, III (1996) Inhibition of complement, evoked antibody, and cellular response prevents rejection of pig-to-primate cardiac xenografts. *Transplantation* 62: 1018–1023

17 de Zwaan C, Kleine AH, Diris JH, Glatz JF, Wellens HJ, Strengers PF, Tissing M, Hack CE, van Dieijen-Visser MP, Hermens WT (2002) Continuous 48-h C1-inhibitor treatment, following reperfusion therapy, in patients with acute myocardial infarction. *Eur Heart J* 23: 1670–1677

18 Fodor WL, Williams BL, Matis LA, Madri JA, Rollins SA, Knight JW, Velander W, Squinto SP (1994) Expression of a functional human complement inhibitor in a transgenic pig as a model for the prevention of xenogeneic hyperacute organ rejection. *Proc Natl Acad Sci USA* 91: 11153–11157

19 Rosengard AM, Cary N, Horsley J, Belcher C, Langford G, Cozzi E, Wallwork J, White DJ (1995) Endothelial expression of human decay accelerating factor in transgenic pig tissue: A potential approach for human complement inactivation in discordant xenografts. *Transplant Proc* 27: 326–327

20 McCurry KR, Kooyman, DL, Diamond LE, Byrne GW, Martin MJ, Logan JS, Platt JL (1995) Human complement regulatory proteins in transgenic animals regulate complement activation in xenoperfused organs. *Transplant Proc* 27: 317–318

21 Waterworth PD, Cozzi E, Tolan MJ, Langford G, Braidley P, Chavez G, Dunning J, Wallwork J, White D (1997) Pig-to-primate cardiac xenotransplantation and cyclophosphamide therapy. *Transplant Proc* 29: 899–900

22 Shiraishi M, Oshiro T, Nozato E, Nagahama M, Taira K, Nomura H, Sugawa H, Muto Y (2002) Adenovirus-mediated gene transfer of triple human complement regulating proteins (DAF, MCP and CD59) in the xenogeneic porcine-to-human transplantation model. Part II: Xenogeneic perfusion of the porcine liver *in vivo*. *Transpl Int* 15: 212–219

23 Rossen RD, Swain JL, Michael LH, Weakley S, Giannini E, Entman ML (1985) Selective accumulation of the first component of complement and leukocytes in ischemic

canine heart muscle. A possible initiator of an extra myocardial mechanism of ischemic injury. *Circ Res* 57: 119–130

24 Mathey D, Schofer J, Schafer HJ, Hamdoch T, Joachim HC, Ritgen A, Hugo F, Bhakdi S (1994) Early accumulation of the terminal complement-complex in the ischaemic myocardium after reperfusion. *Eur Heart J* 15: 418–423

25 Yasojima K, Kilgore KS, Washington RA, Lucchesi BR, McGeer PL (1998) Complement gene expression by rabbit heart: Upregulation by ischemia and reperfusion. *Circ Res* 82: 1224–1230

26 Yasojima K, Schwab C, McGeer EG, McGeer PL (1998) Human heart generates complement proteins that are upregulated and activated after myocardial infarction. *Circ Res* 83: 860–869

27 Vakeva A, Laurila P, Meri S (1993) Co-deposition of clusterin with the complement membrane attack complex in myocardial infarction. *Immunology* 80: 177–182

28 McManus LM, Kolb WP, Crawford MH, O'Rourke RA, Grover FL, Pinckard RN (1983) Complement localization in ischemic baboon myocardium. *Lab Invest* 48: 436–447

29 Langlois PF, Gawryl MS (1988) Detection of the terminal complement complex in patient plasma following acute myocardial infarction. *Atherosclerosis* 70: 95–105

30 Yasuda M, Kawarabayashi T, Akioka K, Teragaki M, Oku H, Kanayama Y, Takeuchi K, Takeda T, Kawase Y, Ikuno Y (1989) The complement system in the acute phase of myocardial infarction. *Jpn Circ J* 53: 1017–1022

31 Semb AG, Vaage J, Sorlie D, Lie M, Mjos OD (1990) Coronary trapping of a complement activation product (C3a des-Arg) during myocardial reperfusion in open-heart surgery. *Scand J Thorac Cardiovasc Surg* 24: 223–227

32 Kilgore KS, Miller BF, Flory CM, Evans VM, Warren JS (1996) The membrane attack complex of complement induces monocyte chemoattractant protein-1 and interkeukin-8 secretion from human umbilical vein endothelial cells. *Am J Pathol* 149: 953–961

33 Kilgore KS, Shen J, Miller BF, Ward PA, Warren JS (1995) Enhancement by the complement membrane attack complex of tumor necrosis factor-induced endothelial cell expression of ICAM-1 and E-selectin. *J Immunol* 155: 1434–1441

34 Hattori R, Hamilton KK, McEver RP, Sims PJ (1989) Complement proteins C5b-9 induce secretion of high molecular weight multimers of endothelial von Willenbrand factor and translocation of granule membrane protein GMP-140 to the cell surface. *J Biol Chem* 264: 9053–9060

35 Werns SW, Lucchesi BR (1990) Free radicals and ischemic tissue injury. *Trends Pharmacol Sciences* 11 (4): 161–166

36 Adlers S, Baker PJ, Johnson RJ, Ochi RF, Pritzl P, Couser WG (1986) Complement membrane attack complex stimulates production of reactive oxygen metabolites by cultured rat mesangial cells. *J Clin Invest* 77: 762–767

37 Hansch GM, Seitz M, Betz M (1987) Effect of the late complement components C5b-9 on human monocytes: release of prostanoids, oxygen radical and of a factor inducing cell proliferation. *Int Arch Allergy Appl Immunol* 82: 317–321

38   Reiter Y, Ciobotariu A, Fishelson Z (1992) Sublytic complement attack protects tumor cells from lytic doses of antibody and complement. *Eur J Immunol* 22: 1207–1213

39   Marchbank KJ, Van Den Berg CW, Morgan BP (1997) Mechanisms of complement resistance induced by non-lethal complement attack and by growth arrest. *Immunology* 90: 647–653

40   Niculescu F, Rus H, Shin ML (1994) Receptor-independent activation of guanine nucleotide-binding regulatory proteins by terminal complement complexes. *J Biol Chem* 269: 4417–4423

41   Carney DF, Lang TJ, Shin ML (1990) Multiple signal messengers generated by terminal complement complexes and their role in terminal complement complex elimination. *J Immunol* 145: 623–629

42   Morgan BP, Campbell AK (1985) A recovery of human polymorphonuclear leukocytes from sublytic complement attack is mediated by changes in intracellular free calcium. *Biochem J* 231: 205–208

43   Carney DF, Hammer CH, Shin ML (1986) Elimination of terminal complement complexes in the plasma membrane of nucleated cells: Influence of extracellular Ca^{2+} and association with cellular Ca^{2+}. *J Immunol* 137: 263–270

44   Tedesco F, Pausa M, Nardon E, Introna M, Mantovani A, Dobrina A (1997) The cytolytically inactive terminal complement complex activates endothelial cells to express adhesion molecules and tissue factor procoagulant activity. *J Exp Med* 185: 1619–1627

45   Tanhehco EJ, Lee H, Lucchesi BR (2000) Sublytic complement attack reduces infarct size in rabbit isolated hearts: Evidence for C5a-mediated cardioprotection. *Immunopharmacol* 49: 391–399

46   Tanhehco EJ, Yasojima K, McGeer PL, McGeer EG, Lucchesi BR (2000) Preconditioning reduces myocardial complement gene expression *in vivo*. *Am J Physiol Heart Circ Physiol* 279: H1157–H1165

47   Tanhehco EJ, Yasojima K, McGeer PL, Washington RA, Lucchesi BR (2000) Free radicals upregulate complement expression in the rabbit isolated heart. *Am J Physiol Heart Circ Physiol* 279: H195–H201

48   Abe J, Berk BC (1998) Reactive oxygen species as mediators of signal transduction in cardiovascular disease. *Trends Cardiovasc Med* 8: 59–64

49   Satriano JA, Shuldiner M, Kazuhiko H, Xing Y, Shan Z, Schlondorff D (1993) Oxygen radicals as second messengers for expression of the monocyte chemoattractant protein, JE/MCP-1, and the monocyte colony-stimulating factor, CSF-1, in response to tumor necrosis factor-alpha and immunoglobulin G: Evidence for involvement of reduced nicotinamide adenine dinucleotide phosphate (NADPH)-dependent oxidase. *J Clin Invest* 92: 1564–1571

50   Moon MR, Parikh AA, Pritts TA, Fischer JE, Cottongim S, Szabo C, Salzman AL, Hasselgren PO (1999) Complement component C3 production in IL-1β-stimulated human intestinal epithelial cells is blocked by NF-κB inhibitors and by transfection with Ser 32/36 mutant IκBa. *J Surg Res* 82: 48–55

51   Vanden Hoek TL, Becker LB, Shao Z, Li C, Schumacker PT (1998) Reactive oxygen

species released from mitochondria during brief hypoxia induce preconditioning in cardiomyocytes. *J Biol Chem* 273: 18092–18098

52 Flynn PJ, Becker WK, Vercellotti GM, Weisdorf DJ, Craddock PR, Hammerschmidt D E, Lillehei RC, Jacob HS (1984) Ibuprofen inhibits granulocyte responses to inflammatory mediators. A proposed mechanism for reduction of experimental myocardial infarct size. *Inflammation* 8: 33–44

53 Venezio FR, DiVincenzo C, PearlmanF, Phair JP (1985) Effects of the newer nonsteroidal anti-inflammatory agents, ibuprofen, fenoprofen, and sulindac, on neutrophil adherence. *J Infect Dis* 152: 690–694

54 Simpson PJ, Mickelson J, Fantone JC, Gallagher KP, Lucchesi BR (1987) Iloprost inhibits neutrophil function *in vitro* and *in vivo* and limits experimental infarct size in canine heart. *Circ Res* 60: 666–673

55 Amsterdam EA, Stahl GL, Pan HL, Rendig SV, Fletcher MP, Longhurst JC (1995) Limitation of reperfusion injury by a monoclonal antibody to C5a during myocardial infarction in pigs. *Am J Physiol* 268: H448–H457

56 Dreyer WJ, Michael LH, Nguyen T, Smith CW, Anderson DC, Entman ML, Rossen RD (1992) Kinetics of C5a release in cardiac lymph of dogs experiencing coronary artery ischemia-reperfusion injury. *Circ Res* 71: 1518–1524

57 Shandelya SM, Kuppusamy P, Herskowitz A, Weisfeldt ML, Zweier JL (1993) Soluble complement receptor type-1 inhibits the complement pathway and prevents contractile failure in the postischemic heart. Evidence that complement activation is required for neutrophil-mediated reperfusion injury. *Circulation* 88: 2812–2826

58 Ivey CL, Williams FM, Collins PD, Jose PJ, Williams TJ (1995) Neutrophil chemoattractants generated in two phases during reperfusion of ischemic myocardium in the rabbit. Evidence for a role for C5a and Interleukin-8. *J Clin Invest* 95: 2720–2728

59 Romson JL, Hook BG, Rigot VH, Schork MA, Swanson DP, Lucchesi BR (1982) The effect of ibuprofen on accumulation of [111]Indium labeled platelets and leukocytes in experimental myocardial infarction. *Circulation* 66: 1002–1011

60 Dreyer WJ, Smith CW, Michael LH, Rossen RD, Hughes BJ, Entman ML, Anderson DC (1989) Canine neutrophil activation by cardiac lymph obtained during reperfusion of ischemic myocardium. *Circ Res* 65: 1751–1762

61 Romson JL, Hook BG, Kunkel SL, Abrams GD, Schork MA, Lucchesi BR (1983) Reduction of the extent of ischemic myocardial injury by neutrophil depletion in the dog. *Circulation* 67: 1016–1023

62 Homeister JW, Satoh P, Lucchesi BR (1992) Effects of complement activation in the isolated heart. Role of the terminal complement components. *Circ Res* 71: 303–319

63 Ito W, Schafer HJ, Bhakdi S, Klask R, Hansen S, Schaarschmidt S, Schofer J, Hugo F, Hamdoch T, Mathey D (1996) Influence of the terminal complement complex on reperfusion injury, no-reflow and arrhythmias: A comparison between C6-competent and C6-deficient rabbits. *Cardiovas Res* 32: 294–305

64 Vanden Hoek TL, Quin Y, Wojcik K, Li CQ, Shao ZH, Anderson T, Becker LB, Hamann

KJ (2002) Reperfusion, not simulated ischemia, initiates intrinsic apoptosis injury in chick cardiomyocytes. *Am J Physiol Heart Circ Physiol* 84: H141–H150

65   Vanden Hoek L, Shao Z, Li P, Zak R, Schumacker PT, Becker LB (1996) Reperfusion injury in cardiac myocytes after simulated ischemia. *Am J Physiol Heart Circ Physiol* 270: H1334–H1341

66   Maroko PR, Carpenter CB, Chiariello M, Fishbein MC, Radvany P, Knostman JD, Hale SL (1978) Reduction by cobra venom factor of myocardial necrosis after coronary artery occlusion. *J Clin Invest* 61: 661–670

67   Vakeva A, Morgan BP, Tikkanen I, Helin K, Laurila P, Meri S (1994) Time course of complement activation and inhibitor expression after ischemic injury of rat myocardium. *Am J Pathol* 144: 1357–1368

68   Gralinski MR, Driscoll EM, Friedrichs GS, DeNardis MR, Lucchesi BR (1996) Reduction of myocardial necrosis after glycosaminoglycan administration: Effects of a single intravenous administration of heparin or N-acetylheparin 2 hours before regional ischemia and reperfusion. *J Cardiovasc Pharmacol Ther* 1: 219–228

69   Rinder CS, Rinder HM, Smith MJ, Tracey JB, Fitch J, Li L, Rollins SA, Smith B (1999) Selective blockade of membrane attack complex formation during simulated extracorporeal circulation inhibits platelet but not leukocyte activation. *J Thorac Cardiovasc Surg* 118: 460–466

70   Fitch JC, Rollins S, Matis L, Alford B, Aranki S, Collard CD, Dewar M, Elefteriades J, Hines R, Kopf G et al (1999) Pharmacology and biological efficacy of a recombinant, humanized, single-chain antibody C5 complement inhibitor in patients undergoing coronary artery bypass graft surgery with cardiopulmonary bypass. *Circulation* 100: 2499–2506

71   Friedrichs GS, Kilgore KS, Manley PJ, Gralinski MR, Lucchesi BR (1994) Effects of heparin and N-acetyl heparin on ischemia/reperfusion-induced alterations in myocardial function in the rabbit isolated heart. *Circ Res* 75: 701–710

72   Black SC, Gralinski MR, Friedrichs GS, Kilgore KS, Driscoll EM, Lucchesi BR (1995) Cardioprotective effects of heparin or N-acetylheparin in an *in vivo* model of myocardial ischaemic and reperfusion injury. *Cardiovasc Res* 29: 629–636

73   Weiler JM, Edens RE, Linhardt RJ, Kapelanski DP (1992) Heparin and modified heparin inhibit complement activation *in vivo*. *J Immunol* 148: 3210–3215

74   Ecker EE, Gross P (1929) Anticomplementary power of heparin. *J Infect Dis* 44: 250–253

75   Baker PJ, Lint TF, McLeod BC, Behrends CL, Gewurz H (1975) Studies on the inhibition of C56-induced lysis (reactive lysis). VI. Modulation of C56-induced lysis polyanions and polycations. *J Immunol* 114: 554–558

76   Loos M, Volanakis JE, Stroud RM (1976) Mode of interaction of different polyanions with the first (C1, C1), the second (C2) and the fourth (C4) component of complement-II. Effect of polyanions on the binding of C2 to EAC4b. *Immunochemistry* 13: 257–261

77   Sharath MD, Merchant ZM, Kim YS, Rice KG, Linhardt RJ, Weiler JM (1985) Small

heparin fragments regulate the amplification pathway of complement. *Immunopharmacology* 9: 73–80

78 Meri S, Pangburn MK (1990) Discrimination between activators and nonactivators of the alternative pathway of complement: Regulation *via* a sialic acid/polyanion binding site on factor H. *Proc Natl Acad Sci USA* 87: 3982–3986

79 Meri S, Pangburn MK (1994) Regulation of alternative pathway complement activation by glycosaminoglycans: Specificity of the polyanion binding site on factor H. *Biochem Biophys Res Commun* 198: 52–59

80 Tyrrell DJ, Horne AP, Holme KR, Preuss JMH, Page CP (1999) Heparin in inflammation: Potential therapeutic applications beyond anticoagulation. In: JT August, MW Anders, F Murad, JT Coyle (eds): *Advances in pharmacology* (vol 46). Academic Press, London, 151–208

81 Saliba M Jr, Covell JW, Bloor CM (1976) Effects of heparin in large doses on the extent of myocardial ischemia after acute coronary occlusion in the dog. *Am J Cardiol* 37: 599–604

82 Gralinski MR, Park JL, Ozeck MA, Wiater BC, Lucchesi BR (1997) LU 51198, a highly sulphated, low-molecular-weight heparin derivative, prevents complement-mediated myocardial injury in the perfused isolated rabbit heart. *J Cardiovasc Pharmacol Therapeut* 282: 554–560

Inflammatory signaling pathways
in cardiac diseases

The role of immune and inflammatory cytokines in ischemic preconditioning of the heart – identification of novel cardiac cell survival signaling programs

Sandrine Lecour[1], Robert M. Smith[1] and Michael N. Sack[2]

[1]Hatter Institute for Cardiology Research and MRC Inter-University Cape Heart Group, University of Cape Town Medical School, Cape Town, 7925, South Africa; [2]Cardiovascular Branch, National Heart Lung and Blood Institute, National Institutes of Health, Bethesda, MD 20892-1650, USA

Introduction

A biologic concept called preconditioning has been described where a transient non-lethal ischemic "trigger" or endogenous molecules produced/released by ischemia enables the tissue to become more resistant/tolerant to subsequent ischemic injury [1]. Preconditioning in humans has been demonstrated in the context of warm-up angina and following repeated percutaneous trans-coronary angioplasty and in patients undergoing coronary artery bypass surgery [2].

Preconditioning, in essence unmasks innate cytoprotective programs that drive this ischemia-tolerant phenotype. Current experimental data support the activation of G_i-protein-coupled receptor mediated signaling as the predominant cellular transduction pathways orchestrating this program [3, 4]. The ischemic preconditioning induced ligands that activate G_i-receptor coupled signaling and are proposed to activate the preconditioning cytoprotective programs include adenosine, bradykinin and opioids [4]. To date, these G_i-protein-coupled receptor mediated signaling events have been shown to activate the mitochondrial ATP sensitive potassium channel (mK_{ATP}), which in turn is thought to promote tolerance against ischemia, *via* mechanisms that have not been completely elucidated [5].

Interestingly, preconditioning has been demonstrated to activate two temporally distinct biological phases of tolerance against ischemia [6, 7]. An initial transient cardioprotection (lasting 1–2 hours) following the preconditioning "trigger" (classical preconditioning) is thought to result from post-translational modification of signaling intermediates activated by the preconditioning [3]. A more prolonged cardioprotection (of 48–72 hours duration) can be activated by preconditioning and is referred to as delayed preconditioning or the "second window of protection" [8]. Delayed preconditioning is regulated at the transcriptional level with the synthesis of heretofore-undefined cytoprotective peptides.

Understanding the biologic programs orchestrating preconditioning would enable us to develop newer strategies to enhance myocardial tolerance against

Inflammation and Cardiac Diseases, edited by Giora Z. Feuerstein, Peter Libby and Douglas L. Mann
© 2003 Birkhäuser Verlag Basel/Switzerland

ischemic injury. Until recently, the role of the innate immune system in preconditioning had not been extensively explored. Interestingly, the pleiotropic cytokine TNF-α that is known to be an apical regulator of innate immunity, has been shown to be modestly elevated in the serum of rabbits and in mouse myocardium following ischemic preconditioning [9, 10]. Moreover, pharmacologic administration and endogenous production of TNF-α has induced preconditioning-like cardioprotection in rabbits, rats and mice [10–13]. Finally, using mice genetically deficient in TNF-α, we have demonstrated that this apical cytokine is required to induce the ischemic preconditioning [10]. In addition, numerous investigators have demonstrated that this cytokine can induce both classical [13, 14] and delayed preconditioning-like cardioprotection [11, 14]. Collectively these data suggest that TNF-α signaling could be an important regulator in preconditioning and may play an important role in promoting innate cardioprotection against cardiac ischemic injury.

Cytokine activation is usually a coordinated induction of numerous pro-inflammatory and anti-inflammatory cytokine cascades and hence TNF-α is unlikely to function in isolation. The induction of multiple cytokines in preconditioning has been recently reviewed [15] and will not be further explored here. Rather, the purpose of this chapter is to explore potentially novel signaling networks that can be induced by the activation of the innate immune system (including TNF-α) that may advance our understanding of the cardioprotective program of preconditioning. The pathways that will be explored include the possible role of TNF-α-mediated sphingolipid signaling [13, 16] in orchestrating preconditioning-like cardioprotection. In addition, putative sphingolipid signaling dependent and independent cytoprotective programs induced by TNF-α [15] are discussed. Figure 1 is a schematic representation of the scope of this chapter.

Sphingolipid signaling: A potential pathway for TNF-α induced cardioprotection

TNF-α is an apical pro-inflammatory cytokine, with a broad spectrum of properties, capable of inducing not only cell survival but also growth, inflammation and apoptosis [17]. These opposing actions are dependent not only upon the amount of TNF-α present, but the cell type involved and the time that the peptide is present [17, 18]. The intracellular signaling pathways involved in induction of cell growth, inflammation and death, with the exception of the sphingolipid signaling described, falls outside the scope of this chapter [19–22].

To date two TNF-α cognate cell surface receptors have been identified and are identified as TNF receptor 1 (TNFR1, or p55) and receptor 2 (TNFR2, p75) [23]. Binding of the inherently trimeric TNF-α to either of these cell surface receptors leads to receptor trimerization and the recruitment of several adaptor proteins to the cytoplasmic domains of the receptors. This then leads to the subsequent activation

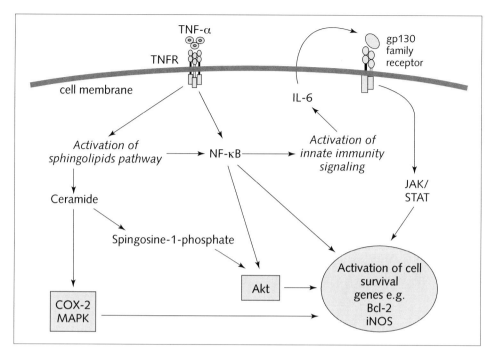

Figure 1
Schematic representation depicting the role of TNF-α signaling in ischemic preconditioning
The TNF-α activated signal transduction discussed in this chapter is shown. Representative cytoprotective signaling molecules are shown in the square boxes and cell-survival promoting proteins are shown in the oval box. Abbreviations: TNFR, tumor necrosis alpha receptor; COX-2, cyclo-oxygenase 2; MAPK, mitogen activated protein kinases; gp130, glycoprotein 130 receptor; IL-6, interleukin 6; JAK, Janus kinase; STAT, signal transduction and activators of transcription; iNOS, inducible nitric oxide synthase.

of numerous signal transduction pathways [17]. TNF-α mediated sphingolipid signaling has only recently been postulated to contribute to the cell survival program activated by preconditioning [13] and this pathway will be explored in the first section of this chapter.

TNF-α activates the sphingolipids pathway

Sphingolipids are a diverse family of phospholipids and glycolipids built upon a long chain sphingoid backbone, generally sphingosine. Over the last few years, many studies provided evidence implicating the sphingolipid ceramide as a second

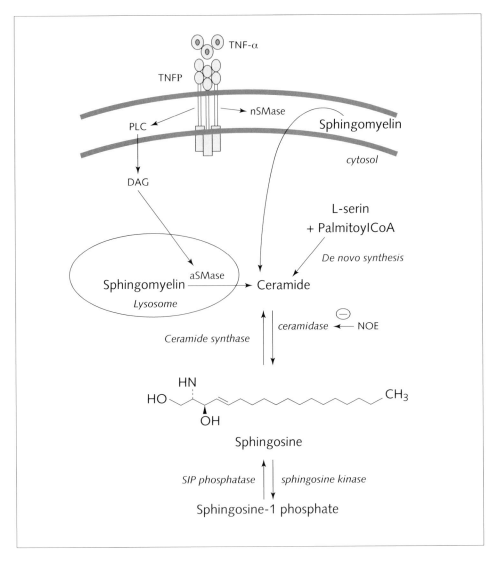

Figure 2

Schematic representation of sphingolipid pathway following TNF-α binding on to its receptor TNF-α binding to its receptors leads to activation of either aSMAse or nSMASE to form ceramide from sphingomyelin. In the presence of ceramidase, ceramide will form sphingosine. In turn, sphingosine kinase generates the signaling intermediate sphingosine-1 phosphate. NOE inhibits the pathway by inhibition of the enzyme ceramidase.

Abbreviations: PLC, phospholipase C; DAG, diacylglycerol; nSMASE, neutral sphingomyelinase; aSMASE, acid sphingomyelinase; NOE, N-oleyl ethanolamine; S1P phosphatase, sphingosine-1-phosphate phosphatase.

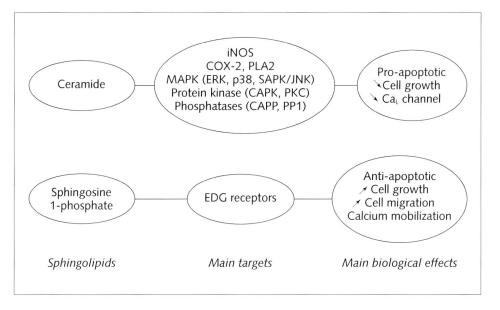

Figure 3
Main targets and biological effects of ceramide and sphingosine-1 phosphate
Abbreviations: iNOS, inducible nitric oxide synthase; COX-2, cyclo-oxygenase 2; PLA2, phospholipase A2; MAPK, mitogen activated protein kinase; CAPK, ceramide activated protein kinase; PKC, protein kinase C; CAPP, ceramidase activated protein phosphatase; PP1, protein phosphatase 1.

messenger in multiple signaling pathways initiated on binding of TNF-α to its TNFR1/p55 receptor [24–26]. A schematic of sphingolipid biochemistry is shown as Figure 2. In brief, ceramides are formed from sphingomyelin *via* two distinct sphingomyelinases, an endosomal acid sphingomyelinase (A-SMase) and a membrane-bound neutral sphingomyelinase (N-SMase) which are present in independent sub-cellular sites [25].

Ceramide, by the action of the enzyme ceramidase, forms sphingosine which in turn can be recycled back to ceramide in the presence of ceramide synthase or forms sphingosine-1-phosphate in the presence of sphingosine kinase (Fig. 3). Of note, *de novo* ceramide biosynthesis from L-serine and palmitoyl CoA catalyzed by the action of serine-palmitoyl transferase and the activation of ceramide synthase, presents an alternative means of generating a signaling pool of ceramide that can also been stimulated by TNF-α. However, it has been speculated that this *de novo* synthesis pathway is more likely involved in long-term effects whereas short-term exposure to TNF induces acute ceramide generation by A-SMase [27].

Main sphingolipids targets

Recent studies have begun to identify key direct targets for sphingolipids action but most of the direct sphingolipid targets remain unknown. However, the pleiotropic effects ascribed to the two major actors within the sphingolipid pathway, namely ceramide and sphingosine-1-phosphate suggest that these two sphingolipids have different downstream cellular biologic targets (Fig. 3).

The most prominent early event after ceramide stimulation is the activation of the mitogen-activated protein kinase (MAPK) cascade, including the SAPK/JNK subfamily, the p38/MAPK subfamily and the ERK/MAPK cascade [28]. Ceramide also up-regulates cyclooxygenase-2 [29] and phospholipase A2 [30] enzymes critically involved in an inflammatory reaction, as well as the inducible nitric oxide synthase [31]. Ceramide, in addition, activates many different proteases including caspases, a family of cysteine proteases involved in the apoptotic pathway such as calpain, a calcium-activated cysteine protease [32] and the metalloproteinases [33]. Additional targets of ceramide includes cytosolic phosphatases, known as the ceramidase activated protein phosphatase (CAPP), protein phosphatase 1 (PP1) and protein kinases such as ceramide activated protein kinase (CAPK), c-Raf and protein kinase C-α,-β or -ζ isoenzymes [34–38].

With regard to sphingosine-1-phosphate, most of its effects are acting *via* the Endothelial Differentiation Gene (EDG) family of G protein-coupled receptors [39]. The sphingosine-1-phosphate sensitive EDG family now includes at least five different isoforms, EDG-1,-3,-5,-6 and 8. While a role for EDG1 has been suggested in cytoskeletal remodeling and motility of endothelial cells, EDG3 and 5 would play a role in cell migration and differentiation. Little is known concerning EDG6 and 8.

Biological effects of sphingolipids

Apoptosis

Ceramide generated either by degradation of sphingomyelin or *de novo* synthesis is thought to trigger apoptosis in many different cell systems. Obeid et al. were the first to show that an exogenously added cell permeable ceramide analog, N-acetyl-sphingosine (c2 ceramide), mimicked TNF-α-induced cell death in promyeloid U937 cell [40]. Several mechanisms by which ceramide triggers apoptosis have been proposed, including an activation of caspases, down-regulation of PI3 kinase activity and Akt which then would decrease phosphorylation of the anti-apoptotic factor Bcl-2 [41]. Ceramide could also promote cell death by direct dephosphorylation of Bcl-2 [42] or by the direct inhibition of the complex III of the mitochondrial respiratory chain [43].

Interestingly, recent data suggests that sphingosine-1-phosphate coupling to its cognate EDG receptors promote cell survival effects and that EDG independent effects of sphingosine-1-phosphate can also promote apoptosis [44].

Cell growth

Addition of sphingolipids to the cells was accompanied by an increased activity of MAPK, a key factor in cell proliferation [45]. Treatment with ceramide has been shown to inhibit cell growth, possibly *via* a decrease of the retinoblastoma protein content and an increase of p53 levels [46]. It has also been speculated that ceramide-induced growth cell arrest may be *via* down-regulation of c-myc [47]. Again, sphingosine-1-phosphate will exert an opposite effect to ceramide and can promote cell proliferation *via* coupling to its cognate cell-surface receptors. In the rat neonatal cardiomyocyte, sphingosine-1-phosphate induces hypertrophy *via* EDG1 receptor signaling [48].

Other biological effect of the sphingolipids

Sphingosine-1-phosphate has also been reported to play a key role in cell migration, possibly *via* activation of a G_i-coupled receptor, phospholipase C mediated calcium signaling and different factors that play a critical role for cell migration response such as rho and rac [49]. Sphingolipids may also play a crucial role in ion fluxes. In myocytes, sphingosine-1-phosphate enhances calcium mobilization possibly *via* the ryanodine receptor and inhibits inward sodium current while ceramide inhibits the L-type calcium channel current [49].

A role for sphingolipids in ischemia reperfusion

Levels of TNF-α and ceramide during ischemia-reperfusion

Myocardial TNF-α production has been well documented during acute myocardial ischemia with or without reperfusion [50, 51]. In classic ischemic preconditioning, the initial ischemic "trigger" or administration of endogenous preconditioning-mimetic adenosine has been shown to attenuate subsequent ischemia-mediated TNF-α production [9, 52] suggesting that a component of the preconditioning "trigger" modulates subsequent ischemia-reperfusion induced TNF-α production.

While Bielawska et al. used an *in vivo* ischemia-reperfusion model and reported an increase of myocardial ceramide during both ischemia and the reperfusion period, Zhang et al. recently found that myocardial ischemia did not alter tissue ceramide levels while myocardial ischemia followed by reperfusion significantly increased tissue ceramide levels [53, 54]. Interestingly, they also reported that this accumulation of ceramide in the reperfused myocardium was not associated with an enhancement of any SMase activity but an inhibition of the ceramidase. Hypoxia reoxygenation conducted in cultured rat cardiac myocytes showed a rapid activation of neutral SMase and accumulation of ceramide within few minutes [55].

All these studies report an increase of TNF-α or ceramide levels during ischemia and/or reperfusion ascribe these perturbations to the resultant cardiac contractile depression, myocyte apoptosis and myocardial structural abnormality associated with ischemia and reperfusion.

A cytoprotective role for TNF-α and ceramide

In our laboratory, we have demonstrated that exogenous TNF-α administration using a preconditioning-like protocol in the isolated perfused rat heart mimics classical ischemic preconditioning and has both an infarct sparing effect and contributes toward improved post-ischemic functional recovery [13]. In order to evaluate the role of the sphingolipids in the cardioprotective effect of TNF-α, we used N-oleoyl ethanolamine (NOE), an inhibitor of the enzyme ceramidase, and demonstrated that NOE abolishes both the cytoprotective effects of TNF-α and that of ischemic preconditioning. Moreover, exogenous ceramide administration using a preconditioning-like protocol in the isolated perfused rat heart mimics classical ischemic preconditioning and this protective effect of ceramide is abolished by NOE. Collectively, these data strongly suggest a protective role of ceramide *via* sphingosine/sphingosine-1-phosphate signaling. Interestingly, our work correlates with other findings described in the central nervous system [56]. Here, Hallenbeck's group reported that hypoxic preconditioning protects cultured neurons against hypoxic stress *via* TNF-α and ceramide [56]. These investigators have also shown that exogenous administration of ceramide reduces infarct size after focal cerebral ischemia [57].

A role for sphingosine-1-phosphate in ischemia-reperfusion has also been explored. Karliner et al. reported that sphingosine-1-phosphate could enhance survival during hypoxia in neonatal rat cardiac myocytes and in the mouse heart through cellular membranes receptors by signaling mechanisms involving protein kinase C and mitochondrial K_{ATP} channels [16, 58]. Moreover, we have confirmed that the administration of sphingosine-1-phosphate could mimic classical ischemic preconditioning and promotes an infarct sparing effect [13].

TNF-α-activated cell-survival signaling

Additional signaling cascades that may be dependent and or independent of sphingolipid signaling probably mediate TNF-α-activated cell survival signaling. In the second half of this chapter we explore the role of TNF-α-induced nuclear regulatory peptides that may orchestrate the preconditioning phenotype. We will discuss the potential role of TNF-α activation of the transcription factors nuclear factor κB (NF-κB) and activating protein-1 (AP-1) (Fig. 4) [59, 60].

We then discuss the activation of the known innate immunity mediator of cytoprotective, namely signal transducer and activator of transcription-3 (STAT3, Fig. 5).

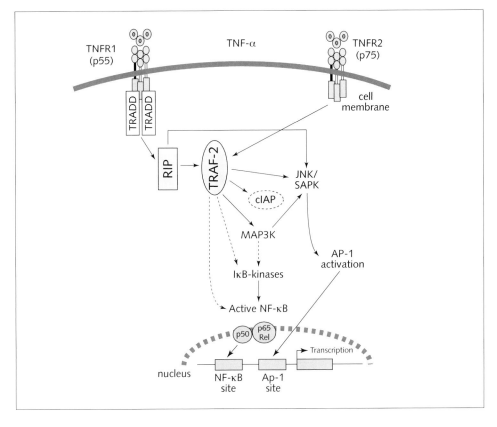

Figure 4
Schematic representation of the pathways involved in the activation of pro-survival genes by the pleiotropic cytokine TNF-α
TNF-α binding to TNFR1 leads to the recruitment of TRADD, RIP and TRAF-2. TRAF-2 and RIP lead to the activation of NF-κB and AP-1, through activation of the protein kinases JNK and IκB kinase. Abbreviations: TNFR1(p55), TNF-α receptor 1; TNFR2(p75), TNF-α receptor 2; TRADD, TNFR1 associated death domain; RIP, receptor interacting protein; TRAF-2, TNF-α receptor associated factor-2; cIAP, cellular inhibitor of apoptosis protein; JNK, c-Jun amino terminal kinases; SAPK, stress activated protein kinase; MAP3K, mitogen activated protein kinase kinase kinase.

NF-κB and AP-1 as a cell-survival target of TNF-α-signaling

NF-κB is a nuclear regulatory peptide responsible for induction of a multitude of genes [61]. It has been shown to be activated by a wide range of intermediates, including reactive oxygen species, hypoxia/anoxia, cytokines, protein kinase C acti-

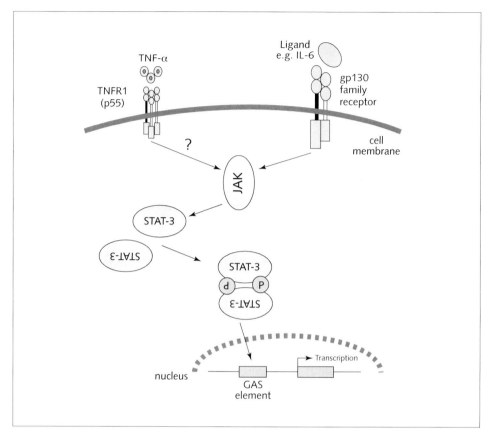

Figure 5
Pathways leading to STAT3 activation of pro-survival genes
TNFR1 activation leads to JAK activation and STAT3 phosphorylation and dimerization.
gp130 receptor activation leads to JAK recruitment and activation, and subsequent STAT3
phosphorylation and dimerization. The phosphorylated STAT3 dimer translocates to the
nucleus where it binds to GAS elements and activates numerous cell survival peptide encod-
ing genes. Abbreviations: TNFR1(p55), TNF-α receptor 1; JAK, Janus kinase; GAS element,
γ-interferon activation site.

vators, mitogen-activated protein kinase activators, bacterial and viral products and UV radiation [62–65]. NF-κB activation is associated with classical and delayed pre-conditioning and pharmacological inhibition of NF-κB activation, in turn, abolish-es these cardioprotective effects [66, 67].

Activation of NF-κB, by the ubiquination of its cytosolic chaperone IκB and the subsequent proteolytic degradation of IκB leads to transfer of the NF-κB complex to the nucleus where it can activate target genes involved in both apoptosis and survival (Fig. 4) [61]. Genes activated by NF-κB that could play a role in promoting cell survival in the setting of preconditioning include:

1. inhibitor of apoptosis protein-1 (IAP-1) [68]
2. X-linked inhibitor of apoptosis protein (XIAP) [69]
3. Bcl-2 [70]
4. manganese superoxide dismutase [71]
5. the inducible isoform of cyclo-oxygenase [72], and
6. inducible nitric oxide synthase [73].

To date the only firmly established candidate peptides that have been validated to be important in the promoting the ischemia-tolerant phenotype of preconditioning include manganese superoxide dismutase, cyclo-oxygenase 2 and inducible nitric oxide synthase [71–73]. In addition NF-κB has also been shown to activate Akt [74], a known cardioprotective signaling kinase [75, 76]. Finally, NF-κB is a pivotal regulatory peptide in the innate immune system and it is known to induce a multitude of pro-inflammatory cytokines (including IL-1β, IL-6 and TNF-α itself) [77, 78] and the anti-inflammatory cytokine interleukin-10 (IL-10) [77]. The role of the innate immune system in promoting cardioprotection has recently been reviewed [15]. Here, the role of TNF-α in activating a potential cardiac survival promoting peptide *via* innate immunity signaling, namely STAT3 will be expanded on later in this chapter.

AP-1 is a heterogeneous collection of dimeric transcription factors, comprising jun, fos and ATF subunits. The activity of the AP-1 complex is regulated by multiple mechanisms, which play a role in cell survival [60]. AP-1 target genes include key cell cycle regulatory proteins (for example Cyclin D1, p21[cip1/waf1], p19[ARF] and p16) and the tumor suppressor protein p53 [79]. The role of AP-1 transactivation cell survival proteins have not been explored in the context of preconditioning, but will probably prove relevant to the generation of this ischemia-tolerant phenotype.

TNF-α activation of STAT3

STAT3 is a member of a unique family of transcription factors with seven known members (STAT1, STAT2, STAT3, STAT4, STAT5A, STAT5B and STAT6), which have been shown to play a critical role in the regulation of multiple genes [80]. Upon recruitment to the receptor signaling complex, STATs are tyrosine phosphorylated by Janus kinases (JAKs). This tyrosine phosphorylation facilitates hetero- or homo-dimerization of STATS, which then translocate to the nucleus and bind to γ-interferon activation site (GAS) motifs, leading to gene transcription (Fig. 5) [80].

There are two possible mechanisms leading to STAT3 activation by TNF-α (Fig. 5). The first results from TNF-α binding to TNFR1. The mechanisms responsible for TNF-α-TNFR1 interaction induced STAT3 activation has not been fully delineated to date, but is thought to involve the Janus kinases JAK1, JAK2 and TYK2 [81]. The second possible mechanism for TNF-α induced activation of STAT3 is due to the function of TNF-α as an apical cytokine. Here TNF-α is known to induce JAK/STAT activating cytokines (including the gp130 receptor family of cytokines such as IL-6) *via* the regulatory kinase – transforming growth factor associated kinase (TAK1) [82, 83].

The glycoprotein 130 (gp130) receptor family of cytokines is a family of cytokines known to be activated by TNF-α [83, 84]. Three members of the gp130 family are produced in the heart, namely leukemia inhibitory factor (LIF), IL-6 and cardiotrophin-1 (CT-1) [85, 86]. These cytokines bind to their own ligand-specific cognate receptor. The ligand-receptor complex then interacts with gp130, a cell surface signaling receptor, which then signal numerous intracellular pathways [87]. Following the activation of gp130, by the cytokine-receptor complex, the gp130 undergoes homo- or hetero-dimerization. Although gp130 and its dimerizing partner possess no intrinsic tyrosine kinase domain, associated cytoplasmic tyrosine kinases are activated, allowing subsequent modification of transcription factors [87]. The downstream pathways activated by the gp130 complex include the JAKs and several members of the STAT family [80, 88–90]. In addition, gp130 signaling is known to activate signaling intermediates that promote cell survival such as the src family of tyrosine kinases, ras, mitogen activated protein kinases (MAPK) and phosphatidylinositol 3-kinase (PI-3 kinase) [91].

Evidence for the involvement in STAT3 in cardioprotection has recently emerged. Experimental studies have shown that pharmacological inhibition of JAK1 and JAK2 abolishes the late phase of preconditioning [92]. Moreover, inhibition of JAK1 can abolish the early phase of preconditioning, and is associated with the diminution of the pro-survival mitochondrial peptide Bcl-2 [93]. Interestingly, STAT3 has also been shown to be necessary for gp-130 cytokine mediated cell survival in neuronal cells [94].

Summary and conclusions

Distinct and divergent temporal and dose effects of cytokines has been well established [17]. The data presented in this chapter support this paradigm, in that the known cytotoxic cytokine TNF-α appears to induce the preconditioning phenotype. In parallel and through as yet undefined mechanisms, the preconditioning program attenuates the subsequent robust (deleterious) production of TNF-α during a subsequent ischemia and reperfusion insult. The mechanisms whereby TNF-α activates the ischemia-tolerant phenotype of preconditioning has not been extensively explored. However, numerous cytoprotective programs have been described in this chapter that warrants investigation. The novel aspects of TNF-α signaling, namely the activation of sphingolipid signaling and the induction of downstream innate immunity orchestrated cellular events have been highlighted in this review. More specifically, the relatively new concept that ceramide and sphingosine-1-phosphate signaling may play a role in cardioprotection is described. In addition, the role of NF-κB, AP-1 and STAT3 in conferring cell-survival benefit in other biological systems need to be further explored in the heart to evaluate if these programs play a role in activating innate cardioprotection.

References

1   Yellon DM, Alkhulaifi AM, Pugsley WB (1993) Preconditioning the human myocardium. *Lancet* 342: 276–277

2   Tomai, F, Crea F, Chiariello L, Gioffre PA (1999) Ischemic preconditioning in humans: Models, mediators, and clinical relevance. *Circulation* 100: 559–563

3   Nakano A, Cohen MV, Downey JM (2000) Ischemic preconditioning: From basic mechanisms to clinical applications. *Pharmacol Ther* 86: 263–275

4   Schulz R, Cohen MV, Behrends M, Downey JM, Heusch G (2001) Signal transduction of ischemic preconditioning. *Cardiovasc Res* 52: 181–189

5   Oldenburg O, Cohen MV, Yellon DM, Downey JM (2002) Mitochondrial K_{ATP} channels: Role in cardioprotection. *Cardiovasc Res* 55: 429–437

6   Murry CE, Jennings RB, Reimer KA (1986) Preconditioning with ischemia: A delay of lethal cell injury in ischemic myocardium. *Circulation* 74: 1124–1136

7   Marber MS, Latchman DS, Walker JM, Yellon DM (1993) Cardiac stress protein elevation 24 hours after brief ischemia or heat stress is associated with resistance to myocardial infarction. *Circulation* 88: 1264–1272

8   Bolli R (2000) The late phase of preconditioning. *Circ Res* 87: 972–983

9   Belosjorow S, Schultz R, Dorge H, Schade FU, Heusch G (1999) Endotoxin and ischemic preconditioning: TNF-α concentration and myocardial infarct development in rabbits. *Am J Physiol* 277: H2470–H2475

10 Smith RM, Suleman N, Mccarthy J, Sack MN (2002) Classic ischemic but not pharmacologic preconditioning is abrogated following genetic ablation of the TNFα gene. *Cardiovasc Res* 55: 553–560

11 Nelson SK, Wong GH, Mccord J.M (1995) Leukemia inhibitory factor and tumor necrosis factor induce manganese superoxide dismutase and protect rabbit hearts from reperfusion injury. *J Mol Cell Cardiol* 27: 223–229

12 Yamashita N, Hoshida S, Otsu K, Taniguchi N, Kuzuya T, Hori M (2000) The involvement of cytokines in the second window of ischaemic preconditioning. *Br J Pharmacol* 131: 415–422

13 Lecour S, Smith RM, Woodward B, Opie LH, Rochette L, Sack MN (2002) Identifica-

tion of a novel role for sphingolipid signaling in TNF alpha and ischemic preconditioning mediated cardioprotection. *J Mol Cell Cardiol* 34: 509–518

14   Hoshida S, Yamashita N, Otsu K, Hori M (2002) Repeated physiologic stresses provide persistent cardioprotection against ischemia-reperfusion injury in rats. *J Am Coll Cardiol* 40: 826

15   Smith RM, Lecour L, Sack MN (2002) Innate immunity and cardiac protection: A putative intrinsic cardioprotective program. *Cardiovasc Res* 474–482

16   Jin ZQ, Zhou HZ, Zhu P, Honbo N, Mochly-Rosen D, Messing RO, Goetzl EJ, Karliner JS, Gray MO (2002) Cardioprotection mediated by sphingosine-1-phosphate and ganglioside GM-1 in wild-type and PKC epsilon knockout mouse hearts. *Am J Physiol Heart Circ Physiol* 282: H1970–H1977

17   Sack MN (2002) TNFa in cardiovascular biology and the potential role for anti-TNFα therapy in heart disease. *Pharmacol Therap* 94: 123–135

18   Sack MN, Smith RM, Opie LH (2000) Tumor necrosis factor in myocardial hypertrophy and ischaemia: An anti-apoptotic perspective. *Cardiovasc Res* 45: 688–695

19   Wallach D (1997) Cell death induction by TNF: A matter of self control. *TIBS* 22: 107–109

20   Beyaert R, Van LG, Heyninck K, Vandenabeele P (2002) Signaling to gene activation and cell death by tumor necrosis factor receptors and Fas. *Int Rev Cytol* 214: 225–72

21   Yokoyama T, Nakano M, Bednarczyk JL, Mcintyre BW, Entman M, Mann DL (1997) Tumor necrosis factor-α provokes a hypertrophic growth response in adult cardiac myocytes. *Circulation* 95: 1247–1252

22   Hanada T, Yoshimura A (2002) Regulation of cytokine signaling and inflammation. *Cytokine Growth Factor Rev* 13: 413

23   Baxter GT, Kuo RC, Jupp OJ, Vandenabeele P, Macewan DJ (1999) Tumor necrosis factor-a mediates both apoptotic cell death and cell proliferation in a human hematopoietic cell line dependent on mitotic activity and receptor subtype expression. *J Biol Chem* 274: 9539–9547

24   Schutze S, Machleidt T, Kronke M (1994) The role of diacylglycerol and ceramide in tumor necrosis factor and interleukin-1 signal transduction. *J Leukoc Biol* 56: 533–41

25   Wiegmann K, Schutze S, Machleidt T, Witte D, Kronke M (1994) Functional dichotomy of neutral and acidic sphingomyelinases in tumor necrosis factor signaling. *Cell* 78: 1005–1015

26   Adam D, Wiegmann K, Adam-Klages S, Ruff A, Kronke M (1996) A novel cytoplasmic domain of the p55 tumor necrosis factor receptor initiates the neutral sphingomyelinase pathway. *J Biol Chem* 271: 14617–22

27   Corda S, Laplace C, Vicaut E, Duranteau J (2001) Rapid reactive oxygen species production by mitochondria in endothelial cells exposed to tumor necrosis factor-alpha is mediated by ceramide. *Am J Respir Cell Mol Biol* 24: 762–768

28   Huwiler A, Kolter T, Pfeilschifter J, Sandhoff K (2000) Physiology and pathophysiology of sphingolipid metabolism and signaling. *Biochim Biophys Acta* 1485: 63–99

29   Subbaramaiah K, Chung WJ, Dannenberg AJ (1998) Ceramide regulates the transcrip-

tion of cyclooxygenase-2. Evidence for involvement of extracellular signal-regulated kinase/c-Jun N-terminal kinase and p38 mitogen-activated protein kinase pathways. *J Biol Chem* 273: 32943–32949

30 Hayakawa M, Jayadev S, Tsujimoto M, Hannun YA, Ito F (1996) Role of ceramide in stimulation of the transcription of cytosolic phospholipase A2 and cyclooxygenase 2. *Biochem Biophys Res Commun* 220: 681–6

31 Pahan K, Sheikh FG, Namboodiri AM, Singh I (1998) Inhibitors of protein phosphatase 1 and 2A differentially regulate the expression of inducible nitric-oxide synthase in rat astrocytes and macrophages. *J Biol Chem* 273: 12219–12226

32 Xie H, Johnson GV (1997) Ceramide selectively decreases tau levels in differentiated PC12 cells through modulation of calpain I. *J Neurochem* 69: 1020–1030

33 Reunanen N, Westermarck J, Hakkinen L, Holmstrom TH, Elo I, Eriksson JE, Kahari VM (1998) Enhancement of fibroblast collagenase (matrix metalloproteinase-1) gene expression by ceramide is mediated by extracellular signal-regulated and stress-activated protein kinase pathways. *J Biol Chem* 273: 5137–5145

34 Dobrowsky RT, Hannun YA (1992) Ceramide stimulates a cytosolic protein phosphatase. *J Biol Chem* 267: 5048–5051

35 Mathias S, Dressler KA, Kolesnick RN (1991) Characterization of a ceramide-activated protein kinase: Stimulation by tumor necrosis factor alpha. *Proc Natl Acad Sci USA* 88: 10009–10013

36 Muller G, Ayoub M, Storz P, Rennecke J, Fabbro D, Pfizenmaier K (1995) PKC zeta is a molecular switch in signal transduction of TNF-alpha, bifunctionally regulated by ceramide and arachidonic acid. *Embo J* 14: 1961–1969

37 Huwiler A, Brunner J, Hummel R, Vervoordeldonk M, Stabel S, Van Den Bosch H, Pfeilschifter J (1996) Ceramide-binding and activation defines protein kinase c-Raf as a ceramide-activated protein kinase. *Proc Natl Acad Sci USA* 93: 6959–6963

38 Huwiler A, Fabbro D, Pfeilschifter J (1998) Selective ceramide binding to protein kinase C-alpha and-delta isoenzymes in renal mesangial cells. *Biochemistry* 37: 14556–14562

39 Fukushima N, Ishii I, Contos JJ, Weiner JA, Chun J (2001) Lysophospholipid receptors. *Annu Rev Pharmacol Toxicol* 41: 507–534

40 Obeid LM, Linardic CM, Karolak LA, Hannun YA (1993) Programmed cell death induced by ceramide. *Science* 259: 1769–71

41 Zundel W, Giaccia A (1998) Inhibition of the anti-apoptotic PI(3)K/Akt/Bad pathway by stress. *Genes Dev* 12: 1941–1946

42 Ruvolo PP, Deng X, Ito T, Carr BK, May WS (1999) Ceramide induces Bcl2 dephosphorylation *via* a mechanism involving mitochondrial PP2A. *J Biol Chem* 274: 20296–20300

43 Gudz TI, Tserng KY, Hoppel CL (1997) Direct inhibition of mitochondrial respiratory chain complex III by cell-permeable ceramide. *J Biol Chem* 272: 24154–24158

44 Davaille J, Li L, Mallat A, Lotersztajn S (2002) Sphingosine 1-phosphate triggers both apoptotic and survival signals for human hepatic myofibroblasts. *J Biol Chem* 277: 37323–37330

45 Auge N, Escargueil-Blanc I, Lajoie-Mazenc I, Suc I, Andrieu-Abadie N, Pieraggi MT, Chatelut M, Thiers JC, Jaffrezou JP, Laurent G et al (1998) Potential role for ceramide in mitogen-activated protein kinase activation and proliferation of vascular smooth muscle cells induced by oxidized low density lipoprotein. *J Biol Chem* 273: 12893–12900

46 Lopez-Marure R, Ventura JL, Sanchez L, Montano LF, Zentella A (2000) Ceramide mimics tumour necrosis factor-alpha in the induction of cell cycle arrest in endothelial cells. Induction of the tumour suppressor p53 with decrease in retinoblastoma/protein levels. *Eur J Biochem* 267: 4325–4333

47 Flamigni F, Faenza I, Marmiroli S, Stanic I, Giaccari A, Muscari C, Stefanelli C, Rossoni C (1997) Inhibition of the expression of ornithine decarboxylase and c-Myc by cell-permeant ceramide in difluoromethylornithine-resistant leukaemia cells. *Biochem J* 324: 783–789

48 Robert P, Tsui P, Laville MP, Livi GP, Sarau HM, Bril A, Berrebi-Bertrand I (2001) EDG1 receptor stimulation leads to cardiac hypertrophy in rat neonatal myocytes. *J Mol Cell Cardiol* 33: 1589–1606

49 Levade T, Auge N, Veldman RJ, Cuvillier O, Negre-Salvayre A, Salvayre R (2001) Sphingolipid mediators in cardiovascular cell biology and pathology. *Circ Res* 89: 957–968

50 Irwin MW, Mak S, Mann DL, Qu R, Penninger JM, Yan A, Dawood F, Wen WH, Shou Z, Liu P (1999) Tissue expression and immunolocalization of tumor necrosis factor-α in postinfarction dysfunctional myocardium. *Circulation* 99: 1492–1498

51 Meldrum DR, Meng X, Dinarello CA, Ayala A, Cain BS, Shames BD, Ao L, Banerjee A, Harken AH (1998) Human myocardial tissue TNFα expression following acute global ischemia *in vivo*. *J Mol Cell Cardiol* 30: 1683–1689

52 Meldrum DR, Dinarello CA, Shames BD, Cleveland JC, Cain BS, Banerjee A, Meng X, Harken AH (1998) Ischemic preconditioning decreases postischemic myocardial tumor necrosis factor-a production. Potential ultimate effector mechanisms of preconditioning. *Circulation* 98: II-214–II-219

53 Bielawska AE, Shapiro JP, Jiang L, Melkonyan HS, Piot C, Wolfe CL, Tomei LD, Hannun YA, Umansky SR (1997) Ceramide is involved in triggering of cardiomyocyte apoptosis induced by ischemia and reperfusion. *Am J Pathol* 151: 1257–1263

54 Zhang DX, Fryer RM, Hsu AK, Zou AP, Gross GJ, Campbell WB, Li PL (2001) Production and metabolism of ceramide in normal and ischemic-reperfused myocardium of rats. *Basic Res Cardiol* 96: 267–274

55 Hernandez OM, Discher DJ, Bishopric NH, Webster KA (2000) Rapid activation of neutral sphingomyelinase by hypoxia-reoxygenation of cardiac myocytes. *Circ Res* 86: 198–204

56 Liu J, Ginis I, Spatz M, Hallenbeck JM (2000) Hypoxic preconditioning protects cultured neurons against hypoxic stress *via* TNF-alpha and ceramide. *Am J Physiol Cell Physiol* 278: C144–C153

57 Furuya K, Ginis I, Takeda H, Chen Y, Hallenbeck JM (2001) Cell permeable exogenous

ceramide reduces infarct size in spontaneously hypertensive rats supporting *in vitro* studies that have implicated ceramide in induction of tolerance to ischemia. *J Cereb Blood Flow Metab* 21: 226–232

58   Karliner JS, Honbo, N, Summers K, Gray MO, Goetzl EJ (2001) The lysophospholipids sphingosine-1-phosphate and lysophosphatidic acid enhance survival during hypoxia in neonatal rat cardiac myocytes. *J Mol Cell Cardiol* 33: 1713–1717

59   Westwick JK, Weitzel C, Minden A, Karin M, Brenner DA (1994) Tumor necrosis factor alpha stimulates AP-1 activity through prolonged activation of the c-Jun kinase. *J Biol Chem* 269: 26396–26401

60   Baud V, Karin M (2001) Signal transduction by tumor necrosis factor and its relatives. *Trends Cell Biol* 11: 372–377

61   Valen G, Yan ZQ, Hansson GK (2001) Nuclear factor kappa-B and the heart. *J Am Coll Cardiol* 38: 307–314

62   Barnes PJ, Adcock IM (1997) NF-kappa-B: a pivotal role in asthma and a new target for therapy. *Trends Pharmacol Sci* 18: 46–50

63   Ghosh S, May MJ, Kopp EB (1998) NF-kappa-B and Rel proteins: Evolutionarily conserved mediators of immune responses. *Annu Rev Immunol* 16: 225–260

64   Li N, Karin M (1998) Ionizing radiation and short wavelength UV activate NF-kappaB through two distinct mechanisms. *Proc Natl Acad Sci USA* 95: 13012–13017

65   Li N, Karin M (2000) Signaling pathways leading to nuclear factor-kappa B activation. *Methods Enzymol* 319: 273–279

66   Xuan YT, Tang XL, Banerjee,S, Takano H, Li R, Han H, QiuY, Li JJ, Bolli R (1999) Nuclear factor-kappaB plays an essential role in the late phase of ischemic preconditioning in conscious rabbits. *Circ Res* 84: 1095–1109

67   Maulik, N, Sato M, Price BD, Das DK (1998) An essential role of NFkappa-B in tyrosine kinase signaling of p38 MAP kinase regulation of myocardial adaptation to ischemia. *FEBS Lett* 429: 365–369

68   Erl W, Hansson GK, De Martin R, Draude G, Weber KS, Weber C (1999) Nuclear factor-kappa-B regulates induction of apoptosis and inhibitor of apoptosis protein-1 expression in vascular smooth muscle cells. *Circ Res* 84: 668–677

69   Stehlik C, De Martin, R, Kumabashiri I, Schmid JA, Binder BR, Lipp J (1998) Nuclear factor (NF)-kappa-B-regulated X-chromosome-linked iap gene expression protects endothelial cells from tumor necrosis factor alpha-induced apoptosis. *J Exp Med* 188: 211–216

70   Maulik N, Goswami S, Galang N, Das DK (1999) Differential regulation of Bcl-2, AP-1 and NF-kappaB on cardiomyocyte apoptosis during myocardial ischemic stress adaptation. *FEBS Lett* 443: 331–336

71   Dana A, Jonassen AK, Yamashita N, Yellon DM. (2000) Adenosine A(1) receptor activation induces delayed preconditioning in rats mediated by manganese superoxide dismutase. *Circulation* 101: 2841–2848

72   Shinmura K, Tang XL, Wang Y, Xuan YT, Liu SQ, Takano H, Bhatnagar A, Bolli R (2000) Cyclooxygenase-2 mediates the cardioprotective effects of the late phase of

ischemic preconditioning in conscious rabbits. *Proc Natl Acad Sci USA* 97: 10197–10202

73   GuoY, Jones WK, Xuan YT, Tang XL, Bao W, Wu WJ, Han H, Laubach VE, Ping P, Yang Z et al (1999) The late phase of ischemic preconditioning is abrogated by targeted disruption of the inducible NO synthase gene. *Proc Natl Acad Sci USA* 96: 11507–11512

74   Meng F, Liu L, Chin PC, D'Mello SR (2002) Akt is a downstream target of NF-kappa-B. *J Biol Chem* 277: 29674–29680

75   Fujio Y, Nguyen T, Wencker D, Kitsis RN, Walsh K (2000) Akt promotes survival of cardiomyocytes *in vitro* and protects against ischemia-reperfusion injury in mouse heart. *Circulation* 101: 660–667

76   Jonassen AK, Sack MN, Mjos OD,Yellon DM (2001) Myocardial protection by insulin at reperfusion requires early administration and is mediated *via* Akt and p70s6 kinase cell-survival signaling. *Circ Res* 89: 1191–1198

77   Haddad JJ (2002) recombinant TNF-alpha mediated regulation of the Ikappa-B-alpha/NF-kappa-B signaling pathway: Evidence for the enhancement of pro- and anti-inflammatory cytokines in alveolar epithelial cells. *Cytokine* 17: 301–310

78   Baldwin AS, Jr (2001) Series introduction: the transcription factor NF-kappaB and human disease. *J Clin Invest* 107: 3–6

79   Shaulian E,.Karin M. (2001) AP-1 in cell proliferation and survival. *Oncogene* 20: 2390–2400

80   Levy DE , Darnell JE (2002) Signalling: Stats: Transcriptional control and biological impact. *Nat Rev Mol Cell Biol* 3: 651–662

81   Guo D, Dunbar JD, Yang CH, Pfeffer LM, Donner DB (1998) Induction of Jak/STAT signaling by activation of the type 1 TNF receptor. *J Immunol* 160: 2742–2750

82   Sakurai H, Miyoshi H, Toriumi W, Sugita T (1999) Functional interactions of transforming growth factor beta-activated kinase 1 with Ikappa-B kinases to stimulate NF-kappaB activation. *J Biol Chem* 274: 10641–10648

83   Craig R, Larkin A, Mingo AM, Thuerauf DJ, Andrews C, Mcdonough PM, Glembotski CC (2000) p38 MAPK and NF-kappa-B collaborate to induce interleukin-6 gene expression and release. Evidence for a cytoprotective autocrine signaling pathway in a cardiac myocyte model system. *J Biol Chem* 275: 23814–23824

84   Gayle D, Ilyin SE, Romanovitch AE, Peloso E, Satinoff E, Plata-Salaman CR (1999) Basal and IL-1beta-stimulated cytokine and neuropeptide mRNA expression in brain regions of young and old Long-Evans rats. *Brain Res Mol Brain Res* 70: 92–100

85   Eiken HG, Oie E, Damas JK, Yndestad A, Bjerkeli V, Aass H, Simonsen S, Geiran OR, Tonnessen T, Christensen G et al (2001) Myocardial gene expression of leukaemia inhibitory factor, interleukin-6 and glycoprotein 130 in end-stage human heart failure. *Eur J Clin Invest* 31: 389–397

86   Sheng Z, Pennica D, Wood WI, Chien KR (1996) Cardiotrophin-1 displays early expression in the murine heart tube and promotes cardiac myocyte survival. *Development* 122: 419–428

87   Hirano T, Ishihara K, Hibi M (2000) Roles of STAT3 in mediating the cell growth, differentiation and survival signals relayed through the IL-6 family of cytokine receptors. *Oncogene* 19: 2548–2556

88   Horvath CM, Darnell JE (1997) The state of the STATs: Recent developments in the study of signal transduction to the nucleus. *Curr Opin Cell Biol* 9: 233–239

89   Darnell JE Jr. (1997) STATs and gene regulation. *Science* 277: 1630–1635

90   Bromberg J, Darnell JE Jr. (2000) The role of STATs in transcriptional control and their impact on cellular function. *Oncogene* 19: 2468–73

91   Negoro S, Oh H, Tone E, Kunisada K, Fujio Y, Walsh K, Kishimoto T, Yamauchi-Takihara K (2001) Glycoprotein 130 regulates cardiac myocyte survival in doxorubicin-induced apoptosis through phosphatidylinositol 3-kinase/Akt phosphorylation and Bcl-xL/caspase-3 interaction. *Circulation* 103: 555–561

92   Xuan YT, Guo Y, Han H, Zhu Y, Bolli R (2001) An essential role of the JAK-STAT pathway in ischemic preconditioning. *Proc Natl Acad Sci USA* 98: 9050–9055

93   Hattori R, Maulik N, Otani H, Zhu L, Cordis G, Engelman RM, Siddiqui MAQ, Das DK (2001) Role of STAT3 in ischemic preconditioning. *J Mol Cell Cardiol* 33: 1929–1936

94   Alonzi T, Middleton G, Wyatt S, Buchman V, Betz UA, Muller W, Musiani P, Poli V, Davies AM (2001) Role of STAT3 and PI 3-kinase/Akt in mediating the survival actions of cytokines on sensory neurons. *Mol Cell Neurosci* 18: 270–282

Stress-activated signals and their role in myocardial ischemia

Masaya Tanno and Michael Marber

The Department of Cardiology, KCL, The Rayne Institute St Thomas' Hospital, London SE1 7EH, UK

Stress activated signalling cascades in myocardial ischemia

Mitogen activated protein kinase (MAPK) pathways are one of the major signal transduction mechanisms involved in cellular homeostasis. Many extracellular stimuli are converted into specific cellular responses through the activation of these serine/threonine protein kinases that can phosphorylate both cytoplasmic and nuclear targets (Fig. 1). Following the discovery of the p42/44 Extracellular signal-Regulated Kinases (ERKs), which are predominantly activated by mitogenic stimuli, other MAPK family members have been identified that are preferentially activated by cellular stresses. These include the c-jun N-terminal kinase/stress activated protein kinase (JNK/SAPK) and the p38 MAPK subfamilies.

The c-Jun N-terminal kinase/stress activated protein kinase (SAPK/JNK)

Historical view

Identification and cloning of JNK/SAPK started in 1990 when a 54-kDa protein activated by intraperitoneal injection of cycloheximide, a protein synthesis inhibitor, was identified [1]. This p54 kinase required concomitant phosphorylation of a Tyr and a Thr residue for activation, a necessity in common with the previously identified ERKs and was therefore termed stress-activated protein kinase (SAPK). Shortly after the discovery of SAPK, another laboratory demonstrated exposure of cells to ultraviolet radiation activated protein kinases of 46 and 54 kDa and called them c-jun N-terminal kinase (JNK) since they phosphorylated c-Jun [2]. In 1994 molecular cloning of these protein kinases revealed SAPK and JNK were identical and encoded by at least three genes: SAPK alpha/JNK2, SAPK beta/JNK3 and SAPK gamma/JNK1 [3, 4]. Alternative splicing further diversifies the expression of these SAPK genes.

Inflammation and Cardiac Diseases, edited by Giora Z. Feuerstein, Peter Libby and Douglas L. Mann
© 2003 Birkhäuser Verlag Basel/Switzerland

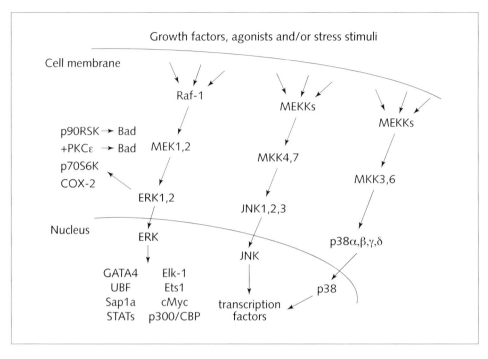

Figure 1
Simplified overview of the 3 most highly characterized MAPK signaling
pathways: ERKs, JNKs, and p38 kinases. Growth factors, agonists, and stress stimuli
facilitate MAPK activation through a network of cytoplasmic membrane bound receptors or
ill defined sensing factors that signal through G proteins to promote activation of MEKKs,
which in turn activate MEKs resulting in activation of ERKs, JNKs, or p38 kinases. On acti-
vation by phosphorylation, ERKs, JNKs, and p38s can translocate to the nucleus where they
phosphorylate mitogenic- or stress-responsive transcription factors (from [88]).

Structure

The defining motif of JNK is the sequence Thr-Pro-Tyr within the activation loop. In common with the other MAPKs, phosphorylation of two key residues (Thr and Tyr) in this motif activates this kinase. The crystal structure of unphosphorylated JNK3, a neuronal specific isoform, revealed the N- and C-terminal domains are rotated relative to their positions in cAMP-dependent protein kinase. This rotation leads to the misalignment of some of the catalytic residues. In addition, the phosphorylation lip of JNK3 partially blocks the substrate-binding site. These structural characteristics may account for the low activity of unphosphorylated JNK [5].

Substrate

SAPK/JNKs were originally identified by their ability to phosphorylate a transcription factor, c-Jun, on Ser 63 and Ser 73 within the N-terminal activation domain. Other physiological substrates for the SAPK/JNKs are the other transcription factors, Elk-1 and ATF-2, which are also substrates for p38-MAPK. These transcription factors, through formation of the activator-protein (AP-1) complex, have been implicated in various cellular processes [6]. AP-1 is a heterodimeric transcription factor typically comprised of c-Jun with c-Fos which in turn is induced by Elk-1, and ATF-2.

Biological functions

SAPK/JNKs mediate apoptosis in response to some stresses. Chemotherapeutic genotoxins (etoposide, tenoposide) or UV irradiation caused apoptosis in Jurkat cells coincident with the transcriptional induction of FasL and its expression on the cell surface [7]. This process is dependent on activation of SAPK/JNK and AP-1, suggesting genotoxic stresses induce apoptosis by FasL induction through activation of SAPK/JNK and AP-1. SAPK/JNKs also play a role in heat shock-dependent apoptosis [8]. Gene disruption studies have revealed JNK1/JNK2 play a pivotal role in appropriate apoptosis in early brain development. Disruption of *sapk-γ*/*sapk-α* allele (which encode JNK2 and 1, respectively) resulted in failure of closure of the hindbrain neural tube, which is an essential step in the process of cephalic neurulation and requires apoptosis [9].

JNK/SAPK in cardiac tissues

Naturally, cellular stresses such as hyperosmotic shock, protein synthesis inhibition (anisomycin), reactive oxygen species (ROS), pro-inflammatory cytokines (IL-1 and TNF), agonists of G protein coupled receptors (ET-1, phenylephrine and angiotensin II) and ischemia/reperfusion, activate JNK/SAPK in cultured cardiac myocytes and perfused hearts as well as in other tissues [10]. The biological consequences of JNK/SAPK activation in cardiac tissues are summarized below.

Cardiomyocyte hypertrophy

Cardiomyocyte hypertrophy is marked by cell enlargement, increased protein synthesis and the expression of embryonic genes such as atrial natriuretic factor. These changes eventually contribute to the contractile abnormalities resulting in clinical heart failure. At the cellular level, mechanical shear stress of cardiomyocytes induced by pressure overload, along with the release of the vasoactive peptides such as endothelin 1 (ET-1) and ANG II, cause the hypertrophy [6]. A Gq mediated pathway is essential for cardiac hypertrophy since mice lacking Gα-q and Gα-11, through which many G protein-coupled receptor agonists activate MAP kinase pathways, show no ventricular hypertrophy in response to pressure overload induced by aortic constriction [11]. Activation of pathways downstream to this G protein play a role in mediating the hypertrophic response to which JNKs contribute, at least in part, together with p42/44 MAPK, p38 MAPK, Akt and p70s6K [12].

Apoptosis

There are few studies indicating involvement of JNK/SAPKs in apoptosis in cardiac tissues. Most information is available for p38-MAPK. For example transfection experiments have implicated p38-alpha MAP kinase as a trigger for apoptosis both in cardiac myocytes [13] and *in vivo* hearts models [14] (and see below). However a recent report suggests not only p38, but also JNK/SAPKs, mediate apoptosis in cardiomyocytes subjected to ischemia/reoxygenation, whereas p42/44 MAP kinase plays a protective role [15].

Ischemia/reperfusion injury, ischemic preconditioning

In contrast to p38 MAPK, which is activated during ischemic injury and remains activated during reperfusion, JNK/SAPKs seem to be activated mainly upon reperfusion in isolated perfused rat hearts [16], although some studies indicate ischemia alone is sufficient to activate p46-JNK in the conscious rabbit [17], or both p46- and p56-JNK in perfused murine hearts (our unpublished data). A brief period of sublethal ischemia protects the heart against subsequent more severe ischemia (ischemic preconditioning). Because of its therapeutic potential, signal transduction pathways underlying the phenomenon of ischemic preconditioning have become a major focus of investigation. Unlike the p38 MAP kinase pathway, only a few studies suggest JNK has a role in cardioprotection [17–19].

The P38 MAP kinases

Historical view

p38 MAPK was originally identified in 1994 as a 38-kDa polypeptide phosphorylated on its Tyr residue in response to endotoxin exposure and osmotic shock [20].

Molecular cloning revealed similarities between p38 and HOG1, the yeast osmo-sensing MAPK [20]. Two independent groups also identified p38α as a kinase activated by IL-1β or physiologic stress which could activate MAPKAP kinase-2 and HSP25/27 phosphorylation [21]. Like other MAPKs, p38 is activated by dual Tyr/Thr phosphorylation in sub-domain VIII of the catalytic domain. p38α was also identified as a target for pyridinyl imidazole anti-inflammatory drugs (cytokine-suppressive anti-inflammatory drugs; CSAIDs). CSAIDs were originally identified as compounds that inhibit the transcriptional induction of TNF and IL-1 during endotoxin shock [22]. The underlying mechanism for the inhibition of inflammation by CSAIDs was their ability to bind and inhibit the catalytic activity of p38 MAPK [22]. As described below, not only is the production of inflammatory cytokines regulated by p38 MAPK, but they also in turn activate p38 MAPK, i.e., pro-inflammatory cytokines lie both upstream and downstream of p38 MAPK in an amplifying autocrine loop. Thus CSAIDs are expected to interrupt this vicious cycle. In addition to the originally identified isoform of p38 (p38α), another three isoforms have been identified and are termed p38β, γ, and δ.

Structure

All p38 isoforms share significant homology at the amino acid level and have a TGY motif in kinase sub-domain VIII [23–26]. More literature are available that describe the crystal structure of p38 MAPK than are available for JNK. p38 MAPK seems to be quite similar to JNK in terms of structure of the unphosphorylated form. The relative orientation of N- and C-terminal lobes of the inactive form of p38 MAPK is different from cAMP-dependent protein kinase, resulting in a relative misalignment of the active site of p38 MAPK to which they both contribute. In addition, the key TGY motif is located on a surface loop that occupies the peptide-binding channel [27]. These findings suggest, upon activation, the orientation of the domains/lobes and location of the surface loop would have to change for catalysis to proceed.

Substrates

Unlike SAPK/JNK, which have only been reported to phosphorylate transcription factors thus far, p38 MAPKs activate other protein kinases as well as transcription factors. MAP kinase-activated protein kinase 2 (MAPKAP-K2) was the first identified p38α substrate [21]. Subsequently, a closely related protein kinase, MAPKAPK-3 was also found to be a substrate of p38α [28]. Both activated MAPKAPK-2 and -3 phosphorylate various substrates including small heat shock protein HSP27 [29]. Transcription factors that have been shown to be phosphorylated by p38 include activating transcription factor-2 (ATF-2), CREB homologous protein (CHOP), myocyte enhancer factor 2C (MEF2C), MEF2A, nuclear factor of activated T cells 4 (NFAT4) and NFATc1 [30].

Biological functions

Inflammation

The p38 MAPK pathway plays an important role in inflammation by stimulating production of pro-inflammatory cytokines such as IL-1β, TNF and IL-6 [31] and inducing adhesion proteins such as VCAM-1 [32]. Several studies in murine models of inflammatory-related disease indicate that the p38-MAPK pathway is a therapeutic target since its inhibition by SB203580 can reduce mortality in a model of endotoxin-induced shock and inhibit the development of collagen-induced arthritis [33]. More relevant to the cardiovascular system the p38-MAPK pathway is also involved in the expression of iNOS [34] which, through high NO output, could play multiple roles including regulation of vasomotor tone, cell adhesion to the endothelium, inhibition of platelet aggregation and vascular smooth muscle cell proliferation [35].

Apoptosis

Numerous studies have shown the activation of p38 is associated with apoptosis initiated by a variety of stresses such as NGF withdrawal and Fas ligation [36, 37]. In cardiomyocytes, p38α and p38β seem to have different roles in apoptosis, since p38 alpha appears to induce apoptosis, whilst p38 beta enhances survival [13, 38].

Cell cycle

The p38 MAPK activated by Cdc42Hs, a Rho family G protein, are required for the transition of quiescent fibroblasts in G_0, into the G_1 phase of the cell cycle [6]. Counterintuitively, in fibroblasts already in G_1 the same signal seems to contribute to the cell cycle inhibition [6].

P38 MAPK in cardiac tissues

Like JNK/SAPK, the p38 MAPKs have been reported to be activated by ROS, hypoxia/reoxygenation, hyperosmotic shock and pro-inflammatory cytokines and ischemia/reperfusion in cardiac myocytes *in vivo* and isolated perfused hearts [10].

The biological responses to activation of the p38 MAPK are involved in a number of pathophysiological processes.

Cardiomyocyte hypertrophy, apoptosis

In response to hemodynamic overload, an adaptive hypertrophic response is triggered in hearts, which is characterized by an increase in the mass and volume of individual cardiomyocytes and induction of an embryonic gene program [39]. In cultured neonatal myocytes, activation of the p38 MAPK beta isoform by upstream MKK6 leads to a hypertrophic response and cell survival, whereas expression of activated MKK3 promotes an apoptotic response mediated through the p38α isoform [13]. These finding are also confirmed *in vivo* by transgenic mice models. Activated mutants of the upstream kinase MKK3 with expression restricted to the hearts cause cardiomyopathy with increased end-systolic volumes and a thinned ventricular wall, associated with heterogeneous myocyte atrophy. In contrast a similar expression pattern of activated MKK6 causes a reduced end-diastolic ventricular volume and no significant myocyte atrophy [14]. These findings indicate a diverse physiological function for different members of the p38 MAPK family, with activation of the p38β contributing to the development of hypertrophy and p38α to the transition to overt heart failure.

Negative inotropic effect, heart failure

In agreement with the above observations in, *in vivo* transgenic mouse hearts [14], a recent study suggested activation of p38 MAPK decreases cell contractility [40]. Specific activation of p38 MAPK by adenovirus mediated gene transfer of MKK3 results in a significant reduction in contractility, which was prevented by co-expressing a p38α dominant negative mutant, and the p38 MAPK pharmacological inhibitor SB203580.

Ischemia/reperfusion injury, ischemic preconditioning

Controversy exists over the role of p38 MAPK in ischemia/reperfusion injury [41]. P38 MAPK and its downstream target MAPKAPK2 have been shown to be activated during ischemia and this activation is sustained during reperfusion [10]. This was thought to represent a possible adaptive phenomenon protecting hearts from ischemia since MAPKAPK2 phosphorylates the cytoprotective HSP25/27, which modulates cytoskeletal integrity [42]. Several studies showed ischemic preconditioning activates p38 MAPK during sustained ischemia and inhibition of this kinase blocked cardioprotection in various experimental models. On the other hand, some recent studies have suggested a deleterious role for p38 MAPK during ischemia [41]. Possible explanations for these discrepant results may be the specificity of the pyridinylimidazole compound SB203580, different biological functions of individual isoforms of the p38 MAPK and the distinction of events occurring during the preconditioning trigger from those occurring during sustained ischemia. Perhaps the most convincing evidence is (1) a study in cultured neonatal myocytes, where preconditioning prevented p38 alpha but not beta activation during sustained simulated ischemia, whilst cells expressing dominant negative p38α were more resistant to lethal ischemia [38] and (2) a study in isolated rat hearts, showing activation of p38 MAPK during multi-cycle ischemic preconditioning protocol attenuates the activation during subsequent sustained ischemia and reperfusion, the latter being responsible for the cardioprotection [43].

The role of cytokines in myocardial ischemic injury

Cytokines are implicated at various stages of the path from atherosclerosis, to plaque rupture, myocardial infarction, post-infarction remodeling and heart failure. For the purposes of this chapter we have separated the role of cytokines into this temporal framework.

Formation of atherosclerosis

Accumulating evidence suggests atherosclerosis is an inflammatory process involving vascular endothelial and smooth muscle cells, monocytes, T-lymphocytes, pro-inflammatory cytokines and growth factors [44]. Primary pro-inflammatory cytokines, such as TNF-α and interleukin-1 (IL-1), activate the endothelium and cause the expression of adhesion molecules that are crucial to the recruitment of inflammatory cells to the vessel wall and their ability to contribute to atherogenesis [44]. However, no studies have been performed so far to establish whether therapy with anti-pro-inflammatory cytokines prevents atherosclerosis. Primary pro-inflammatory cytokines stimulate the production of IL-6, a secondary pro-inflammatory cytokine, which in turn accelerates the production of acute phase proteins such as C-reactive protein (CRP) and fibrinogen [45]. Both IL-6 and acute phase proteins can be used as markers of inflammation.

Plaque instability and plaque rupture

Accumulating evidence suggests that inflammation within the atherosclerotic plaque contribute to its destabilization and subsequent disruption [44]. A systemic inflammatory response often accompanies acute coronary syndromes, and its presence has been widely recognized as an index of further events [46]. A recent study identified serum concentration of IL-18, as well as IL-6, high-sensitivity CRP and fibrinogen, as strong independent predictors of death from cardiovascular causes in patients with coronary artery disease [47]. However, the focus of inflammation may reside not within the vasculature itself but in injured myocardium distal to the disrupted plaque [48].

Preconditioning, apoptosis

Production of TNF-α during myocardial ischemia has been documented [49]. Signalling mediated by TNF-α seems to be bifunctional, because it could result either in cell survival through activation of NF-κB, or in caspase activation-dependent apoptosis [50]. Consistent with this signalling mechanism, the role of TNF-α in ischemia/reperfusion injury has been controversial. Mice lacking both Type 1 and Type 2 TNF-α receptors had significantly greater apoptosis compared with their wild type counterparts after acute coronary occlusion and reperfusion, suggesting TNF-α may give rise to a cytoprotective signal that prevents and/or delays the development of cardiac myocyte apoptosis after acute ischemic injury [51]. In addition, TNF-α production during ischemia was necessary for ischemic preconditioning-induced cardioprotection [52]. Furthermore, exogenous low concentrations of TNF-α (0.5 ng/ml) induced myocardial tolerance to ischemia/reperfusion injury [52, 53]. On the other hand, Meldrum et al. [54] reported ischemic preconditioning or adenosine pretreatment reduces TNF-α peptide appearance in the ischemic/reperfused myocardium, whilst a deficiency in TNF-α signalling results in reduced myocardial infarction by preventing activation of NF-κB at an early stage of reperfusion [55]. A possible explanation of these divergent results would be that TNF-α may activate an intrinsic protective mechanism during ischemia, but that this protection is overwhelmed by the detrimental signalling cascade triggered by TNF-α during reperfusion.

Early post-ischemia/reperfusion

Accumulating evidences demonstrates that an open infarct related coronary artery promotes myocardial repair even after large myocardial infarction [56, 57]. Reperfusion induces neutrophil-, monocyte- and lymphocyte-infiltration, which ultimately leads to healing and repair of injured territory through the release of cytokines and growth factors [58]. In reperfused myocardium, resident mast cells release histamine and TNF-α, which result in ICAM-1 expression in myocytes through IL-6 synthesis. ICAM-1 facilitates emigration of neutrophils to the reperfused myocardium and their concomitant adhesion-dependent cytotoxic effect such as microvascular obstruction and release of proteolytic enzymes and reactive oxygen species [58]. Infiltrating monocytes differentiate into macrophages and contribute to fibroblast proliferation by secreting a variety of growth factors and cytokines. Expression of metalloproteinases, responsible for myocardial extracellular protein degradation, is regulated by IL-10, which is also produced by infiltrating lymphocytes and macrophages [58].

Remodeling, heart failure

In 1990, a strong association between the level of circulating TNF-α and the degree of heart failure was demonstrated [59]. After this report, high blood levels of proinflammatory cytokines such as IL-1 and IL-6 as well as TNF-α were observed after myocardial infarction [60–62], and implicated in the left ventricular remodeling through the promotion of myocyte hypertrophy and alteration of gene expression in the non-infarcted myocardium [63, 64]. The extensive literature linking TNF to heart failure is reviewed within an accompanying chapter.

Stress activated signaling, dissecting causation from association

Thus the p38 or JNK pathways are associated with many cardiac pathologies. In some of the studies summarized above, the key has been dissection of causation from association. In the remainder of this chapter we outline the tools available to achieve this.

Mechanisms of signaling specificity

G proteins/MKKKs/MKKs/MAPKs

MAPK pathways are composed of three-kinase cascades acting in series. MAPKs are activated directly by MAPK/extracellular signal-regulated kinase kinases (MKKs or MEKs), which are dual specificity protein kinases that recognize only certain MAPKs as substrates. MKKs are activated by MKK kinases (MKKKs) that have less specificity. In the SAPK/JNK pathway, this MAPK is activated by MKK4 and MKK7, which in turn are phosphorylated by MKKK1/2/3, mixed lineage kinases (MLKs), such as ASK and TAK1 at the MKKK level [65]. MKK3 and 6 have been reported to activate p38 MAPK, where MKK6 can activate all four p38 isoforms, while MKK3 preferentially activates only p38α and γ. Upstream of the MKK3/6, several MKKs have been shown to cause p38 activation. These include MLK2/3, ASK1, TAK1 [30].

Regulation by scaffold protein

Scaffolding proteins, by definition, organize other proteins into a complex but lack enzymatic activity. This "organizer" was first identified for the Ste5 scaffold in the yeast pheromone-responsive pathway with organization of components in the MAPK signal complex to increase specificity, and signal amplitude [66]. JNK-interacting protein 1 (JIP-1) has been identified as a scaffolding protein for JNK [67], which interacts specifically with JNK/SAPK and its upstream kinases but not other MAPKs and facilitates signal transmission [67, 68]. However, the action of JIP seems to be complicated since it can also inhibit consequent biological activity by preventing JNK/SAPK from translocating from cytoplasm to nucleus, where phosphorylation of downstream transcription factors occurs [67]. A scaffolding protein associated with p38 MAPK has also been identified recently. Ge et al. showed a protein called TAB1, binds to p38α and stimulates phosphorylation of the kinase itself (autophosphorylation) on the two key residues in the phosphorylation lip. In response to certain stresses, TAB1 binds exclusively to p38α. In addition, the triggered autophosphorylation is likely to be intra-molecular event [69]. These finding clearly showed MKKK-MKK-MAPK module is not the only regulator of these signal cascades.

Interrogation of signal specificity

Pharmacological tools

The most extensive activity in MAPK inhibitor development has revolved around p38 MAPK. Significantly, a series of pyridinyl imidazoles, represented by SB203580, which were originally identified by their ability to suppress inflammatory cytokine synthesis, have been shown to inhibit p38 MAPK by binding to the ATP pocket [70]. Three amino acids within the ATP binding pocket, Thr-106, His-107 and Leu-108 shared by p38α and β but not δ, γ, JNK or ERK, play a major role in determining the specificity of this compound for p38α and β. Because of this specificity, many studies have used SB203580 during myocardial ischemia to infer that activation of p38 MAPK is either beneficial or detrimental to myocardial ischemic injury [41]. However, despite this specificity for p38α and β, at a higher concentrations SB203580 inhibits thromboxane synthase, cyclo-ocygenases 1 and 2, PI3 kinase/protein kinase B and JNKs, all of which could also affect ischemic injury [71–73]. This could be one of the reasons why p38 MAPK inhibition has been reported to have variable effects in myocardial ischemia/reperfusion [41]. Substitution of the three amino acids in the ATP binding pocket, from Thr106, His 107 and Leu108 to Met, Pro and Phe respectively, in combination with the use of SB203580, is a powerful tool to investigate the exact role of p38 MAPK in myocardial tolerance against ischemia. These mutants have effects that are indistinguishable from wild type p38α except they are inherently resistant to SB203580. This has enabled us to conclude, at least in a myoblast cell line and adult rat cardiomyocytes, that activation of p38 during simulated ischemia is detrimental [74].

As described above, SB203580 inhibits p38 MAPK activity by preventing ATP binding. Thus SB203580 should not inhibit the dual phosphorylation of p38 MAPK (Fig. 2) since it does not block the ATP binding properties, or the catalytic activity, of the upstream MKK3/6 [75]. However, Ge et al. were able to demonstrate that in response to some stimuli, SB203580 did prevent p38 MAPK phosphorylation and that this was because it blocked the autophosphorylation of p38 MAPK induced by association with the scaffold protein TAB1 [69]. These data suggest SB203580 can also be a useful tool with which to distinguish the mechanism of p38 activation.

The JNK/SAPK pathway has also been targeted pharmacologically. SP600125 has been reported to selectively inhibit JNK2 at 100 nM *in vitro* [76]. Another inhibitor of JNK/SAPK pathway, CEP1347, has also been developed. This agent targets the JNK pathway *via* inhibition of MLK1, 2 and 3, a specific MKKKs upstream of JNK/SAPKs [77]. However, these agents have not been investigated as extensively as the p38 MAPK inhibitors.

Genetic tools

JNK/SAPK pathway

In mammalian systems, the targeting of alleles encoding individual proteins within the JNK/SAPK pathways has been used to evaluate their biological roles. Combined disruption of JNK1 and JNK2 causes early embryonic death associated with defects in brain development [9]. However, mice deficient in either JNK1 or JNK2 appear morphologically normal, suggesting JNK1 and JNK2 are able to functionally complement one another. Targeted disruption of upstream kinases has also indicated possible roles of JNK/SAPK pathway. Deficiency of MKK4 causes embryonic death caused by increased apoptosis in the developing liver and consequent hepatic failure [9]. MKK7 is also required for embryonic viability, although the cause of death has remained unclear [78]. Data from mice deficient in components further upstream are also available. The role of MKKK1-JNK/SAPK pathway in pressure-overloaded hearts has been examined using MKKK1 knockout mice [79]. MKKK1-JNK/SAPK pathway appears to be required for pressure overload-induced cytokine up-regulation, but not for cardiac hypertrophy. However, the low specificity of such upstream kinases complicates the interpretation of the results. Another approach to evaluate the signal pathway is targeted activation of an allele. Recently, a study, using targeted activation of JNK in transgenic hearts with expression of MKK7 in ventricular myocardium *via* a Cre-LoxP-mediated gene switch

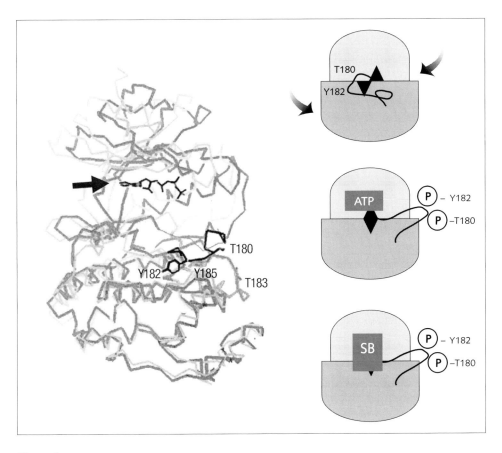

Figure 2
Left: crystal structures of p38 MAP kinase (dark gray) superimposed with ERK (light gray) at their C-terminal domains (from [89]). The phosphorylation lip of p38 is in black. The side chains of residues Thr180 and Tyr182 in p38 and Thr183 and Tyr185 in ERK are shown and labeled. For reference, the position of ATP (arrow) from the structure of cAPK is shown after superimposition of the N-terminal domain of cAPK and p38. Right: schematic structures of p38 MAP kinase to depict the conformational transitions involved in the regulation of kinase activity. In inactive, unphosphorylated p38, the relative orientation of the two domains is different from that observed in ERK. The twist results in misalignment of the catalytic site and the phosphorylation lip occupies the substrate binding site (top). Upon phosphorylation of two key residues, Thr180 and Tyr182, conformational changes occur in the lip and catalysic site. These involve refolding of the loop and crankshaft-like motions in the N-terminal lobe, resulting release of steric hinderence and alignment of the catalytic site. At this stage, with ATP binding to its binding pocket, p38 is ready to phosphorylate downstream targets (middle). However, SB203580 can occupy the ATP binding pocket and inhibit the catalysis despite the dual phosphorylation on the loop (bottom).

strategy, showed JNK was responsible for the down-regulation of connexin 43 expression and loss of gap junction-mediated intracellular communication, which may contribute to the cardiac dysfunction and premature death phenotype [80].

P38 MAPK pathway

Just like disruption of JNK, attempts to elucidate the action of p38 MAPK by targeted disruption has so far failed. Several groups derived p38 alpha null germ-line transmutation. However all resulted in an embryonic lethal phenotype due to variable deficiencies in vascularization of the embryo and yolk sac and growth retardation [81], forcing alternative strategies. As mentioned above, MKK3 and -6 are specific activators of p38 MAPK, with MKK3, which preferentially activates p38α MAPK, increasing myocyte death [13]. MKK3 deficient mice have a normal macro- and microscopic phenotype. Macrophages derived from these mice have been studied in detail. In response to lipopolysaccharide, peak p38 MAPK activation is markedly reduced whilst in response to TNF it is absent [82, 83]. However, in response to sorbitol, the amplitude of the p38 MAPK peak is unchanged but it is delayed [83]. Within myocardium it has not been known whether the activation of p38 MAPK will be reduced, delayed or may be even normal in response to various stimuli. However, our preliminary data suggested global ischemia phosphorylates p38 MAPK normally in MKK3$^{-/-}$ murine hearts, while TNF fails to phosphorylated p38 on this background.

Mechanisms of signaling specificity based on crystal structure

How does the cell keep the signaling pathways of all the related MAP kinases distinct from one another? Multiple mechanisms have been reported to exist to ensure the specificity of the MAP kinase signaling cascades. One way that MAPKs keep their specificity is to physically interact with specific docking sites in transcription factors, protein kinases, protein phosphatases, scaffolding proteins and substrates [84]. MAP kinases contain the common docking (CD) site and the ED site, which function together with the CD domain to regulate docking specificity [85]. In addition to those docking sites on MAP kinases, MAPK interacting proteins also have a docking site, termed the D domain [84]. D domains were first identified in c-jun, MEF2 and Elk-1, and have been shown to be important for recognition, binding, specificity and phosphorylation [86]. Recent work, resolving the crystal structure of p38α with its binding partners, revealed many details about these interactions and their subsequent events [87]. Comparison of the crystal structures of p38 with, and without, MEF2A, a p38 substrate, or MKK3, a p38 activator, revealed these peptides interact with p38 at the same site, termed the docking groove. Despite binding to the same site, the crystal structure suggested different conformations may occur in the docking groove, catalytic site and phosphorylation lip, which may be responsible for the different responses induced by these docked proteins or peptides [87].

Conclusions

There is no doubt that the JNK and p38-MAPK pathways play an integral role in myocardial biology. At present there is compelling evidence that activation of kinases within these pathways can have both beneficial and detrimental consequences. This diversity is likely to reside in nuances of signaling specificity beyond our current knowledge level. It is only through further knowledge and continued observation that these current inconsistencies will be resolved.

References

1   Kyriakis JM, Avruch J (1990) pp54 microtubule-associated protein 2 kinase. A novel serine/threonine protein kinase regulated by phosphorylation and stimulated by poly-L-lysine. *J Biol Chem* 265: 17355–17363

2   Hibi M, Lin A, Smeal T, Minden A, Karin M (1993) Identification of an oncoprotein- and UV-responsive protein kinase that binds and potentiates the c-Jun activation domain. *Genes Dev* 7: 2135–2148

3   Derijard B, Hibi M, Wu IH, Barrett T, Su B, Deng T, Karin M, Davis RJ (1994) JNK1: A protein kinase stimulated by UV light and Ha-Ras that binds and phosphorylates the c-Jun activation domain. *Cell* 76: 1025–1037

4   Kyriakis JM, Banerjee P, Nikolakaki E, Dai T, Rubie EA, Ahmad MF, Avruch J, Woodgett JR (1994) The stress-activated protein kinase subfamily of c-Jun kinases. *Nature* 369: 156–160

5   Xie X, Gu Y, Fox T, Coll JT, Fleming MA, Markland W, Caron PR, Wilson KP, Su MS (1998) Crystal structure of JNK3: A kinase implicated in neuronal apoptosis. *Structure* 6: 983–991

6   Kyriakis JM, Avruch J (2001) Mammalian mitogen-activated protein kinase signal transduction pathways activated by stress and inflammation. *Physiol Rev* 81: 807–869

7   Kasibhatla S, Brunner T, Genestier L, Echeverri F, Mahboubi A, Green DR (1998) DNA damaging agents induce expression of Fas ligand and subsequent apoptosis in T lymphocytes *via* the activation of NF-kappa-B and AP-1. *Mol Cell* 1: 543–551

8   Zanke BW, Boudreau K, Rubie E, Winnett E, Tibbles LA, Zon L, Kyriakis J, Liu FF, Woodgett JR (1996) The stress-activated protein kinase pathway mediates cell death following injury induced by cis-platinum, UV irradiation or heat. *Curr Biol* 6: 606–613

9   Davis RJ (2000) Signal transduction by the JNK group of MAP kinases. *Cell* 103: 239–252

10   Sugden PH, Clerk A (1998) "Stress-responsive" mitogen-activated protein kinases (c-Jun N-terminal kinases and p38 mitogen-activated protein kinases) in the myocardium. *Circ Res* 83: 345–352

11   Wettschureck N, Rutten H, Zywietz A, Gehring D, Wilkie TM, Chen J, Chien KR, Offermanns S (2001) Absence of pressure overload induced myocardial hypertrophy after conditional inactivation of Galphaq/Galpha11 in cardiomyocytes. *Nat Med* 7: 1236–1240

12   Robert P, Tsui P, Laville MP, Livi GP, Sarau HM, Bril A, Berrebi-Bertrand I (2001) EDG1 receptor stimulation leads to cardiac hypertrophy in rat neonatal myocytes. *J Mol Cell Cardiol* 33: 1589–1606

13   Wang Y, Huang S, Sah VP, Ross J Jr, Brown JH, Han J, Chien KR (1998) Cardiac muscle cell hypertrophy and apoptosis induced by distinct members of the p38 mitogen-activated protein kinase family. *J Biol Chem* 273: 2161–2168

14   Liao P, Georgakopoulos D, Kovacs A, Zheng M, Lerner D, Pu H, Saffitz J, Chien K, Xiao RP, Kass DA et al (2001) The *in vivo* role of p38 MAP kinases in cardiac remodeling and restrictive cardiomyopathy. *Proc Natl Acad Sci USA* 98: 12283–12288

15   Yue TL, Wang C, Gu JL, Ma XL, Kumar S, Lee JC, Feuerstein GZ, Thomas H, Maleeff B, Ohlstein EH (2000) Inhibition of extracellular signal-regulated kinase enhances ischemia/reoxygenation-induced apoptosis in cultured cardiac myocytes and exaggerates reperfusion injury in isolated perfused heart. *Circ Res* 86: 692–699

16   Bogoyevitch MA, Gillespie-Brown J, Ketterman AJ, Fuller SJ, Ben-Levy R, Ashworth A, Marshall CJ, Sugden PH (1996) Stimulation of the stress-activated mitogen-activated protein kinase subfamilies in perfused heart. p38/RK mitogen-activated protein kinases and c-Jun N-terminal kinases are activated by ischemia/reperfusion. *Circ Res* 79: 162–173

17   Ping P, Zhang J, Huang S, Cao X, Tang XL, Li RC, Zheng YT, Qiu Y, Clerk A, Sugden P et al (1999) PKC-dependent activation of p46/p54 JNKs during ischemic preconditioning in conscious rabbits. *Am J Physiol* 277: H1771–1785

18   Fryer RM, Patel HH, Hsu AK, Gross GJ (2001) Stress-activated protein kinase phosphorylation during cardioprotection in the ischemic myocardium. *Am J Physiol* 281: H1184–1192

19   Sato M, Cordis GA, Maulik N, Das DK (2000) SAPKs regulation of ischemic preconditioning. *Am J Physiol* 279: H901–907

20   Han J, Lee JD, Bibbs L, Ulevitch RJ (1994) A MAP kinase targeted by endotoxin and hyper-osmolarity in mammalian cells. *Science* 265: 808–811

21   Freshney NW, Rawlinson L, Guesdon F, Jones E, Cowley S, Hsuan J, Saklatvala J (1994) Interleukin-1 activates a novel protein kinase cascade that results in the phosphorylation of Hsp27. *Cell* 78: 1039–1049

22   Lee JC, Laydon JT, McDonnell PC, Gallagher TF, Kumar S, Green D, McNulty D, Blumenthal MJ, Heys JR, Landvatter SW (1994) A protein kinase involved in the regulation of inflammatory cytokine biosynthesis. *Nature* 372: 739–746

23   Cuenda A, Cohen P, Buee-Scherrer V, Goedert, M (1997) Activation of stress-activated

protein kinase-3 (SAPK3) by cytokines and cellular stresses is mediated *via* SAPKK3 (MKK6); comparison of the specificities of SAPK3 and SAPK2 (RK/p38). *Embo J* 16: 295–305

24   Lechner C, Zahalka MA, Giot JF, Moller NP, Ullrich A (1996) ERK6, a mitogen-activated protein kinase involved in C2C12 myoblast differentiation. *Proc Natl Acad Sci USA* 93: 4355–4359

25   Li Z, Jiang Y, Ulevitch RJ, Han J (1996) The primary structure of p38 gamma: A new member of p38 group of MAP kinases. *Biochem Biophys Res Commun* 228: 334–34

26   Wang XS, Diener K, Manthey CL, Wang S, Rosenzweig B, Bray J, Delaney J, Cole CN, Chan-Hui PY, Mantlo N et al (1997) Molecular cloning and characterization of a novel p38 mitogen-activated protein kinase. *J Biol Chem* 272: 23668–23674

27   Wilson KP, Fitzgibbon MJ, Caron PR, Griffith JP, Chen W, McCaffrey PG, Chambers SP, Su MS (1996) Crystal structure of p38 mitogen-activated protein kinase. *J Biol Chem* 271: 27696–27700

28   McLaughlin MM, Kumar S, McDonnell PC, Van Horn S, Lee JC, Livi GP, Young PR (1996) Identification of mitogen-activated protein (MAP) kinase-activated protein kinase-3, a novel substrate of CSBP p38 MAP kinase. *J Biol Chem* 271: 8488–8492

29   Stokoe D, Engel K, Campbell DG, Cohen P, Gaestel M (1992) Identification of MAP-KAP kinase 2 as a major enzyme responsible for the phosphorylation of the small mammalian heat shock proteins. *FEBS Lett* 313: 307–313

30   Ono K, Han J (2000) The p38 signal transduction pathway: activation and function. *Cell Signal* 12: 1–13

31   Perregaux DG, Dean D, Cronan M, Connelly P, Gabel CA (1995) Inhibition of interleukin-1 beta production by SKF86002: Evidence of two sites of *in vitro* activity and of a time and system dependence. *Mol Pharmacol* 48: 433–442

32   Pietersma A, Tilly BC, Gaestel M, de Jong N, Lee JC, Koster JF, Sluiter W (1997) p38 mitogen activated protein kinase regulates endothelial VCAM-1 expression at the post-transcriptional level. *Biochem Biophys Res Commun* 230: 44–48

33   Badger AM, Bradbeer JN, Votta B, Lee JC, Adams JL, Griswold DE (1996) Pharmacological profile of SB 203580, a selective inhibitor of cytokine suppressive binding protein/p38 kinase, in animal models of arthritis, bone resorption, endotoxin shock and immune function. *J Pharmacol Exp Ther* 279: 1453–1461

34   Da Silva J, Pierrat B, Mary JL, Lesslauer W (1997) Blockade of p38 mitogen-activated protein kinase pathway inhibits inducible nitric-oxide synthase expression in mouse astrocytes. *J Biol Chem* 272: 28373–28380

35   Andrew PJ, Mayer B (1999) Enzymatic function of nitric oxide synthases. *Cardiovasc Res* 43: 521–531

36   Xia Z, Dickens M, Raingeaud J, Davis RJ, Greenberg ME (1995) Opposing effects of ERK and JNK-p38 MAP kinases on apoptosis. *Science* 270: 1326–1331

37   Kummer JL, Rao PK, Heidenreich KA (1997) Apoptosis induced by withdrawal of trophic factors is mediated by p38 mitogen-activated protein kinase. *J Biol Chem* 272: 20490–20494

38   Saurin AT, Martin JL, Heads RJ, Foley C, Mockridge JW, Wright MJ, Wang Y, Marber MS (2000) The role of differential activation of p38-mitogen-activated protein kinase in preconditioned ventricular myocytes. *FASEB J* 14: 2237–2246

39   Simpson PC (1989) Proto-oncogenes and cardiac hypertrophy. *Annu Rev Physiol* 51: 189–202

40   Liao P, Wang SQ, Wang S, Zheng M, Zhang SJ, Cheng H, Wang Y, Xiao RP (2002) p38 Mitogen-activated protein kinase mediates a negative inotropic effect in cardiac myocytes. *Circ Res* 90: 190–196

41   Ping P, Murphy E (2000) Role of p38 mitogen-activated protein kinases in preconditioning: A detrimental factor or a protective kinase? *Circ Res* 86: 921–922

42   Clerk A, Michael A, Sugden PH (1998) Stimulation of multiple mitogen-activated protein kinase sub-families by oxidative stress and phosphorylation of the small heat shock protein, HSP25/27, in neonatal ventricular myocytes. *Biochem J* 333: 581–589

43   Marais E, Genade S, Huisamen B, Strijdom JG, Moolman JA, Lochner A (2001) Activation of p38 MAPK induced by a multi-cycle ischaemic preconditioning protocol is associated with attenuated p38 MAPK activity during sustained ischaemia and reperfusion. *J Mol Cell Cardiol* 33: 769–778

44   Ross R (1999) Atherosclerosis – an inflammatory disease. *N Engl J Med* 340: 115–126

45   Gabay C, Kushner I (1999) Acute-phase proteins and other systemic responses to inflammation. *N Engl J Med* 340: 448–454

46   Toss H, Lindahl B, Siegbahn A, Wallentin L (1997) Prognostic influence of increased fibrinogen and C-reactive protein levels in unstable coronary artery disease. FRISC Study Group. Fragmin during instability in coronary artery disease. *Circulation* 96: 4204–4210

47   Blankenberg S, Tiret L, Bickel C, Peetz D, Cambien F, Meyer J, Rupprecht HJ (2002) Interleukin-18 is a strong predictor of cardiovascular death in stable and unstable angina. *Circulation* 106: 24–30

48   Cusack MR, Marber MS, Lambiase PD, Bucknall CA, Redwood SR (2002) Systemic inflammation in unstable angina is the result of myocardial necrosis. *J Am Coll Cardiol* 39: 1917–1923

49   Meldrum DR, Meng X, Dinarello CA, Ayala A, Cain BS, Shames BD, Ao L, Banerjee A, Harken AH (1998) Human myocardial tissue TNF alpha expression following acute global ischemia *in vivo*. *J Mol Cell Cardiol* 30: 1683–1689

50   Haunstetter A, Izumo S (1998) Apoptosis: Basic mechanisms and implications for cardiovascular disease. *Circ Res* 82: 1111–1129

51   Kurrelmeyer KM, Michael LH, Baumgarten G, Taffet GE, Peschon JJ, Sivasubramanian N, Entman ML, Mann DL (2000) Endogenous tumor necrosis factor protects the adult cardiac myocyte against ischemic-induced apoptosis in a murine model of acute myocardial infarction. *Proc Natl Acad Sci USA* 97: 5456–5461

52   Smith RM, Suleman N, McCarthy J, Sack MN (2002) Classic ischemic but not pharmacologic preconditioning is abrogated following genetic ablation of the TNF alpha gene. *Cardiovasc Res* 55: 553–560

53 Lecour S, Smith RM, Woodward B, Opie LH, Rochette L, Sack MN (2002) Identification of a novel role for sphingolipid signaling in TNF alpha and ischemic preconditioning mediated cardioprotection. *J Mol Cell Cardiol* 34: 509–518

54 Meldrum DR, Dinarello CA, Shames BD, Cleveland JC Jr, Cain BS, Banerjee A, Meng X, Harken AH (1998) Ischemic preconditioning decreases post-ischemic myocardial tumor necrosis factor-alpha production. Potential ultimate effector mechanism of preconditioning. *Circulation* 98 (19 Suppl): II214–218; discussion II218–219

55 Maekawa N, Wada H, Kanda T, Niwa T, Yamada Y, Saito K, Fujiwara H, Sekikawa K, Seishima M (2002) Improved myocardial ischemia/reperfusion injury in mice lacking tumor necrosis factor-alpha. *J Am Coll Cardiol* 39: 1229–1235

56 Late Assessment of Thrombolytic Efficacy (LATE) study with alteplase 6–24 hours after onset of acute myocardial infarction. *Lancet* 342: 759–766

57 Reimer KA, Vander Heide RS, Richard VJ (1993) Reperfusion in acute myocardial infarction: Effect of timing and modulating factors in experimental models. *Am J Cardiol* 72: 13G–21G

58 Frangogiannis NG, Smith CW, Entman ML (2002) The inflammatory response in myocardial infarction. *Cardiovasc Res* 53: 31–47

59 Levine B, Kalman J, Mayer L, Fillit HM, Packer M (1990) Elevated circulating levels of tumor necrosis factor in severe chronic heart failure. *N Engl J Med* 323: 236–241

60 Munkvad SJ, Gram J, Jespersen J (1991) Interleukin-1 and tumor necrosis factor-alpha in plasma of patients with acute ischemic heart disease who undergo thrombolytic therapy: A randomized, placebo-controlled study. *Lymphokine Cytokine Res* 10: 325–327

61 Guillen I, Blanes M, Gomez-Lechon MJ, Castell JV (1995) Cytokine signaling during myocardial infarction: Sequential appearance of IL-1 beta and IL-6. *Am J Physiol* 269: R229–235

62 Latini R, Bianchi M, Correale E, Dinarello CA, Fantuzzi G, Fresco C, Maggioni AP, Mengozzi M, Romano S, Shapiro L (1994) Cytokines in acute myocardial infarction: Selective increase in circulating tumor necrosis factor, its soluble receptor, and interleukin-1 receptor antagonist. *J Cardiovasc Pharmacol* 23: 1–6

63 Ono K, Matsumori A, Shioi T, Furukawa Y, Sasayama S (1998) Cytokine gene expression after myocardial infarction in rat hearts: Possible implication in left ventricular remodeling. *Circulation* 98: 149–156

64 Swynghedauw B (1999) Molecular mechanisms of myocardial remodeling. *Physiol Rev* 79: 215–262

65 Barr RK, Bogoyevitch MA (2001) The c-Jun N-terminal protein kinase family of mitogen-activated protein kinases (JNK MAPKs). *Int J Biochem Cell Biol* 33: 1047–1063

66 Choi KY, Satterberg B, Lyons DM, Elion EA (1994) Ste5 tethers multiple protein kinases in the MAP kinase cascade required for mating in S. cerevisiae. *Cell* 78: 499–512

67 Dickens M, Rogers JS, Cavanagh J, Raitano A, Xia Z, Halpern JR, Greenberg ME, Sawyers CL, Davis RJ (1997) A cytoplasmic inhibitor of the JNK signal transduction pathway. *Science* 277: 693–696

68   Whitmarsh AJ, Cavanagh J, Tournier C, Yasuda J, Davis RJ (1998) A mammalian scaffold complex that selectively mediates MAP kinase activation. *Science* 281: 1671–1674

69   Ge B, Gram H, Di Padova F, Huang B, New L, Ulevitch RJ, Luo Y, Han J (2002) MAPKK-independent activation of p38alpha mediated by TAB1-dependent autophosphorylation of p38 alpha. *Science* 295: 1291–1294

70   Young PR, McLaughlin MM, Kumar S, Kassis S, Doyle ML, McNulty D, Gallagher TF, Fisher S, McDonnell PC, Carr SA et al (1997) Pyridinyl imidazole inhibitors of p38 mitogen-activated protein kinase bind in the ATP site. *J Biol Chem* 272: 12116–12121

71   Clerk A, Sugden PH (1998) The p38-MAPK inhibitor, SB203580, inhibits cardiac stress-activated protein kinases/c-Jun N-terminal kinases (SAPKs/JNKs). *FEBS Lett* 426: 93–96

72   Borsch-Haubold AG, Pasquet S, Watson SP (1998) Direct inhibition of cyclooxygenase-1 and -2 by the kinase inhibitors SB 203580 and PD 98059. SB 203580 also inhibits thromboxane synthase. *J Biol Chem* 273: 28766–28772

73   Lali FV, Hunt AE, Turner SJ, Foxwell BM (2000) The pyridinyl imidazole inhibitor SB203580 blocks phosphoinositide-dependent protein kinase activity, protein kinase B phosphorylation, and retinoblastoma hyperphosphorylation in interleukin-2-stimulated T cells independently of p38 mitogen-activated protein kinase. *J Biol Chem* 275: 7395–7402

74   Martin JL, Avkiran M, Quinlan RA, Cohen P, Marber MS (2001) Antiischemic effects of SB203580 are mediated through the inhibition of p38alpha mitogen-activated protein kinase: Evidence from ectopic expression of an inhibition-resistant kinase. *Circ Res* 89: 750–752

75   Kumar S, Jiang MS, Adams JL, Lee JC (1999) Pyridinylimidazole compound SB 203580 inhibits the activity but not the activation of p38 mitogen-activated protein kinase. *Biochem Biophys Res Commun* 263: 825–831

76   Han Z, Boyle DL, Chang L, Bennett B, Karin M, Yang L, Manning AM, Firestein GS (2001) c-Jun N-terminal kinase is required for metalloproteinase expression and joint destruction in inflammatory arthritis. *J Clin Invest* 108: 73–81

77   Maroney AC, Glicksman MA, Basma AN, Walton KM, Knight E Jr, Murphy CA, Bartlett BA, Finn JP, Angeles T, Matsuda Y et al (1998) Motoneuron apoptosis is blocked by CEP-1347 (KT 7515), a novel inhibitor of the JNK signaling pathway. *J Neurosci* 18: 104–111

78   Dong C, Yang DD, Tournier C, Whitmarsh AJ, Xu J, Davis RJ, Flavell RA (2000) JNK is required for effector T-cell function but not for T-cell activation. *Nature* 405: 91–94

79   Sadoshima J, Montagne O, Wang Q, Yang G, Warden J, Liu J, Takagi G, Karoor V, Hong C, Johnson GL et al (2002) The MEKK1-JNK pathway plays a protective role in pressure overload but does not mediate cardiac hypertrophy. *J Clin Invest* 110: 271–279

80   Barker RJ, Gourdie RG (2002) JNK bond regulation: Why do mammalian hearts invest in connexin 43? *Circ Res* 91: 556–558

81   Ihle JN (2000) The challenges of translating knockout phenotypes into gene function. *Cell* 102: 131–134

82   Lu HT, Yang DD, Wysk M, Gatti E, Mellman I, Davis RJ, Flavell RA (1999) Defective IL-12 production in mitogen-activated protein (MAP) kinase kinase 3 (Mkk3)-deficient mice. *Embo J* 18: 1845–1857

83   Wysk M, Yang DD, Lu HT, Flavell RA, Davis RJ (1999) Requirement of mitogen-activated protein kinase kinase 3 (MKK3) for tumor necrosis factor-induced cytokine expression. *Proc Natl Acad Sci USA* 96: 3763–3768

84   Sharrocks AD, Yang SH, Galanis A (2000) Docking domains and substrate-specificity determination for MAP kinases. *Trends Biochem Sci* 25: 448–453

85   Tanoue T, Maeda R, Adachi M, Nishida E (2001) Identification of a docking groove on ERK and p38 MAP kinases that regulates the specificity of docking interactions. *Embo J* 20: 466–479

86   Weston CR, Lambright DG, Davis RJ (2002) Signal transduction. MAP kinase signaling specificity. *Science* 296: 2345–2347

87   Chang CI, Xu B, Akella R, Cobb MH, Goldsmith EJ (2002) Crystal Structures of MAP Kinase p38 complexed to the docking sites on its nuclear substrate MEF2A and activator MKK3b. *Mol Cell* 9:1241–1249

88   Bueno OF, Molkentin JD (2002) Involvement of extracellular signal-regulated kinases 1/2 in cardiac hypertrophy and cell death. *Circ Res* 91: 776–781

89   Wilson KP, Fitzgibbon MJ, Caron PR, Griffith JP, Chen W, McCaffrey PG, Chambers SP, Su MS (1996) Crystal structure of p38 mitogen-activated protein kinase. *J Biol Chem* 271: 27696–27700

p38 MAPK in cardiac remodeling and failure: cytokine signaling and beyond

Thomas M. Behr, Christopher P. Doe, Haisong Ju and Robert N. Willette

Department of Investigative and Cardiac Biology, GlaxoSmithKline, King of Prussia, PA 19406-0939, USA

Introduction

Compelling evidence suggests that a complex interplay between various mitogen-activated protein kinases (MAPK) mediate adaptive and maladaptive changes in the myocardium. MAPKs are serine-threonine protein kinases that co-ordinate, in part, the myocardial response to inflammatory, ischemic, mechanical, oxidative, neuro-humoral and pharmacological stressors. The three major subgroups of MAPKs include the extracellular signal-regulated kinase (ERK), c-jun-NH2-terminal kinase (JNK), and p38 MAPK. Several excellent articles are available which provide a general description of these MAPK signaling pathways [1–3]. The well-established role of p38 MAPK in inflammatory cytokine signal-transduction and generation make this an attractive anti-inflammatory target. In addition, the role of p38 MAPK in the signal-transduction of cardiovascular patho-mediators suggests new a therapeutic approach to the treatment of cardiovascular disease. The current review focuses on p38 MAPK and its role in cardiac biology and pathology. The regulation and action of p38 MAPK are described separately at the level of the cell, organ and system. The emerging pharmacology of selective p38 MAPK inhibitors is also discussed briefly in the context of cardiac structure and function.

The identification and cloning of p38 MAPK was a simultaneous achievement by two groups working independently. It was first cloned from a murine pre-B cell line in 1994 [4]. A 38-kDa protein was tyrosine phosphorylated in response to bacterial LPS and extracellular changes in osmolarity. A GENBANK search showed that the 38-kDa protein shared sequence identity with the yeast MAPK family member encoded by the HOG1 gene [4, 5]. Soon after the discovery of murine p38 MAPK, the human homologue of p38 MAPK was purified and cloned. Using radio-photoaffinity techniques, Lee et al. (1994) reported a target binding protein for anti-inflammatory pyridinylimidazole compounds known to inhibit inflammatory cytokine production. They named the binding protein CSBP2 (for cytokine-suppresive anti-inflammatory drug binding protein 2) which was identical to p38 MAPK [6]. In addition to the original isoform of p38 MAPK (or p38α), three more isoform

Inflammation and Cardiac Diseases, edited by Giora Z. Feuerstein, Peter Libby and Douglas L. Mann
© 2003 Birkhäuser Verlag Basel/Switzerland

of p38 MAPK (p38β, p38γ, and p38δ) were identified and they share 74%, 60%, and 54% homology, respectively, to human p38α [7–10]. The gene expression patterns for p38α&β MAPK isoforms can be generally regarded as ubiquitous, however, p38γ is enriched in skeletal muscle and p38δ is enriched in kidney, testis, pancreas, small intestine and lung [10]. Only p38α and p38β MAPKs are inhibited by available pyridinylimidazole compounds, which bind in the p38 MAPK pocket to inhibit their kinase activity.

The p38 MAPKs contain 11 conserved kinase domains and required consensus sequences for a serine/threonine protein kinase. In addition, p38 MAPKs contain the Thr-Gly-Tyr dual phosphorylation motif at positions 180–182, which is known to be a regulatory site [6]. The predicted amino acid sequence of p38 MAPK has 52% identity with that of HOG1 in yeast [4]. p38 MAPK is highly conservative among mammalian species, e.g., the murine p38 MAPK has only two difference in amino acid to human CSBP2/p38 at positions 48 (Leu to His) and 263 (Thr to Ala) [6].

A variety of stress stimuli, e.g., osmolarity, UV, oxidative stress, growth factors, and cytokines, regulate p38 MAPK by dual phosphorylation of Thr and Tyr in the Thr-Gly-Tyr activation motif. It has well been documented that p38 MAPK is activated by a cascade of three kinases composed of MAP3K (MAP kinase kinase kinase), MAPKK (MKK3/6) and MAPK [1]. Evidence suggests that MKKs distinct from MKK3 and MKK6 can also activate p38δ [10]. In general, the stress-induced intermediates responsible for p38 MAPK activation are largely unknown.

In addition to the classical activation pathway, recent results indicate that p38 MAPK can be activated by an alternative pathway independent of the kinase cascade. For example, p38 MAPK can be activated by interaction with a scaffolding protein TAB1 (transforming growth factor-β-activated protein kinase 1 (TAK1)-binding protein 1) [11].

The efficiency of MAPK signal transduction is also dependent upon collateral activation of positive feed-forward mechanisms (e.g., cytoplasmic phospholipase A_2) and negative feed-back mechanisms (e.g., the activity of MAPK phosphatases that serve to limit MAPK activity and is itself regulated by MAPK activity) [12]. Dual-dephosphorylation of p38 MAPK is mediated by protein phosphatase 2A and MKP-1&5 (see Okabato et al. for review and [13, 14]). However, the substrate specificities and pathophysiologic control of these regulatory mechanisms have not yet been elucidated for p38 MAPK in the heart.

p38 MAPK has been shown to play an important role in the transduction and production of inflammatory cytokines as well as expression of numerous genes [1–3]. Specifically, p38 MAPK plays a role in the production of TNF-α, IL-1, IL-4, IL-6, IL-8 and IL-12 [15]. p38 MAPK regulates gene expression by phosphorylating/activating a variety of transcription factors, e.g., ATF-1/2, CHOP/GADD153, CREBs, ELK-1, Ets-1, MAX, MEF-2A&2C, NF-κB (indirect), HSF and SAP-1 [16].

294

p38 MAPK actions in the cardiomyocyte

Differentiation

Recently, several reports have demonstrated that p38 MAPK plays an important regulatory role in a number of cellular functions unrelated to the stress responses. These include developmental processes in flies and mice, as well as proliferation, differentiation, and survival in several vertebrate cell types [17, 18]. P19 cells have been used to study the role of p38 MAPK in the differentiation of cardiomyocytes. P19 cells are malignant stem cells of teratocarcinoma and resemble the pluripotent stem cells from the inner mass of early mouse pre-implantation embryos [19]. The PC19 cell line provides a useful model to study molecular and cellular changes during embryonic differentiation, since the cells can differentiate into cell types from different germ layers. In response to aggregation and dimethyl sulfoxide, P19 cells differentiate into cardiomyocyte-like cells. It was shown that p38 MAPK was activated in a sustained manner during the development of P19 cells into cardiomyocyte-like cells and the kinetics of p38 MAPK activation were similar to the induced DNA binding activity of the transcription factor, activator protein 1 (AP-1). AP-1 is composed of the members of the Jun and Fos families and may have a role in cardiomyocyte differentiation. The inhibition of p38 MAPK prevented increased c-Jun and Fra-2 expression and thus prominently inhibited the AP-1 DNA binding activity. As a consequence, the inhibition of the p38 MAPK pathway completely prevented the formation of beating cardiomyocytes, and the expression of myosin heavy chain, c-actin and desmin [20, 21]. This suggests that p38 MAPK functions as a regulator of AP-1 activity by inducing certain AP-1 encoding genes [20]. This was the first *in vivo* evidence that p38 MAPK may play a role in cardiac development [22].

Cardiomyocyte hypertrophy

Cultured neonatal and adult ventricular myocytes have served as a model system for studies aimed at gaining a better understanding of cell growth. Primary myocardial cells respond to a variety of stimuli by undergoing a hypertrophic growth program virtually identical to that observed in the developing neonate and the pathologic adult myocardium [23–26]. The first evidence of p38 MAPK involvement in the cardiac hypertrophic growth program was provided by Zechner et al. 1997 [28]. Activation of p38 MAPK by transfection with the specific upstream activator MKK6 resulted in unique features of the cardiomyocyte growth program, i.e., an increase in cell size, sarcomeric organization, and the induction of certain cardiac specific genes, namely ANP, BNP and skeletal α-actin (α-SkA) [28]. At this time, the role of different isoforms of p38 MAPK was not known, but evidence suggested that simultaneous activation of different isoforms may result in more complex responses. For example, when p38 MAPK was activated by another upstream activator kinase, MKK3, features of hypertrophy and apoptosis were observed. The differences in phenotype observed with MKK3 and MKK6 activation are believed to reflect the actions of different p38 MAPK isoforms [29]. Surprisingly, coactivation of p38 MAPK by MKK3 and JNK activation by MKK7, did not lead to synergy of the hypertrophic response, but resulted in cell death. Moreover, MKK7 and MKK6 co-expression inhibited any hypertrophic response. These findings suggest an intricate crosstalk between the different MAPKs in the growth and cell death program of cardiomyocytes [29].

At least four enzymes have been identified in the mammalian family of p38 MAPKs [30, 34]. Infection of cardiomyocytes with adenoviral vectors expressing upstream activators for the p38 MAPKs, activated mutants of MKK3b and MKK6b, elicited characteristic hypertrophic responses, including an increase in cell size, enhanced sarcomeric organization, and elevated atrial natriuretic factor expression. Over-expression of the activated MKK3b in cardiomyocytes also led to an increase in apoptosis. The hypertrophic response and cell survival were enhanced by co-infection of an adenoviral vector expressing wild type p38β, and was suppressed by the p38β negative mutant. In contrast, the MKK3b-induced cell death was increased by co-infection of an adenovirus expressing wild type p38α, and was suppressed by the dominant negative p38α mutant. These findings provided the first evidence in any cell system for divergent physiological functions for different members of the p38 MAPK family. The distinct phenotypes of hypertrophy and cell death in MKK3b infected cardiomyocytes appears to be dictated by the balance of the relative activity between two different p38 MAPK isoforms. Thus, the p38β isoform seems to be more potent in inducing hypertrophy, whereas p38α appears to be more important in cardiomyocyte apoptosis.

However, in these studies signaling pathways stimulated by constitutive over-expression are chronically activated. The effects of transient activation under physiological conditions may not be adequately reproduced by prolonged over-expression. The temporal effects of p38 MAPK activation can be studied with the use of specific inhibitors, e.g., SB-203580. Studies with SB-203580 have demonstrated its lack of effect on the early changes in cell size between 4 and 24 hours stimulated by phenylephrine or endothelin-1, however, it decreased the myofibrillar organization at 48 hours. This implied that the role of p38 MAPKs may actually be in the maintenance of the hypertrophic response over a longer period of time [35]. Unfortunately, currently available p38 MAPK inhibitors are potent inhibitors of both p38α and p38β isoforms, with little or no activity at p38γ and p38δ.

More support for a role of p38 MAPK in cardiomyocyte hypertrophy came from studies using mechanical stretch on cardiomyocytes *in vitro*. The cardiomyocytes were cultured on flexible wells and subjected to cyclical stretch. The stretch produced a time-dependent increase in p38 MAPK activity and hBNP promotor activity [36, 37]. Inhibition of p38 MAPK activity by treatment with SB203580 produced a dose-dependent reduction in stretch activated hBNP promoter activity. Co-transfection with a dominant negative MKK6 had the same downregulating effect [38]. Recent evidence suggests that integrins act as the stretch sensors in cardiomyocytes and are responsible for the activation of p38 MAPK through the integrin-FAK-Src-Ras pathway [39]. Indirect autocrine/paracrine stimuli, involving the sequential production of angiotensin II and endothelin, may also play a role in mechanically induced cardiomyocyte hypertrophy [40]. It was shown that about 50% of the strain dependent increment in hBNP promoter activity was dependent on the sequential stimulation of angotensin II and endothelin production in the cardiac myocyte [37]. The autocrine/paracrine dependent and independent pathways may involve the activation and signaling pathways of several different MAPKs, perhaps in a redundant fashion that lead to increased BNP gene transcription and, ultimately, myocyte hypertrophy [40].

The role of p38 MAPK in cardiomyocyte hypertrophy is not without considerable controversy. It was shown that the specific inhibitor SB-203580 failed to inhibit phenylephrine-induced ANF gene expression in low-density myocyte cultures but did inhibit gene expression in higher density cultures. Dense myocyte cultures also had a higher metabolic activity and contraction rate than cells plated at low density. When this effect was mimicked by rapid electrical pacing, ANF gene expression was activated and this expression was inhibited by p38 MAPK inhibition. However, addition of SB-203580 at time points ranging between one and 72 hours suggested that the effect of p38 MAPK on the ANF promoter may be both direct and indirect. Electrical pacing induced a small, but consistent, increase in p38 phosphorylation (phospho-p38) at time points ranging from 30 minutes to four hours, but at later times phospho-p38 levels were reduced. When myocytes were treated with phenylephrine or electrically paced in the presence of the p38 inhibitor, there was little discernible change in morphology or rates of protein synthesis from DMSO-treated cells at 48 or 72 hours. These data indicate that cell density and myocyte contraction may modulate p38-dependent pathways for ANF gene expression, but these pathways may not be direct and have limited effects on hypertrophic morphology [41]. In addition, it was shown that by blocking JNK by a dominant negative mutant of its upstream activator, endothelin-1 dependent hypertrophy was markedly inhibited without affecting p38 MAPK or ERK activity [42].

Differences in study design and limitations of cardiomyocyte cell culture are important to consider when examining the role of p38 MAPK in hypertrophy. Most of the data relating to the hypertrophic response have been obtained in cardiomyocytes after 48 hours of transfection or agonist stimulation. However, hypertrophic responses, as mentioned earlier, appear as early as four hours. The inhibition of p38α/β with SB203580 had no effect on these changes over the first 24 hours [35]. This may suggest that p38 MAPK is not involved in the initiation of hypertrophy but rather in its maintenance over a longer period of time [43]. Furthermore, when control cardiomyocytes are cultured in serum free medium over the 48 hour period, they become progressively smaller [43] and eventually undergo apoptosis [44]. Thus the p38-dependent hypertrophy beyond 48 hours may reflect cell survival rather than true hypertrophy.

Role of p38 MAPK in cell survival and apoptosis

Ample evidence suggests a correlation between the activation of the p38 MAPK pathway and apoptosis in a variety of cell types. However, information regarding the involvement of p38 MAPK in cardiomyocyte apoptosis is surprisingly scarce and largely correlative. Many activators of p38 MAPK, like proinflammatory cytokines and Reactive Oxygen Species (ROS) [42–45], have been shown to cause apoptosis in cardiomyocytes [47, 48]. The role of ROS in p38 MAPK activation and apoptosis will be discussed in the ischemia/reperfusion section of this review. The role of p38 MAPK in the signal transduction of cytokine pathways leading to apoptosis remains unclear in cardiomyocytes.

The most compelling evidence for the role of p38 MAPK in myocyte apoptosis is provided by transfection experiments using constitutively active MKKs to activate different p38 MAPK isoforms and their dominant negative mutants. As mentioned above, these experiments have shown a convincing role of p38 MAPK in myocyte survival and apoptosis. The over expression of p38 MAPK, in the setting of upstream activation, resulted in myocyte apoptosis.

In addition, there is accumulating evidence that p38 MAPK, together with other MAPKs, is involved in the presumed continuum of cardiac hypertrophy to failure due to apoptosis. It was shown that constitutively active $G\alpha q$, over-expressed in cardiomyocytes, is followed by a robust activation of p38 MAPK which results in apoptosis [49]. It should be noted that the effects of p38 MAPK inhibition have not been reported in this model. Hence the role of of p38 MPAPK activation in $G\alpha q$ mediated apoptosis is unclear in cardiomyocytes.

Direct evidence for an involvement of p38 MAPK in cardiomyocyte apoptosis could be shown in daunomycin-induced apoptosis. Daunomycin and adriamycin are widely used antineoplastic agents, with cardiotoxicity as a prominent serious adverse effect. Daunomycin was able to activate MAPKs through ROS and Ca^{2+}. Pretreatment of cardiomyocytes with SB203580 significantly reduced daunomycin-induced apoptosis, suggesting that p38 MAPK plays an important role in this cardiotoxicity [50].

Hypoxia and simulated ischemia in cardiomyocytes

Ischemia and reperfusion in myocardium is a subject worthy of considerable attention, given its routine manifestations in clinical practice. In particular, preconditioning, the phenomenon whereby brief episodes of ischemia or pharmacological agents protect the heart against subsequent ischemic injury is under intense investigation.

Following ischemic preconditioning, there are two phases of protection: An early (short lived) phase termed early or classic preconditioning [51] and a late (more prolonged) phase termed late preconditioning or the second window of protection [52].

Ischemia and reperfusion are major stresses on the heart and it is not surprising that p38 MAPK has been considered to be a major player in the response of the cardiomyocyte. Unfortunately, results are conflicting. This is usually explained by variability in the circumstances of the trigger, simulation of ischemia, *in vitro* maintenance conditions, cell type, and species of origin [53]. In addition, a second plausible explanation for the p38 MAPK controversy may be the differential actions of individual isoforms of the p38 MAPK family.

Reports have demonstrated that p38 MAPK is activated for a prolonged period of time period during lethal hypoxia in neonatal rat cardiomyocytes and if p38 MAPK is inhibited by SB203580, then cellular injury is reduced [54]. Furthermore, the p38 isotype preferentially activated by simulated ischemia *in vitro* is p38α [53], reinforcing the known role of this isotype in mediating cell death in this model [29]. Also in adult rabbit cardiomyocytes, there is a period of early and prolonged p38 MAPK activation for 60 minutes following ischemia [55]. In cell pellets that have been preconditioned, p38 MAPK activation is significantly enhanced at 30-minutes, but not significantly diminished at the 60-minutes time point. The p38 MAPK inhibitor, SB203580, also sensitized cells to simulated ischemia, suggesting that p38 MAPK activation is protective, but this did not correlate with changes in phosphorylation/translocation of the downstream substrate hsp27. Hsp27 is a heat shock protein that is considered to be cardioprotective. Moreover, it is not clear which p38 isotype contributed to the different activation levels found in that study. Thus, it is not clear whether or not these results in adult rabbit cardiomyocytes conflict with the proposed detrimental effects of p38α activation in neonatal rat cardiomyocytes [29, 54, 56].

Mechanotransduction in cardiomyocytes

There are two distinct patterns of hypertrophic response dependent on the type of mechanical insult. First, increased afterload on the heart (pressure-overload) is associated with concentric hypertrophy and parallel sarcomere deposition. In contrast, volume overload is associated with enlarged chamber dimensions and wall thickness resulting from the serial depositon of sarcomeres along the myocyte long axis, eccentric hypertrophy [57]. These findings alone suggest potential differences in mechanotransduction and effector mechanisms in the heart. Evidence for different MAPK transduction pathways in response to different modes of strain-induced myocyte stress has been explored using paced cardiomyocytes attached to a stretchable membrane [58]. Based on phosphorylation experiments, it was demonstrated that ERK activation was more sensitive to systolic strain, whereas p38 MAPK activation occurred within 10 minutes regardless of whether strain was applied during systole or diastole. Phosphorylation of JNK was also independent of whether the cells were loaded during diastole or systole, however the JNK response was more delayed. Although these studies are far removed from the more complex effects of chronic pressure/volume overload in the intact heart, they do demonstrate the potential for activation of p38 MAPK in response to strain and also that differential modes of cardiac myocyte strain can differentially modulate the MAPKs.

p38 MAPK regulation and actions in the heart

Effects of non-ischemic and overload stress

The effect of different forms of stress have been investigated in the isolated amphibian heart. Aggeli et al. [59] investigated the effects of mechanical overload in a Langendorf perfused frog heart preparation. Pressure overload, induced by increased perfusion pressure was associated with increased phosphorylation of ERK 1/2 after only one minute of the mechanical insult, this later declined. This was inhibitable with PD-98059 suggesting that p43-Erk was involved in this process. JNK1 was also activated within 30 seconds of increased perfusion pressure, reaching a maximum at 15 minutes. In addition, p38 MAPK phosphorylation was increased immediately on increasing perfusion pressure. However, this activation was not maintained, returning back to control levels within 15 minutes. In a separate study this group also demonstrated marked activation of p38 MAPK in the amphibian heart in response to hyperosmotic stress induced by sorbitol perfusion [60]. Clerk and colleagues [61] looked at the effects of increased aortic perfusion pressure, peroxide induced oxidative stress and 20 minute zero-flow ischemia on MAPK activity in the isolated perfused rat heart. They demonstrated marked activation of p38 MAPK by oxidative stress, ischemia and increased aortic pressure. In addition, the activation of MAPKAPK-2, a down stream substrate of p38 MAPK, induced by ischemia or H_2O_2, was abolished by the p38 MAPK inhibitor SB-203580. Importantly, ischemia-induced MAPKAPK-2 activity was abolished with a free radical scavenger, implicating the p38 MAPK pathway in the cardiac response to reactive oxygen species (ROS). A recent study demonstrated a progressive increase in myocardial NADPH oxidase, a potent source of ROS, during the development of pressure overload hypertrophy in the guinea pig [62]. In parallel with this were activation of myocardial p38 MAPK and ERK1/2 and 5 and myocardial hypertrophy. These authors suggest that ROS may activate myocardial redox-sensitive MAPK pathways and that the activation of p38 MAPK and ERK5 was temporally related to the transition from compensated to decompensated heart failure.

The activation of p38 MAPK in the heart has also been examined in stroke prone spontaneously hypertensive rats (SHRSP) maintained on high fat/salt diet [63]. This is a model of accelerated hypertensive end-organ damage characterized by premature mortality/moribidity, endothelial and renal dysfunction, stroke, microthrombosis and concentric constrictive left ventricular hypertrophy. After three weeks of implementing the diet, phosphorylated p38 MAPK and MAPKAP-K2 activity were concomitantly increased in the left ventricle in association with compensatory hypertrophy. Activation of p38 MAPK was initially sustained, but began to decrease with deterioration of LV function. In one of the few studies of chronic treatment, p38 MAPK inhibitors afforded profound protection in the SHRSP myocardium. LV hypertrophy was reduced and measures of LV function were improved. However, treatment with the p38 MAPK inhibitor also reduced circulating cytokines, reduced endothelial and renal dysfunction and improved survival. Thus, direct and/or indirect effects of p38 MAPK may contribute to changes in myocardial structure and function in this hypertensive model.

The concept that cardiac hypertrophy may be adaptive, such as following exercise training, has long been recognized. A recent study demonstrated activation of cardiac p38 MAPK, ERK1/2 and calcineurin, but not JNK, in mice following exercise training. However, further studies using selective blockers will be required to determine the relative roles and functional consequences of the cardiac MAPK in response to exercise [64].

Ischemic preconditioning, ischemia, and reperfusion

Ischemia represents a complex stress on the intact heart involving not only changes in cardiac mechanical stress, but also alterations in the redox state, intracellular pH, and in the longer term recruitment and activation of macrophages. There have been several excellent reviews on the subject concerning the differential effects of ischemia or hypoxia on activation of MAP kinase pathways in cardiomyocytes and in isolated hearts [61, 65]. However, comparatively fewer studies have addressed directly the role p38 MAPK in cardioprotection and myocardial damage in the intact heart.

Marias et al. [66] investigated the effects of sustained ischemia in normal isolated working rat hearts and hearts pre-conditioned with brief episodes of ischemia. They observed a robust activation of p38 MAPK after only five minutes of global ischemia. This activation was reduced if the hearts had been pre-conditioned. In addition, pre-conditioned hearts demonstrated a faster decline in p38 MAPK activity during reperfusion, which was associated with improved coronary flow, aortic flow, systolic pressure, heart rate and total work. Although these data suggest that pre-conditioning the intact heart results in decreased p38 MAPK activation associated with cardioprotection, these data alone do not establish a causal link between the two. Indeed, the association between reduced p38 MAPK activity and cardioprotection has not been the experience of other investigators using isolated rat hearts and rabbit cardiomyocytes [67, 68]. Marais et al. [69] also investigated the effects of different modes of inducing pre-conditioning on the p38 MAPK in the isolated working rat heart. Like ischemic preconditioning, preconditioning *via* β-adrenergic stimulation with isoproterenol reduced p38 MAPK activation and improved cardiac function during a subsequent prolonged ischemic event. Pretreatment with a p38 MAPK inhibitor, SB-203580, prior to and during β-adrenergic stimulation, blocked the cardioprotective effect. In contrast, inhibition of p38 MAPK during ischemic pre-conditioning did not abolish cardioprotection. These results suggest that activation of p38 MAPK during ischemic pre-conditioning was not the trigger for the cardioprotection.

Conflicting results were obtained by Nakano et al. [70] who investigated the role of p38 MAPK using a rabbit model of regional ischemia which was induced *in vitro* by coronary artery ligation. They found that treatment with SB-203580 blocked the beneficial reduction in infarct/area at risk ratio afforded by ischemic pre-conditioning. In addition, these authors could only demonstrate an increase in p38 MAPK activity during ischemia when the heart had been pre-conditioned [71]. Although there is no easy explanation for these contrasting results, they may reflect differences in experimental preparations rabbit *versus* rat, degrees of stress observed in global *versus* regional ischemia, endpoints for cardioprotection and regimens of drug administration.

Mocanu et al. [72] also investigated the effect of SB-203580 during the pre-conditioning cycle, after pre-conditioning and in the absence of pre-conditioning in the Langendorff perfused rat heart. In summary, the administration of SB-203580 during pre-conditioning did not prevent the reduction in infarct size associated with pre-conditioning alone. SB-203580 administration after pre-conditioning abolished the cardioprotection. Finally, administration of SB-203580 during the prolonged ischemic event had no effect on infarct size. These results suggest that activation of p38 MAPK is not involved with the initiation of ischemic pre-conditioning, but may play a role in sustaining the cardioprotective effects of pre-conditioning.

It is interesting to note that chronic hypoxia has also been associated with cardioprotection in the hypoxic rabbit [73]. Increased activity of p38 MAPK, JNK and protein kinase C has been demonstrated in these hearts and inhibition of these signaling pathways abolishes this cardioprotective effect, but only in chronically hypoxic hearts.

Direct evidence for the involvement and relative importance of any MAPK pathways is difficult to demonstrate due to the cross-talk between the various families. In addition to the experimental conditions, sampling methods can all influence the experimental interpretation. Thus, controversy surrounds the role of p38 MAPK activation in mediating the cardioprotective response to ischemic pre-conditioning.

Bogoyevitch et al. [65] investigated the effects of 30 minutes of global ischemia and reperfusion on the activities of p38 MAPK, JNK and ERK in the isolated perfused heart. They demonstrated increased phosphorylation of p38 MAPK after only ten minutes of ischemia, which remained activated after 20 minutes of reperfusion. Further evidence to support p38 MAPK activation was provided by the parallel increase in MAPKAPK-2 activity, its down-stream effector. Interestingly ERK was not activated and JNK/SAPKs were activated only following reperfusion. These data suggest that the p38 MAPK signal transduction pathway is associated with ischemic insult and highlight differences in ishemic regulation of p38 MAPK, JNK/SAPKs and ERK pathways.

In models of myocardial ischemia/repserfusion, Ma et al. [74] and Gao et al. [75] examined the functional significance of p38 MAPK activation by using selective p38 MAPK inhbitors, SB-203580 and SB-239063. In Langendorff-perfused rabbit hearts, ischemia and reperfusion again produced a robust activation of p38 MAPK. Treatment with SB-203580 significantly decreased cardiomyocyte apoptosis and improved post-ischemic cardiac function. The cardioprotective effects of SB-203580 were closely related to its inhibition of p38 MAPK. Treatment was not cardioprotective when administered ten minutes after reperfusion. These investigators then evaluated the effects of a p38 MAPK inhibitor, SB-239063, on myocardial injury in a murine ischemia/reperfusion (I/R) model. Treatment with the p38 MAPK inhibitor reduced PMN accumulation in the reperfused myocardial and markedly attenuated myocardial reperfusion injury (myocardial infarct size). The up-regulation of endothelial adhesion molecules (P-selectin and ICAM-1) in the myocardium was also reduced. Several groups have published similar results with p38 MAPK inhibitors in isolated hearts. These results suggest that p38 MAPK plays a pivotal role in the signal transduction pathway mediating post-ischemic myocardial apoptosis and inflammation. It is likely that p38 MAPK is acting at the level of the cardiomyocyte and the endothelium to mediate these effects.

Transgenic analysis of cardiac hypertrophy

Perturbations including transgenic activation and de-activation of the up-stream regulators and substrates of various MAPK targets have been used in a targeted approach to determine the relative roles of p38 MAPK, ERK and JNK/SAP families in the mediating the hypertrophic response *in vivo*.

Bueno et al. [76] have provided indirect support for a role of MAPKs in the development of hypertrophy by using transgenic mice over-expressing MKP-1, a phosphatase that prevents activation of p38 MAPK, ERK1/2 and JNK1/2. In wild type mice phenylephrine administration was associated with increased cardiac p38 MAPK, JNK1/2 and ERK 1/2 activity. However, over-expression of MKP-1 blocked the phenylephrine-induced increase in all three MAPKs. In addition, over-expression of MKP-1 was associated with lethality (7–15 days), ventricular dilation, and small disorganized myofibrils, suggesting reduced MAPK activity was associated with impaired development of the myocardium. Transgenic mice with lower levels of expression of MKP-1 had reduced myofibril cross-sectional area and showed a marked reduction in hypertrophy to aortic banding when compared to wild type mice. Although this study did not discriminate between the signaling pathways involved, it does suggest that MAPKs play a pivotal role in the neonatal development of the heart and in the development of hypertrophy to pressure overload.

In another study Bueno et al. [77] used a transgenic mouse which over-expressed cardiac MEK1 (upstream activation kinase for ERK1/2). This was found to selectively stimulate the ERK1/2 signaling pathway in the absence of changes in p38 MAPK or JNK1/2. At eight weeks of age these transgenic mice exhibited a concentric hypertrophy characterized by increased heart weight-body weight ratios and myofibrillar cross-sectional area. Furthermore hearts isolated from transgenic animals exhibited greater contractility and systolic function when examined in both Langendorff and working heart mode. These data demonstrate that increased p38 MAPK and JNK activity are not absolutely required for developmental hypertrophy. These studies do not rule out the involvement of p38 MAPK in mediating the reactive hypertrophic response to stressors such as pressure overload.

Esposito et al. [78] examined transgenic mice over-expressing a carboxy-terminal peptide (tggqi) which inhibits Gαq signaling in this mouse (dominant-negative Gαq mutant). Stimulation of Gαq is known to be a potent upstream stimulus of the ERK MAPK pathway, but can also stimulate p38 MAPK. Both wild type and transgenic mice were subject to aortic banding and MAPK activity was determined at seven hours, three and seven days. JNK was elevated at all time points in wild type mice, but not in the transgenic mice. ERK was elevated at seven days in the wild type but was unaltered in the transgenics and p38 MAPK was elevated after three days in wild type, but the increase was delayed in the transgenics. Hypertrophy was attenuated, but not prevented in the transgenic G(tggqi) mice suggesting that increased ERK and JNK activity due to pressure overload is mediated by Gq coupled receptors. However these data suggest that pressure overload can activate p38 MAPK *via* non-Gαq receptor-mediated mechanisms. In a separate study, transgenic inactivation of Gαq and Gα11 abolished the hypertrophic response to pressure overload [79]. Also, mice lacking Gαq failed to elicit the expression of fetal genes, a hall mark of the hypertrophic response. Unfortunately, MAPK activities were not measured in this study.

Taken together these studies strongly implicate the activation in ERK 1/2 pathway as an important pathway in the development of hypertrophy, but do not preclude a role for p38 MAPK activation in response to pressure overload. Liao et al. [80] used gene switch transgenic mice to more closely examine the role of p38 MAPK activation. In these mice genes encoding for the upstream kinases, MKK3BE and MKK6BE, of p38 MAPK were permanently switched on in cardiac tissue. These mice exhibited a cardiac phenotype similar to that associated with heart failure including myocardial fibrosis, fetal gene expression, systolic and diastolic depression and an increase in chamber stiffness. These mice also exhibited signs of congestion (pulmonary edema and dyspnea) and increased mortality. However, differences in the cardiac phenotype between the two transgenic strains were observed. MKK3BE activation was associated with myocyte atrophy, end-systolic dilation and cardiac chamber thinning. In contrast, MKK6BE activation was associated with reduced end-diastolic chamber dimensions and a moderate increase in myocyte size. Neither strain exhibited significant alterations in right or left ventricular weight. Although it was not the aim of this study to determine the effects of MKK3BE and MKK6BE over-expression on the down-stream signaling pathways, differences in the cardiac phenotype may be associated with differences in substrate for these two kinases. A significant finding from this study was that both phenotypes exhibited extensive cardiac remodeling, in the absence of significant cardiac hypertrophy. These data suggest that activation of p38 MAPK may be associated with deleterious changes associated with the development of cardiomyopathy typical of end-stage heart failure. Indeed, Bueno et al. speculate that selective activation of ERK 1/2 pathway may mediate the beneficial adaptive hypertrophic response, whereas activation of p38 MAPK and or JNK may be involved in maladaptive changes leading to cardiomyopathies and decompensation. Further support for this idea comes from studies indicating that transgenic over expression of RAS in the mouse heart is associated with cardiac hypertrophy accompanied by cardiomyopathy. RAS is known to activate both MEK1 pathways and also other MAPK pathways including JNK and p38 MAPK.

Patel et al. [81] investigated the possibility of reversing the hypertrophic and fibrotic remodeling in the ventricles of rabbits with a genetically modified β-myosin heavy chain Q. The phenotype of this rabbit is one of hypertrophic cardiomyopathy similar to the human condition. The transgenic rabbits had elevated levels of activated ERK1/2; however p38 MAPK was not elevated in this model compared to non-transgenic controls. Treatment with simvastatin was associated with regression of the hypertrophy, reduced fibrosis and an improvement in left ventricular filling. Treatment was also associated with a decrease in ERK activity, but p38 MAPK and JNK remained unchanged. Whilst these data support the notion that elevated ERK may be linked with hypertrophy they do not suggest that p38 MAPK or JNK have a major role to play in the maintenance of the cardiomyopathic state. Therefore, the relative role of ERK and other MAPK in maladaptive remodeling may be more complex than the initial conclusions derived from the transgenic mouse studies (above).

Evidence in human cardiomyopathies

Several studies have investigated the effects of cardiomyopathies on MAPK activity in failing human hearts. The effects of unloading of the chronically failing left ventricle on MAPK activation was examined by Flesch et al. [82]. The use of a left ventricular assist device (LVAD), resulted in a reduction in ERK1/2 and JNK1/2 activity, however, p38 MAPK activity was significantly increased. Interestingly, myocyte cell size was reduced and myocyte apoptosis was reduced following LVAD support suggesting that activation of p38 MAPK was associated with beneficial effects on cardiac function. Consistent with these findings, Takeishi et al. [83] compared p38 MAPK activity in tissues taken from hearts with dilated cardiomyopathy compared to normal donor hearts and found depressed p38 MAPK activity in the failing hearts. ERK1/2 activity was increased in failing hearts and JNK was unchanged. In a separate study, p38 MAPK activity was assessed in non-failing human hearts and failing hearts obtained from patients with idiopathic or ischemic end-stage failure [84]. This study demonstrated a decrease in p38 MAPK activity and in MAPKAPK-2 activity in cardiomyocytes in failing hearts regardless of whether the heart failure was ischemic or idiopathic in origin. Although the effects of concomitant drug therapy cannot be ruled out, these three studies indicate that p38 MAPK activity is reduced during the advanced stages of heart failure. However, little is known regarding the regulation and role of p38 MAPK in the progression of heart failure.

Conclusions

The findings reviewed herein strongly suggest that p38 MAPK plays a critical role in the heart's "stress-response" to a variety of stimuli. The regulation of p38 MAPK activity in the heart is unequivocal. However, whether or not activation of p38 MAPK in the myocardium portends favorable or unfavorable changes seems to depend critically on the physiological/pathological context. Fortunately, good pharmacologic tools are now becoming available to help clarify this vague conclusion. The use of selective p38 MAPK inhibitors in appropriate models of cardiac injury, remodeling and failure will help define future therapeutics and contribute to our understanding of the pathophysiological role of p38 MAPK in the heart.

References

1   Chang L, Karin M (2001) Mammalian MAP kinase signalling cascades. *Nature* 410: 37–40
2   Kyriakis JM, Avruch J (2001) Mammalian mitogen-activated protein kinase signal transduction pathways activated by stress and inflammation. *Physiol Rev* 81: 807–869
3   Widmann C, Gibson S, Jarpe MB, Johnson GL (1999) Mitogen-activated protein kinase: conservation of a three-kinase module from yeast to human. *Physiol Rev* 79: 143–180
4   Han J, Lee JD, Bibbs L, Ulevitch RJ (1994) A MAP kinase targeted by endotoxin and hyperosmolarity in mammalian cells. *Science* 265: 808–811

5   Brewster JL, de Valoir T, Dwyer ND, Winter E, Gustin MC (1993) An osmosensing signal transduction pathway in yeast. *Science* 259: 1760–1763

6   Lee JC, Laydon JT, McDonnell PC, Gallagher TF, Kumar S, Green D, McNulty D, Blumenthal MJ, Heys JR, Landvatter SW (1994) A protein kinase involved in the regulation of inflammatory cytokine biosynthesis. *Nature* 372: 739–746

7   Jiang Y, Gram H, Zhao M, New L, Gu J, Feng L, Di Padova F, Ulevitch RJ, Han J (1997) Characterization of the structure and function of the fourth member of p38 group mitogen-activated protein kinases, p38delta. *J Biol Chem* 272: 30122–30128

8   Lechner C, Zahalka MA, Giot JF, Moller NP, Ullrich A (1996) ERK6, a mitogen-activated protein kinase involved in C2C12 myoblast differentiation. *Proc Natl Acad Sci USA* 93: 4355–4359

9   Stein B, Yang MX, Young DB, Janknecht R, Hunter T, Murray BW, Barbosa MS (1997) p38-2, a novel mitogen-activated protein kinase with distinct properties. *J Biol Chem* 272: 19509–19517

10   Wang XS, Diener K, Manthey CL, Wang S, Rosenzweig B, Bray J, Delaney J, Cole CN, Chan-Hui PY et al (1997) Molecular cloning and characterization of a novel p38 mitogen-activated protein kinase. *J Biol Chem* 272: 23668–23674

11   Ge B, Gram H, Di Padova F, Huang B, New L, Ulevitch RJ, Luo Y, Han J (2002) MAPKK-independent activation of p38alpha mediated by TAB1-dependent autophosphorylation of p38alpha. *Science* 295: 1291–1294

12   Bhalla US, Ram PT, Iyengar R (2002) MAP kinase phosphatse as a locus of flexibility in a mitogen-activated protein kinase signaling network. *Science* 297: 1018–1023

13   Sundaresan P, Farndale RW (2002) P38 mitogen-activated protein kinase dephosphylation is regulated by protein phosphatase 2A in human platelets activated by collagen. *FEBS Lett* 528: 139–144

14   Obalu T, Brown GE, Yaffe MB (2000) MAP Kinase pathways activated by stress: The p38 MAPK pathway. *Crit Care Med* 28: N67–N77

15   Lee JC, Kumar S, Griswold DE, Underwood DC, Votta BJ, Adams JL (2000) Inhibition of p38 MAP kinase as a therapeutic strategy. *Immunopharmacology* 47: 185–201

16   Nebreda AR, Porras A (2000) p38 MAP kinases: beyond the stress response. *Trends Biochem Sci* 25: 257–260

17   Davis RJ (2000) Signal transduction by the JNK group of MAP kinases. *Cell* 103: 239–252

18   Nebreda AR, Porras A (2000) p38 MAP kinases: Beyond the stress response. *Trends Biochem Sci* 25: 257–260

19   McBurney MW, Jones-Villeneuve EM, Edwards MK, Anderson PJ (1982) Control of muscle and neuronal differentiation in a cultured embryonal carcinoma cell line. *Nature* 299: 165–167

20   Eriksson M, Leppa S (2002) Mitogen-activated protein kinases and activator protein 1 are required for proliferation and cardiomyocyte differentiation of P19 embryonal carcinoma cells. *J Biol Chem* 277: 15992–16001

21 Davidson SM, Morange M (2000) Hsp25 and the p38 MAPK pathway are involved in differentiation of cardiomyocytes. *Dev Biol* 218:146–160

22 Adams RH, Porras A, Alonso G, Jones M, Vintersten K, Panelli S, Valladares A, Perez L, Klein R, Nebrada AR (2000) Essential role of p38alpha MAP kinase in placental but not embryonic cardiovascular development. *Mol Cell* 6: 109–116

23 Schneider MD, McLellan WR, Black FM, Parker TG (1992) Growth factors, growth factor response elements, and the cardiac phenotype. *Basic Res Cardiol* 87 (Suppl 2): 33–48

24 van Bilsen M, Chien KR (1993) Growth and hypertrophy of the heart: Towards an understanding of cardiac specific and inducible gene expression. *Cardiovasc Res* 27: 1140–1149

25 Lembo G, Hunter JJ, Chien KR (1995) Signaling pathways for cardiac growth and hypertrophy. Recent advances and prospects for growth factor therapy. *Ann NY Acad Sci* 752:115–127

26 Van Heugten HA, De Jonge HW, Bezstarosti K, Sharma HS, Verdouw PD, Lamers JM (1995) Intracellular signaling and genetic reprogramming during agonist-induced hypertrophy of cardiomyocytes. *Ann NY Acad Sci* 752:343–352

27 Yamazaki T, Komuro I, Yazaki Y (1995) Molecular mechanism of cardiac cellular hypertrophy by mechanical stress. *J Mol Cell Cardiol* 27:133–140

28 Zechner D, Thuerauf DJ, Hanford DS, Mcdonough PM, Glembotski CC (1997) A role for the p38 mitogen-activated protein kinase pathway in myocardial cell growth, sarcomeric organization, and cardiac-specific gene expression. *J Cell Biol* 139:115–127

29 Wang YB, Huang SA, Sah VP, Ross J, Heller Brown J, Han J, Chien KR (1998) Cardiac muscle cell hypertrophy and apoptosis induced by distinct members of the p38 mitogen-activated protein kinase family. *J Biol Chem* 273: 2161–2168

30 Han J, Lee JD, Bibbs L, Ulevitch RJ (1994) A MAP kinase targeted by endotoxin and hyperosmolarity in mammalian cells. *Science* 265: 808–811

31 Lee JC, Laydon JT, McDonnell PC, Gallagher TF, Kumar S, Green D, McNulty D, Blumenthal MJ, Heys JR, Landvatter SW et al (1994) A protein kinase involved in the regulation of inflammatory cytokine biosynthesis. *Nature* 372:739–746

32 Jiang Y, Chen C, Li Z, Guo W, Gegner JA, LIn S, Han J (1996) Characterization of the structure and function of a new mitogen-activated protein kinase (p38beta). *J Biol Chem* 271: 17920–17926

33 Li Z, Jiang Y, Ulevitch RJ, Han J (1996) The primary structure of p38 gamma: A new member of p38 group of MAP kinases. *Biochem Biophys Res Commun* 228:334–340

34 Kumar S, McDonnell PC, Gum RJ, Hand AT, Lee JC, Young PR (1997) Novel homologues of CSBP/p38 MAP kinase: activation, substrate specificity and sensitivity to inhibition by pyridinyl imidazoles. *Biochem Biophys Res Commun* 235: 533–538

35 Clerk A, Michael A, Sugden PH (1998) Stimulation of the p38 mitogen-activated protein kinase pathway in neonatal rat ventricular myocytes by the g protein-coupled receptor agonists, endothelin-1 and phenylephrine – A role in cardiac myocyte hypertrophy. *J Cell Biol* 142:523–535

36   Liang F, Wu J, Garami M, Gardner DG (1997) Mechanical strain increases expression of the brain natriuretic peptide gene in rat cardiac myocytes. *J Biol Chem* 272: 28050–28056

37   Liang F, Gardner DG (1998) Autocrine/paracrine determinants of strain-activated brain natriuretic peptide gene expression in cultured cardiac myocytes. *J Biol Chem* 273: 14612–14619

38   Liang F, Gardner DG (1999) Mechanical strain activates BNP gene transcription through a p38/NF-kappaB-dependent mechanism. *J Clin Invest* 104:1603–1612

39   Aikawa R, Nagai T, Kudoh S, Zou Y, Tanaka M, Tamura M, Akazawa H, Takano H, Nagai R, Komuro I (2002) Integrins play a critical role in mechanical stress-induced p38 MAPK activation. *Hypertension* 39: 233–238

40   Liang F, Lu S, Gardner DG (2000) Endothelin-dependent and -independent components of strain-activated brain natriuretic peptide gene transcription require extracellular signal regulated kinase and p38 mitogen-activated protein kinase. *Hypertension* 35: 188–192

41   Hines WA, Thorburn J, Thorburn A (1999) Cell density and contraction regulate p38 MAP kinase-dependent responses in neonatal rat cardiac myocytes. *Am J Physiol* 277: H331–H341

42   Choukroun G, Hajjar R, Kyriakis JM, Bonventre JV, Rosenzweig A, Force T (1998) Role of the stress-activated protein kinases in endothelin-induced cardiomyocyte hypertrophy. *J Clin Invest* 102: 1311–1320

43   Sugden PH, Clerk A (1998) Stress-responsive mitogen-activated protein kinases (C-jun n-terminal kinases and p38 mitogen-activated protein kinases). In the myocardium [Review]. *Circ Res* 83: 345–352

44   Yamazaki T, Komuro I, Kudoh S, Zou Y, Kudoh S, Tanaka M, Shiojima I, Hiroi Y, Mizuno T, Maemura K, Kurihara H, Aikawa R et al (1996) Endothelin-1 is involved in mechanical stress-induced cardiomyocyte hypertrophy. *J Biol Chem* 271: 3221–3228

45   Clerk A, Fuller SJ, Michael A, Sugden PH (1998) Stimulation of stress-regulated mitogen-activated protein kinases (stress-activated protein kinases c-jun n-terminal kinases and p38-mitogen-activated protein kinases). In perfused rat hearts by oxidative and other stresses. *J Biol Chem* 273: 7228–7234

46   Clerk A, Sugden PH (1997) Mitogen-activated protein kinases are activated by oxidative stress and cytokines in neonatal rat ventricular myocytes. *Biochem Soc Trans* 25: S

47   Aikawa R, Komuro I, Yamazaki T, Zou Y, Kudo S, Tanaka M, Shiojima I, Hiroi Y, Yazaki Y (1997) Oxidative stress activates extracellular signal-regulated kinases through Src and Ras in cultured cardiac myocytes of neonatal rats. *J Clin Invest* 100: 1813–1821

48   Krown KA, Page MT, Nguyen C, Zechner D, Gurierrez V, Comstock KL, Glembotski CC, Quintana PJE, Sabbadini RA (1996) Tumor necrosis factor alpha-induced apoptosis in cardiac myocytes. Involvement of the sphingolipid signaling cascade in cardiac cell death. *J Clin Invest* 98: 2854–2865

49   Adams JW, Sakata Y, Davis MG, Sah VP, Wang Y, Liggett SB, Chien KR, Heller Brown

J, Dorn GW (1998) Enhanced g-alpha-q signaling – a common pathway mediates cardiac hypertrophy and apoptotic heart failure. *Proc Natl Acad Sci USA* 95: 10140–10145

50 Zhu W, Zou Y, Aikawa R, Harada K, Kudoh S, Uozumi H, Hayashi D, Gu Y, Yamazaki T, Nagai R et al (1999) MAPK superfamily plays an important role in daunomycin-induced apoptosis of cardiac myocytes. *Circulation* 100: 2100–2107

51 Murry CE, Jennings RB, Reimer KA (1986) Preconditioning with ischemia: A delay of lethal cell injury in ischemic myocardium. *Circulation* 74: 1124–1136

52 Marber MS, Latchman DS, Walker JM, Yellon DM (1993) Cardiac stress protein elevation 24 hours after brief ischemia or heat stress is associated with resistance to myocardial infarction. *Circulation* 88:1264–1272

53 Marber MS (2000) Ischemic preconditioning in isolated cells. *Circ Res* 86:926–931

54 Mackay K, Mochly-Rosen D (1999) An inhibitor of p38 mitogen-activated protein kinase protects neonatal cardiac myocytes from ischemia. *J Biol Chem* 274: 6272–6279

55 Armstrong SC, Delacey M, Ganote CE (1999) Phosphorylation state of hsp27 and p38 MAPK during preconditioning and protein phosphatase inhibitor protection of rabbit cardiomyocytes. *J Mol Cell Cardiol* 31: 555–567

56 Saurin AT, Martin JL, Heads RJ, Foley C, Mockridge JW, Wright MJ, Wang Y, Marber MS (2000) The role of differential activation of p38-mitogen-activated protein kinase in preconditioned ventricular myocytes. *FASEB J* 14: 2237–2246

57 Nicol RL, Frey N, Pearson G, Cobb M, Richardson J, Olson EN (2001) Activated MEK5 induces serial assembly of sarcomeres and eccentric cardiac hypertrophy. *Embo J* 20: 2757–2767

58 Yamamoto K, Dang QN, Maeda Y, Huang H, Kelly RA, Lee RT (2001) Regulation of cardiomyocyte mechanotransduction by the cardiac cycle. *Circulation* 103: 1459–1464

59 Aggeli IK, Gaitanaki C, Lazou A, Beis I (2001) Stimulation of multiple MAPK pathways by mechanical overload in the perfused amphibian heart. *Am J Physiol Regul Integr Comp Physiol* 281: R1689–1698

60 Aggeli IK, Gaitanaki C, Lazou A, Beis I (2002) Hyperosmotic and thermal stresses activate p38-MAPK in the perfused amphibian heart. *J Exp Biol* 205: 443–454

61 Clerk A, Fuller SJ, Michael A, Sugden PH (1998) Stimulation of 'stress-regulated' mitogen-activated protein kinases (stress-activated protein kinases/c-Jun N-terminal kinases and p38-mitogen-activated protein kinases) in perfused rat hearts by oxidative and other stresses. *J Biol Chem* 273: 7228–7234

62 Li JM, Gall NP, Grieve DJ, Chen M, Shah AM (2002) Activation of NADPH oxidase during progression of cardiac hypertrophy to failure. Hypertension 40: 477–484

63 Behr TM, Nerurkar SS, Nelson AH, Coatney RW, Woods TN, Sulpizio A, Chandra S, Brooks DP, Kumar S, Lee JC et al (2001) Hypertensive end-organ damage and premature mortality are p38 mitogen-activated protein kinase-dependent in a rat model of cardiac hypertrophy and dysfunction. *Circulation* 104: 1292–1298

64 Nakamura A, Yoshida K, Takeda S, Dohi N, Ikeda S (2002) Progression of dystrophic features and activation of nitrogen-activated protein kinases and calcineuron by physical exercise, in hearts of mdx mice. *FEBS Lett* 520: 18–24

65   Bogoyevitch MA, Gillespie-Brown J, Ketterman AJ, Fuller SJ, Ben-Levy R, Ashworth A, Marshall CJ, Sugden PH (1996) Stimulation of the stress-activated mitogen-activated protein kinase subfamilies in perfused heart. p38/RK mitogen-activated protein kinases and c-Jun N terminal kinases are activated by ischemia/reperfusion. *Circ Res* 79: 162–173

66   Marais E, Genade S, Huisamen B, Strijdom JG, Moolman JA, Lochner A (2001) Activation of p38 MAPK induced by a multi-cycle ischaemic preconditioning protocol is associated with attenuated p38 MAPK activity during sustained ischaemia and reperfusion. *J Mol Cell Cardiol* 33: 769–778

67   Maulik N, Yoshida T, Zu YL, Sato M, Banerjee A, Das DK (1998) Ischemic preconditioning triggers tyrosine kinase signaling: a potential role for MAPKAP kinase 2. *Am J Physiol* 275: H1857–1864

68   Weinbrenner C, Liu GS, Cohen MV, Downey JM (1997) Phosphorylation of tyrosine 182 of p38 mitogen-activated protein kinase correlates with the protection of preconditioning in the rabbit heart. *J Mol Cell Cardiol* 29: 2383–2391

69   Marais E, Genade S, Strijdom H, Moolman JA, Lochner A (2001) p38 MAPK activation triggers pharmacologically-induced beta-adrenergic preconditioning, but not ischaemic preconditioning. *J Mol Cell Cardiol* 33: 2157–2177

70   Nakano A, Cohen MV, Critz S, Downey JM (2000) SB 203580, and inhibitor of p38 MAPK, abolishes infarct-limiting effect of ischemic preconditioning in isolated rabbit hearts. *Basic Res Cardiol* 95: 466–471

71   Nakano A, Baines CP, Kim SO, Pelech SL Downey JM, Cohen MV, Critz SD (2000) Ischemic preconditioning activates MAPKAPK2 in the isolated rabbit heart: evidence for involvement of p38 MAPK. *Circ Res* 86: 144–151

72   Mocanu MM, Baxter GF, Yue Y, Critz SD, Yellon DM (2000) The p38 MAPK inhibitor, SB203580, abrogates ischemic preconditioning in rat heart but timing of administration is critical. *Basic Res Cardiol* 95: 472–478

73   Raifee P, Shi Y, Kong X, Pritchard KA, Jr., Tweddell JS, Litwin SB, Mussatto K, Jaquiss RD, Su J, Baker JE (2002) Activation of protein kinases in chronically hypoxic infant human and rabbit hearts: Role in cardioprotection. *Circulation* 106: 239–245

74   Ma XL, Kumar S, Gao F, Louden CS, Lopez BL, Christopher TA, Wang C, Lee JC, Feuerstein GZ, Yue TL (1999) Inhibition of p38 mitogen-activated protein kinase decreases cardiomyocyte apoptosis and improves cardia function after myocardial ischemia and reperfusion. *Circulation* 13: 1685–1691

75   Gao F, Yue TL, Shi DW, Christopher TA, Lopez BL, Ohlstein EH, Barone FC, Ma XL (2002) p38 MAPK inhibition reduces myocardial reperfusion injury *via* inhibition of endothelial adhesion molecule expression and blockade of PMN accumulation. *Cardiovasc Res* 153 (2): 414–422

76   Bueno OF, De Windt LJ, Lim HW, Tymitz KM, Witt SA, Kimball TR, Molkentin JD (2001) The dual-speciificity phosphatase MKP-1 limits the cardiac hypertrophic response *in vitro* and *in vivo*. *Circ Res* 88: 88–96

77   Bueno OF, De Windt LJ, Tymitz KM, Witt SA, Kimball TR, Klevitsky R, Hewett TE,

Jones SP, Lefer DJ, Peng CF et al. (2000) The MEK1-ERK1/2 signaling pathway promotes compensated cardiac hypertrophy in transgenic mice. *Embo J* 19: 6341–6350

78 Esposito G, Prasad SV, Rapacciuolo A, Mao L, Koch WJ, Rockman HA (2001) Cardiac overexpression of a G(q) inhibitor blocks induction of extracellular signal-regulated kinase and c-Jun NH(2)-terminal kinase activity in *in vivo* pressure overload. *Circulation* 103: 1453–1458

79 Wettschureck N, Rutten H, Zywietz A, Gehring D, Wilkie TM, Chen J, Chien KR, Offermanns S (2001) Absence of pressure overload induced myocardial hypertrophy after conditional inactivation of Galphaq/Galpha 11 in cardiomyocytes. *Nat Med* 7: 1236–1240

80 Liao P, Georgakopoulos D, Kovacs A, Zheng M, Lerner D, Pu H, Saffitz J, Chien K, Xiao RP, Kass DA et al (2001) The *in vivo* role of p38 MAP kinases in cardiac remodeling and restrictive cardiomyopathy. *Proc Natl Acad Sci USA* 98: 12283–12288

81 Patel R, Nagueh SF, Tsybouleva N, Abdellatif M, Lutucuta S, Kopelen HA, Quinones MA, Zoghbi WA, Entman ML, Roberts R et al (2001) Simvastatin induces regression of cardiac hypertrophy and fibrosis and improves cardiac function in a transgenic rabbit model of human hypertrophic cardiomyopathy. *Circulation* 104: 317–324

82 Flesch M, Margulies KB, Mochmann HC, Engel D, Sivasubramanian N, Mann DL (2001) Differential regulation of mitogen-activated protein kinases in the failing human heart in response to mechanical unloading. *Circulation* 104: 2273–2276

83 Takeishi Y, Huang Q, Abe J, Che W, Lee JD, Kawakatsu H, Hoit BD, Berk BC, Walsh RA (2002) Activation of mitogen-activated protein kinases and p90 ribosomal S6 kinase in failing human hearts with dilated cardiomyopathy. *Cardiovasc Res* 53: 131–137

84 Lemke LE, Bloem LJ, Fouts R, Esterman M, Sandusky G, Vlahos CJ (2001) Decreased p38 MAPK activity in end-stage failing human myocardium: p38 MAPK alpha is the predominant isoform expressed in human heart. *J Mol Cell Cardiol* 33: 1527–1540

Inflammation and myocarditis

Inflammation and myocarditis

Jay W. Mason

Cardiovascular Sciences, Covance Central Diagnostics, Reno, NY 89502, USA

Introduction

Myocarditis means, literally, inflammation of the myocardium. There are numerous known causes including viral infection, infection by other agents (bacteria, fungi, protozoa and metazoa), hypersensitivity to drugs and chemicals, and systemic autoimmune disorders. Other forms of myocarditis have poorly defined etiologies, such as giant-cell myocarditis and peripartum myocarditis.

Among the poorly defined forms of myocarditis, the most common form of the disorder in the western world, lymphocytic myocarditis, must be included. It is not poorly defined because of a lack of information about it. Extraordinarily extensive research into the nature of lymphocytic myocarditis has yielded vast knowledge, but virtually all of the work has been carried out in animal models and *in vitro*. Truly definitive work in humans has not been accomplished, leaving uncertainty as to which animal and fundamental observations are relevant to the human disease. Lymphocytic myocarditis, which is diagnosed in humans by endomyocardial biopsy or at autopsy, is believed to be usually the result of viral infection of the myocardium, or less commonly to other undefined myocyte injury processes, that in either case result in immune and autoimmune responses, producing the typical histology and contributing to further injury.

The purpose of this review is to provide physicians with a clinical framework for management of patients with suspected lymphocytic myocarditis as well as an understanding of the limitations of our current knowledge.

A disease of three phases

Lymphocytic myocarditis can be viewed as a disease of three phases [1]. These phases have been observed in a variety of animal models and in humans. In the simplest case, which might be more the exception than the rule, the disease passes chrono-

Inflammation and Cardiac Diseases, edited by Giora Z. Feuerstein, Peter Libby and Douglas L. Mann
© 2003 Birkhäuser Verlag Basel/Switzerland

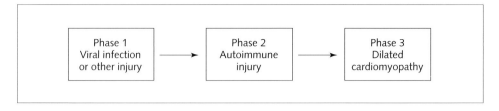

Figure 1

In its simplest form, lymphocytic myocarditis in humans passes through three successive phases. In Phase 1 a viral infection, or some other insult to the myocardium, results in myocyte damage which usually does not result in clinical heart failure. The infection is ultimately contained by an effective immune response, but autoimmunity resulting from myocyte damage and, presumably, presentation of cross-reacting antigens, develops in Phase 2. Injurious cytokines may play an important role in this phase. Though autoimmunity may eventually regress, dilated cardiomyopathy may develop as a result of adverse remodeling. Appropriate diagnosis and treatment of myocarditis requires knowledge of the phase of disease at the time of the patient's presentation. Unfortunately, this simple pattern may be greatly complicated by overlapping of the disease mechanisms of each phase as a result of viral persistence. This complexity is portrayed in Figure 2.

logically through the three phases shown in Figure 1, with the mechanisms operative in each phase turning off before the succeeding phase begins.

Typically, congestive heart failure does not bring the patient to medical attention in phase 1. Furthermore, it seems likely that most cases of viral infection of the heart end in phase 1, as a result of an effective immune response, without subsequent development of autoimmunity, cardiac dilatation or congestive heart failure. When the initial viral infection is very aggressive, it may cause sufficient myocardial damage to lead to heart failure and even death during phase 1. For patients presenting during phase 1, the diagnosis is made by detection of the offending virus. Antiviral therapies, though currently limited in scope and availability, are expected to have the greatest efficacy in this phase of the disease. Immune modulation or suppression may also be helpful in selected cases during this stage, if the immune response itself is responsible for a significant portion of ongoing myocyte injury. Unfortunately, we have no reliable means for recognizing this pathophysiology. As a result, manipulation of immunity is reserved as an investigational therapy or a heroic clinical measure during phase 1 of the disease.

In humans the diagnosis of congestive heart failure due to active myocarditis is thought to be made most commonly during phase 2. Autoimmunity triggered by the initial viral infection leads to further myocardial damage and finally to clinically overt failure. Several mechanisms of autoimmunity have been identified in animal models, including molecular mimicry [2] and cytokine responses [3]. Immune suppression or modulation would be expected to be effective during this phase of disease. Several such therapies have been tested in clinical trials. Immunosuppressive drug therapy has appeared to be effective in individual cases, most convincingly in patients with recurrent myocarditis in whom therapy repeatedly improves inflammation and ventricular function, while withholding it is associated with deterioration. However, no randomized trial has yet demonstrated efficacy of immunosuppression in groups. The largest completed trial, the US Myocarditis Treatment Trial [4], showed no improvement in left ventricular function or survival in subjects receiving prednisone and cyclosporine. Other strategies to modulate the immune system may have promise (see "New therapies" below).

Diagnosis of phase 2, at present, depends on endomyocardial biopsy, as there is no other reliable means by which to demonstrate the presence in the myocardium of the auto-reactive lymphocytic infiltrate that characterizes this phase. The Dallas criteria [5] were used in the US Myocarditis Treatment Trial for histological diagnosis of myocarditis. These criteria provided uniformity of diagnosis for the trial, but have never been tested for accuracy against a gold standard, in large part because one does not exist. The Dallas criteria may have permitted patients into the trial who were not likely to respond to immunosuppression, while excluding others who might have benefited. An accurate and less cumbersome means of diagnosis is needed (see "New diagnostic techniques" below).

After the injuries sustained in phases 1 and 2, the myocardium responds in phase 3 with dilatation and deterioration of contractile function. This remodeling process may be identical to that which occurs in idiopathic dilated cardiomyopathy (IDC). In fact, there is evidence that a substantial proportion of cases of IDC [6–11], and of unexpected sudden death [12, 13], including sudden infant death [14], is the result of sub-clinical or undiagnosed viral myocarditis. However, when IDC is the end result of myocarditis, other mechanisms may be active, accounting for continued ventricular dysfunction and further deterioration (see "Multiple causes of CHF" below). Treatment in phase 3 is largely directed at unloading the left ventricle and repopulating myocyte beta receptors, therapy that is common to all forms of IDC.

Multiple causes of CHF

There are numerous potential causes of congestive heart failure (CHF) in patients with myocarditis. While these many causes bring complexity to the management of myocarditis, they also afford opportunities. Figure 2 diagrams these multiple influences and indicates that they occur in a chronological sequence.

The importance of viral persistence in the later stages of the disease is not clear, but may be considerable [15, 16]. Persistence may take one of several forms. Truly latent viruses produce no progeny. However, they may elaborate viral proteins capa-

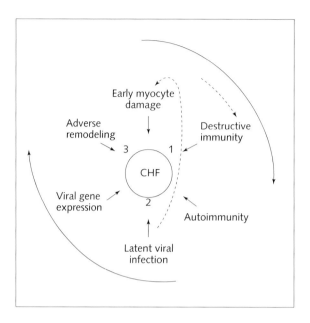

Figure 2
Myocarditis may cause Congestive Heart Failure (CHF) through numerous mechanism. The diagram indicates six general mechanisms. These may occur in the chronological sequence shown by the solid arrows in the diagram, in association with the three phases of myocarditis indicated around the center circle. Activation of latent virus may reinitiate earlier phases of disease while the later phases are still active (dashed arrows).

ble of stimulating a destructive immune response, which could further worsen cardiac function. Wessely and colleagues [17] recently demonstrated that Coxsackie provirus can impair ventricular function through transcriptional expression without immune activation. Latent viruses may intermittently activate and fully reinitiate the phasic cycle of myocarditis, or they may produce a very low level of progeny leading to a chronic, low grade immune response.

New therapies

Table 1 is an incomplete list of promising new therapies of myocarditis that have been proposed or tested.

The complexity of the disease and its multiple pathophysiologies of CHF offer numerous points of therapeutic attack. Prevention of initial viral infection is the most appealing approach. Despite the fact that dozens of viruses may cause

Table 1 - Promising new therapies for myocarditis

Therapy	Comment	Phase*
Tested in humans		
Hyperimmune globulin [31, 32]	Possibly effective in IDC but not in myocarditis	2, 3
Immunoadsorption [33, 34]	Possibly effective in IDC; not tested in myocarditis	2, 3
Ganciclovir for CMV [35, 36]	Effective in case reports; preventive post transplant	1
Tested in animals		
Anti-TNF-α antibody [37, 38]	Effective in mice to prevent or treat early myocarditis	1
TCR-based DNA vaccines [39]	Effective in autoimmune myocarditis in mice	2
Antigen-induced tolerance [40]	Nasal myosin prevents myosin-induced murine myocarditis	2
Coxsackievirus vaccine [41, 42]	Effective in preventing myocarditis in mice	Before 1
Tested in vitro *or proposed*		
Anti-CAR or tyrosine kinase p^{56} [18–21]		Before 1
Multivalent childhood vaccination		Before 1

Phase of disease in which therapy could be applied. CMV, cytomegalovirus; IDC, idiopathic dilated cardiomyopathy; TNF, tumor necrosis factor; TCR, T-cell receptor; CAR, Coxsackie/adenovirus receptor

myocarditis, a large minority, if not a majority, of cases could be prevented by a vaccine again the cardiotropic Coxsackie viruses. A multivalent vaccine covering cardiotropic enteroviruses and adenoviruses might prevent most cases. Interestingly, some enteroviruses and adenoviruses share a receptor that permits them to gain entrance to human cells [18–21]. The Coxsackie-adenovirus receptor, co-receptors and intracellular components might serve as a target for prevention of infection that would be as effective as a vaccine.

New diagnostic techniques

Though many consider histology to be the gold standard for diagnosis of myocarditis, its use as such has not been validated, and it is clear that histology alone cannot detect all forms of myocardial inflammation both because of sampling error and the unavailability of histologic markers for some agents and outcomes of inflammation. Furthermore, endomyocardial biopsy is too cumbersome. It is not readily available to all clinicians, it has to be scheduled well in advance, it requires a hospital stay, it carries a risk of significant complications and it is uncomfortable for the patient.

A reliable serological marker would be ideal. Although circulating antibodies to components of cardiac tissue have been known to be present in myocarditis, they are also present in other forms of cardiac and non-cardiac disease. More specific auto-antibodies are under study and may provide the needed specificity which was lacking in previous markers. Antibodies specific to atrial or ventricular myocardium [22], and IgG3 cardiac myosin auto-antibodies [23] are not only sensitive to the presence of immune or autoimmune mediated cardiac inflammation, but may carry prognostic information.

Greater awareness of the viruses capable of causing myocarditis will also improve diagnosis. Hepatitis C virus is an example of a previously unsuspected, but possibly common cause of myocarditis and subsequent dilated cardiomyopathy [24].

A number of imaging techniques have been explored. Echocardiographic tissue features may be helpful in detecting myocarditis, though there has been no update concerning this approach in several years [25]. Ultrasound energy has been used to fracture microbubbles engulfed by active white cells, with subsequent imaging as a novel means for detecting inflammation in myocardium [26, 27]. The clinical value of this technique remains to be clarified.

Using pre- and post-Gadolinium imaging with T1- and T2-weighted sequences as well as serial T1-weighted turbo fast low-angle shot acquisition, Laissy and colleagues [28] found MRI to be perfectly sensitive and specific for detection of myocarditis, and to provide information on chronicity of the inflammation [28]. This method has not yet been tested prospectively in a typical clinical setting.

Future

No comprehensively applicable single diagnostic tool or therapy for myocarditis should be expected. The etiologic agents and pathophysiologic mechanisms are too diverse. However, an ability to understand the complex disease process in individual patients may be provided in the future by micro-array analyses. Host responses to the viral infection can be monitored over time by this technique [29]. Eventually, certain patterns of mRNA expression will have diagnostic value in humans, both for making a diagnosis of myocarditis as well as determining the phase of the disease process. Even overlapping of phases could be identified by a cDNA "fingerprint". Eventually it should be possible to use genetic expression data to study any patient with heart failure and determine if myocarditis is active or if it played a role in the development of CHF [30].

References

1   Liu PP, Mason JW (2001) Advances in the understanding of myocarditis. *Circulation* 104: 1076–1082

2   Gauntt CJ, Arizpe HM, Higdon AL et al (1995) Molecular mimicry, anti-Coxsackie virus B3 neutralizing monoclonal antibodies, and myocarditis. *J Immunol* 154: 2983–2995

3   Matsumori A, Yamada T, Suzuki H, Matoba Y, Sasayama S (1994) Increased circulating cytokines in patients with myocarditis and cardiomyopathy. *British Heart Journal* 72: 561–566

4   Mason JW, O'Connell JB, Herskowitz A et al (1995) A clinical trial of immunosuppressive therapy for myocarditis. *N Engl J Med* 333: 269–275

5   Aretz HT, Billingham ME, Edwards WD et al (1987) Myocarditis, a histopathologic definition and classification. *Am J Cardiovasc Pathol* 1: 3–14

6   Fujioka S, Kitaura Y, Ukimura A et al (2000) Evaluation of viral infection in the myocardium of patients with idiopathic dilated cardiomyopathy [In Process Citation]. *J Am Coll Cardiol* 36: 1920–1926

7   Giacca M, Severini GM, Mestroni L et al (1994) Low frequency of detection by nested polymerase chain reaction of enterovirus ribonucleic acid in endomyocardial tissue of patients with idiopathic dilated cardiomyopathy. *J Am Coll Cardiol* 24: 1033–1040

8   Schwaiger A, Umlauft F, Weyrer K et al (1993) Detection of enteroviral ribonucleic acid in myocardial biopsies from patients with idiopathic dilated cardiomyopathy by polymerase chain reaction. *Am Heart J* 126: 406–410

9   Vasiljevic JD, Kanjuh V, Seferovic P (1990) The incidence of myocarditis in endomyocardial biopsy samples from patients with congestive heart failure. *Am Heart J* 120: 1370–1377

10 Wee L, Liu P, Penn L et al (1992) Persistence of viral genome into late stages of murine myocarditis detected by polymerase chain reaction. *Circulation* 86: 1605–1614

11 Why HJ, Meany BT, Richardson PJ et al (1994) Clinical and prognostic significance of detection of enteroviral RNA in the myocardium of patients with myocarditis or dilated cardiomyopathy. *Circulation* 89: 2582–2589

12 Wisten A, Forsberg H, Krantz P, Messner T (2002) Sudden cardiac death in 15–35-year olds in Sweden during 1992–99. *J Intern Med* 252: 529–536

13 Cioc AM, Nuovo GJ (2002) Histologic and *in situ* viral findings in the myocardium in cases of sudden, unexpected death. *Mod Pathol* 15: 914–922

14 Rasten-Almqvist P, Eksborg S, Rajs J (2002) Myocarditis and sudden infant death syndrome. *Apmis* 110: 469–480

15 Lenzo JC, Fairweather D, Cull V, Shellam GR, James Lawson CM (2002) Characterisa-

tion of murine cytomegalovirus myocarditis: Cellular infiltration of the heart and virus persistence. *J Mol Cell Cardiol* 34: 629–640

16   Mason JW (2002) Viral latency: A link between myocarditis and dilated cardiomyopathy? *J Mol Cell Cardiol* 34: 695–698

17   Wessely R, Klingel K, Santana LF et al (1998) Transgenic expression of replication-restricted enteroviral genomes in heart muscle induces defective excitation-contraction coupling and dilated cardiomyopathy. *J Clin Invest* 102: 1444–1453

18   Liu P, Aitken K, Kong YY et al (2000) Essential role for the tyrosine kinase p56lck in Coxsackie virus B3 mediated heart disease. *Nat Med* 6: 429–434

19   Liu PP, Opavsky MA (2000) Viral myocarditis: Receptors that bridge the cardiovascular with the immune system? *Circ Res* 86: 253–254

20   Martino T, Petric M, Weingartl H et al (2000) The Coxsackie-adenovirus receptor (CAR) is used by reference strains and clinical isolates representing all 6 serotypes of Coxsackie virus group B, and by swine vescicular disease virus. *J Virol* 271: 99–108

21   Opavsky MA, Penninger J, Aitken K et al (1999) Susceptibility to myocarditis is dependent on the response of alphabeta T lymphocytes to Coxsackie viral infection. *Circ Res* 85: 551–558

22   Caforio AL, Mahon NJ, Tona F, McKenna WJ (2002) Circulating cardiac autoantibodies in dilated cardiomyopathy and myocarditis: Pathogenetic and clinical significance. *Eur J Heart Fail* 4: 411–417

23   Warraich RS, Noutsias M, Kasac I et al (2002) Immunoglobulin G3 cardiac myosin auto-antibodies correlate with left ventricular dysfunction in patients with dilated cardiomyopathy: Immunoglobulin G3 and clinical correlates. *Am Heart J* 143: 1076–1084

24   Matsumori A, Yutani C, Ikeda Y, Kawai S, Sasayama S (2000) Hepatitis C virus from the hearts of patients with myocarditis and cardiomyopathy. *Lab Invest* 80: 1137–1142

25   Lieback E et al (1996) Clinical value of echocardiographic tissue characterization in the diagnosis of myocarditis. *Eur Heart J* 17: 135–142

26   Lindner JR, Song J, Xu F et al (2000) Noninvasive ultrasound imaging of inflammation using microbubbles targeted to activated leukocytes. *Circulation* 102: 2745–2750

27   Lindner JR, Dayton PA, Coggins MP et al (2000) Noninvasive imaging of inflammation by ultrasound detection of phagocytosed microbubbles. *Circulation* 102: 531–538

28   Laissy JP, Messin B, Varenne O et al (2002) MRI of acute myocarditis: A comprehensive approach based on various imaging sequences. *Chest* 122: 1638–1648

29   Taylor LA, Carthy CM, Yang D et al (2000) Host gene regulation during Coxsackie virus B3 infection in mice: Assessment by microarrays. *Circ Res* 87: 328–334

30   Hwang JJ, Dzau VJ, Liew CC (2001) Genomics and the pathophysiology of heart failure. *Curr Cardiol Rep* 3: 198–207

31   Bozkurt B, Villanueva FS, Holubkov R et al (1999) Intravenous immune globulin in the therapy of peripartum cardiomyopathy. *J Am Coll Cardiol* 34: 177–180

32   Gullestad L, Aass H, Fjeld JG et al (2001) Immunomodulating therapy with intravenous immunoglobulin in patients with chronic heart failure. *Circulation*; 103: 220–225

33 Muller J, Wallukat G, Dandel M et al (2000) Immunoglobulin adsorption in patients with idiopathic dilated cardiomyopathy. *Circulation* 101: 385–391

34 Felix SB, Staudt A, Dorffel WV et al (2000) Hemodynamic effects of immunoadsorption and subsequent immunoglobulin substitution in dilated cardiomyopathy: Three-month results from a randomized study. *J Am Coll Cardiol* 35: 1590–1598

35 Macdonald PS, Keogh AM, Marshman D et al (1995) A double-blind placebo-controlled trial of low-dose ganciclovir to prevent cytomegalovirus disease after heart transplantation. *J Heart Lung Transplant* 14: 32–38

36 Ng TT, Morris DJ, Wilkins EG (1997) Successful diagnosis and management of cytomegalovirus carditis. *J Infect* 34: 243–247

37 Matsumori A, Crumpacker CS, Abelmann WH (1987) Prevention of viral myocarditis with recombinant human leukocyte interferon alpha A/D in a murine model. *J Am Coll Cardiol* 9: 1320–1325

38 Yamada T, Matsumori A, Sasayama S (1994) Therapeutic effect of anti-tumor necrosis factor-alpha on the murine model of viral myocarditis induced by encephalomyocarditis virus. *Circulation* 89: 846–851

39 Matsumoto Y, Jee Y, Sugisaki M (2000) Successful TCR-based immunotherapy for autoimmune myocarditis with DNA vaccines after rapid identification of pathogenic TCR. *J Immunol* 164: 2248–2254

40 Wang Y, Afanasyeva M, Hill SL, Kaya Z, Rose NR (2000) Nasal administration of cardiac myosin suppresses autoimmune myocarditis in mice [In Process Citation]. *J Am Coll Cardiol* 36: 1992–1999

41 Fohlman J, Ilback NG, Friman G, Morein B (1990) Vaccination of Balb/c mice against enteroviral mediated myocarditis. *Vaccine* 8: 381–384

42 Fohlman J, Pauksen K, Morein B, Bjare U, Ilback NG, Friman G (1993) High yield production of an inactivated Coxsackie B3 adjuvant vaccine with protective effect against experimental myocarditis. *Scand J Infect Dis* (Suppl) 88: 103–108

The inflammatory process in experimental myocarditis

Noel R. Rose[1,2] and Marina Afanasyeva[1]

[1]Department of Pathology, [2]Department of Molecular Microbiology and Immunology, The Johns Hopkins Medical Institutions, Bloomberg School of Public Health, 615 North Wolfe Street, Baltimore, MD 21205, USA

Introduction

Myocarditis is defined by inflammation of the heart muscle which is usually associated with myocyte necrosis. Although it was first described in 1812 by Corvisart [1], the diagnosis of myocarditis remained relatively uncommon until the introduction of endomyocardial biopsies in 1962 by Sakakibara and Konno [2]. The true incidence of myocarditis is unknown because of the difficulty in diagnosis. This is partly due to the mild and self-limited nature of disease in most cases. However, it is a major cause of heart failure and sudden death, especially in children, adolescents and young adults. The five-year survival of biopsy-confirmed myocarditis in adults is 56%, and the prognosis is even worse in children [3]. Moreover, myocarditis is suspected to be a precursor of dilated cardiomyopathy (DCM), an often fatal condition frequently requiring cardiac transplantation. DCM has been reported to account for most cases of heart failure, particularly among young adults [4].

Often myocarditis and DCM occur in association with an antecedent febrile illness, especially an upper respiratory tract infection. The virus most commonly associated with myocarditis in the United States is Coxsackie virus B3 (CB3) [5]. Although CB3 can often be isolated from the heart during the early stages of acute myocarditis, infectious virus is seldom found in later, chronic stages and in DCM. Based on these observations, it has been postulated that the late stage of myocarditis is the result of the host's autoimmune response to a cardiac-specific antigen [6].

To test this hypothesis and to explore the mechanisms underlying the development of late stage myocarditis, we developed a mouse model of CB3-induced myocarditis [7]. Following infection, most strains of mice developed a severe, but time-limited, myocarditis, recovering completely in about three weeks. Infectious virus could be isolated from the heart for about nine days after infection, resembling the course of events in most human cases. A few strains of mice, such as A/J and BALB/c, failed to recover from this acute disease, but progressed to an on-going, chronic myocarditis mimicking the rare but clinically important cases in humans. These mice produced heart-specific IgG antibodies, with α-cardiac myosin (CM) heavy chain being identified as the primary cardiac antigen. Subsequently, we reproduced the cardinal pathologic features of chronic myocarditis by immunizing susceptible strains of mice with purified murine CM in the absence of virus [8]. Myocarditis, therefore, can be regarded as a prototype of infection-induced autoimmune disease.

Most of the work described in this chapter will be based on CM-induced experimental autoimmune myocarditis (EAM). The advantage of this model is the ability to study the inflammatory process in a purely autoimmune disease without complications associated with the viral component. Thus, it provides a system which is easier to manipulate and interpret.

Cellular mediators

Experiments by Smith and Allen [9] showed that CD4+ T-helper (Th) cells play a central role in the pathogenesis of CM-induced EAM. Depletion of CD4+ T-cells with monoclonal antibody prevented the development of disease. Furthermore, EAM could be reproduced in immunologically deficient SCID mice by transfer of CD4+ T-cells isolated from immunized mice. We were able to reproduce the disease in immunologically competent but sub-lethally irradiated recipient A/J mice by transfer of splenocytes isolated from immunized A/J mice and cultured *in vitro* for three days in the presence of CM [10]. The role of CD8+ T-cells in EAM is less defined. It has been demonstrated that CD8+ deficiency in mice leads to exacerbation of both CM-induced [11] and CB3-induced [12] myocarditis. However, depleting CD8+ T-cells with a monoclonal antibody reduced the severity of CM-induced EAM [13, 14]. Supporting the importance of CD4+ T-cell subset in the pathogenesis of EAM, we found greater numbers of CD4+ T-cells compared to CD8+ T-cells in the heart infiltrate on day 21 post-immunization as assessed by immunohistochemistry [15]. These finding were confirmed by flow cytometric analysis of the heart infiltrate from the enzymatically digested hearts collected on day 21 post-immunization, which demonstrated CD4+/CD8+ ratios ranging from two to six in both A/J and BALB/c mice (unpublished observations).

In addition to T-cells, the heart infiltrate also contains a large number of macrophages, few B cells and some granulocytes. The percentage of granulocytes in the heart infiltrate correlates with the severity of myocarditis (unpublished observations). Severe cases of CM-induced EAM are characterized by the presence of abundant neutrophils and eosinophils, as well as scattered giant cells [10].

Pro-inflammatory cytokines

Experiments in our laboratory showed that interleukin (IL)-1 and tumor necrosis factor (TNF)-α are necessary, but not sufficient, for the development of autoimmune myocarditis. Strains of mice that are normally resistant to autoimmune myocarditis developed the disease if they were co-treated with IL-1 or TNF-α in conjunction with CB3 infection or immunization with CM [16, 17]. Conversely, susceptible strains of mice did not develop disease if IL-1 or TNF-α were blocked [18, 19]. Thus, pro-inflammatory cytokines produced during the initial stages of viral infection determine whether a mouse will later develop a pathogenic autoimmune response. The pathogenic role of TNF-α has been demonstrated not only in the CB3-induced model but also in CM-induced autoimmune myocarditis. Furthermore, Bachmaier et al. [20] have shown that mice deficient in TNF receptor p55 are resistant to the induction of CM-induced disease suggesting the importance of TNF-α-triggered signaling.

Th1 cytokines

Current research has focused a great deal of attention on the differing roles of the Th1 and Th2 subsets of CD4+ T-cells and their signature cytokines, IFN-γ and IL-4, respectively [21]. It has been shown that IL-12 is critical for promoting Th1 responses, whereas IL-4 is important in favoring Th2 responses. We undertook to investigate the relative contributions of Th1 and Th2 cytokines to the heart muscle inflammation characteristic of EAM. To examine the role of IL-12, we used BALB/c mice deficient in IL-12 receptor signaling, IL-12 receptor knockout (KO) and STAT4 KO [22]. Both types of genetic deficiency produced a phenotype resistant to CM-induced EAM. To confirm the importance of IL-12 in the initiation of disease, we treated BALB/c mice with recombinant IL-12 during disease induction. IL-12 treatment exacerbated disease as evidenced by both gross appearance of the hearts and increased heart-to-body weight ratio. IL-12, however, did not significantly change the degree of myocardial inflammation as assessed by microscopic examination of heart sections. Okura et al. [23] demonstrated in Lewis rats that IL-12 treatment exacerbated myocarditis induced with a rat cardiac myosin-derived peptide. The authors also found that addition of IL-12 to the T-cell culture increased the severity of myocarditis upon T-cell transfer. Furthermore, mice deficient in the p40 subunit of IL-12 were shown to be resistant to the development of myocarditis [24].

Since IFN-γ is believed to be responsible for downstream effects of IL-12, its role was investigated using three approaches: depleting IFN-γ with a monoclonal antibody, using IFN-γ KO mice, or treating mice with exogenous recombinant IFN-γ [10, 22]. Mice treated with anti-IFN-γ antibody and mice genetically deficient in this cytokine demonstrated markedly exacerbated disease upon CM immunization. The hearts were extensively infiltrated by mononuclear cells and granulocytes including abundant eosinophils. Administration of recombinant IFN-γ to A/J mice in conjunction with CM immunization markedly reduced the severity of myocarditis or even completely prevented its development. These findings demonstrated that IFN-γ plays a disease-limiting role in EAM and is not responsible for the disease-promoting action of IL-12.

Many hearts from IFN-γ deficient mice immunized with CM demonstrated morphologic features characteristic of DCM: Enlargement of the hearts and dilatation of left and right ventricular cavities, frequently accompanied by the dilation of both atria. Increased frequency of progression to DCM and greater cardiac dysfunction was demonstrated in IFN-γ KO mice as compared to the wild type (WT) by *in vivo* left-ventricular catheterization and pressure-volume analysis, a method first described in mice by Georgakopoulos et al. [25]. The KO mice with DCM demonstrated increased left ventricular volumes, decreased end-systolic pressure, decreased cardiac output, pronounced depression of systolic function manifested by reduced slope and rightward shift of the end-systolic pressure-volume relation (ESPVR), reduced maximal rate of pressure development (dP/dt_{max}), and reduced stroke work-end diastolic volume relation. Such systolic dysfunction was accompanied by impairment of lusitropic properties of the heart resulting in increased passive stiffness (β), prolonged relaxation (tau), decreased peak filling rate, and increased end-diastolic pressure [26]. Furthermore, longitudinal studies employing cardiac echocardiographic examination in a cohort of these mice revealed increased left ventricular chamber dimensions, decreased fractional shortening, and global left ventricular wall hypokinesis, classic hallmarks of DCM. These studies demonstrated that progression from a normal to dilated phenotype occurs within a ten-day period. The functional changes found in a large proportion of IFN-γ KO mice were virtually identical to those seen in human DCM.

The immunologic mechanisms by which IFN-γ suppresses disease are still under investigation. IFN-γ KO mice have increased spleen cellularity with increased percentages of T-cells of both CD4 and CD8 types [22]. Additionally, there was an expansion of activated CD44[high] CD3+ T-cells in the peripheral blood in IFN-γ KO mice. Percentages of activated T-cells in the KO mice were already significantly higher on day three post-immunization with the difference increasing at later time points. We hypothesized that the increase in the population of activated T-cells may be due to impaired activation-induced cell death. In support of this hypothesis, we found the KO mice had reduced percentages of CD3+ T-cells undergoing apoptosis (Annexin V+/7AAD−) in the peripheral blood on day nine post-immunization [26]. Furthermore, reduced apoptosis was observed in CD4+ T-cell population in the spleen and axillary lymph nodes from the KO mice on day 16 post-immunization. IFN-γ KO mice exhibited a higher proportion of CD4+, but not CD8+, T-cells among the heart-infiltrating leukocytes, further suggesting the contribution of CD4+ T-cells to the severity of disease in these mice. Similar to the findings in the peripheral blood, T-cells from the heart infiltrate of the KO mice expressed higher levels of CD44 as was assessed by flow cytometry (unpublished observations).

Th2 cytokines

Presence of abundant eosinophils in the heart infiltrate in A/J mice, correlation of disease with CM-specific IgG1 but not IgG2a responses, and elevated total IgE levels upon CM immunization suggested the importance of IL-4 in the disease process. A similar histologic picture and antibody profile in response to CM immunization were characteristic of a less susceptible strain, BALB/c. IgG1 response remained predominant even when immunizations were repeated in the absence of a potentially "pro-Th2" co-adjuvant pertussis toxin. Consequently, we studied the effect of depleting IL-4 on the disease. Administration of anti-IL-4 monoclonal antibody significantly reduced the severity of myocarditis, especially in the numbers of infiltrating eosinophils [10]. Anti-IL-4 treated groups had a substantial reduction in the total IgE levels and in CM-specific IgG1 response as well as a significant increase in CM-specific IgG2a response. To analyze further the effect of anti-IL-4 treatment on cytokine production, splenocytes were collected on day 21 post-immunization and cultured in the presence of CM. Splenocyte supernatants from mice treated with anti-IL-4 showed decreased levels of Th2 cytokines: IL-4, IL-5, and IL-13, but dramatically increased levels of IFN-γ compared to both the isotype and vehicle buffer control groups. These findings demonstrated that the reduction of disease severity upon IL-4 blockade was associated with a switch from a Th2-like to a Th1-like phenotype. Since anti-IL-4 treatment reduced the severity but not prevalence of disease, it is likely that IL-4 is important in the progression to a more severe disease but may be dispensable for disease initiation. Increased production of a disease-limiting cytokine, IFN-γ, may also explain the reduced severity of disease in response to anti-IL-4 treatment.

IL-10 is frequently classified as a Th2 cytokine but there is a growing body of evidence that it does not follow the classic Th1/Th2 paradigm. It may be grouped into a category of regulatory cytokines. To investigate the effect of IL-10 in the pathogenesis of autoimmune myocarditis, we blocked IL-10 with monoclonal antibody during either early or late phase of disease development of CM-induced EAM in A/J mice [27]. Mice treated with anti-IL-10 antibody during the early stage of the disease (between the day of the first immunization and day 12) showed no significant change in disease prevalence or severity compared with controls. However, when anti-IL-10 was administered during the later phase starting on day 10, the prevalence and severity were significantly increased. In addition, mice treated with anti-IL-10 had increased levels of CM-specific IgG1 and IgG2b antibody. These findings are consistent with our observation that the production of IL-10 is greatest during the recovery phase of the disease. Blocking IL-10 during the later phase was accompanied by increased IL-2, IL-4, and TNF-α production, all of which appear to promote or prolong inflammation. We have also demonstrated that IL-10 blockade with a monoclonal antibody prevented suppression of disease through nasal tolerance induced by intra-nasal administration of CM before immunization, implicating IL-10 as a mediator of mucosal tolerance [27, 28]. Watanabe et al. [29] demonstrated the disease-suppressive effect of IL-10 in a rat model of autoimmune myocarditis (see Chapter by Watanabe et al. in this book).

Discussion

This chapter describes some of the cytokines that either promote or suppress autoimmune myocarditis and DCM. Key cytokines generated during the initial immune response determine the later development of myocarditis. They include the pro-inflammatory cytokines, IL-1 and TNF-α, and a Th1 cytokine, IL-12. In murine viral myocarditis, IL-12 has been shown to be protective by reducing viral replication and mortality [30]. Therefore, IL-12 may be beneficial during the early viral disease but detrimental during later autoimmune phase. From a clinical point of view, it would be hard to predict the outcome of any potential IL-12-modulating therapy without knowing whether a viral or autoimmune component predominates. The down-stream effects of IL-12 are frequently attributed to another Th1 cytokine, IFN-γ; yet, IFN-γ suppresses disease development in the CM-induced model of myocarditis. Interestingly, it has been shown that IFN-γ plays a protective role in murine acute myocarditis caused by encephalomyocarditis virus [31] and over-expression of IFN-γ in the pancreas prevents the development of CB3-induced myocarditis in NOD mice [32]. The unique combination of anti-viral and anti-inflammatory effects of IFN-γ may be useful in a clinical setting.

We found that blocking a classic Th2 cytokine, IL-4, with monoclonal antibody reduced the severity of myocarditis. This finding somewhat contradicts those in other models of organ-specific autoimmune diseases where IL-4 has been shown to play a protective/regulatory role. Our observation may be unique to the model or the A/J strain of mice, which is considered a Th2-prone strain. However, a similar phenotype suggestive of a Th2 response has been observed in BALB/c mice. Eosinophils, a hallmark of a Th2 process, are commonly present in severe cases of human myocarditis, possibly contributing to local damage. It is plausible that factors such as genetic background, type of autoimmune disease, or even different phases of the same pathologic condition affect how a certain cytokine or its absence will influence the outcome of disease.

We found that another Th2 cytokine, IL-10, plays a protective, anti-inflammatory role. This accords with findings in other autoimmune disease models. In addition to cytokines, other soluble or cell-surface molecules contribute to the pathogenesis of autoimmune myocarditis by either promoting disease initiation, such as complement component C3 and its receptors, CR1(CD35) and CR2 (CD21) [33, 34] or suppressing disease progression, such as CTLA-4 ([35], unpublished observations).

The future directions of our research include the dissection of the mechanisms by which the above-mentioned cytokines and other mediators contribute to the heart inflammation. It is of particular interest to determine how IL-12 promotes disease in an IFN-γ-independent manner and what underlying immunologic mechanisms explain the disease-limiting effect of IFN-γ, a cytokine with frequently ascribed pro-inflammatory effects. We need to gain a deeper understanding of how cardiac inflammation leads to cardiac dysfunction and consequently cardiomyopathy and heart failure. A detailed study of the effects of inflammatory mediators on cardiomyocyte function, cardiac chamber remodeling, and overall performance of a heart as a pump may lead to new improved treatments of heart failure.

Acknowledgements
The authors thank Mrs Hermine Bongers for her excellent secretarial assistance. Their research is supported by NIH research grants HL67290, HL70729, and AI51835.

References

1   Corvisart JN (1812) Essai sur les maladies et les lesions organiques du coeur. *Gates J MMMS* 182–189, 299–303 [Cited by Gravanis MB, Sternby NH (1991) *Arch Pathol Lab Med* 115: 390–392]

2   Sakakibara S, Konno S (1962) Endomyocardial biopsy. *Jpn Heart J* 3: 357–543

3   Grogan M, Redfield MM, Bailey KR, Reeder GS, Gersh BJ, Edwards WD, Rodeheffer RJ (1995) Long-term outcome of patients with biopsy-proved myocarditis: Comparison with idiopathic dilated cardiomyopathy. *J Am Coll Cardiol* 26: 80–84

4   Towbin JA, Bowles NE (2002) The failing heart. *Nature* 415: 227–233

5   Grist NR, Bell EJ (1969) Coxsackie viruses and the heart. *Am Heart J* 77: 295–300

6   Huber SA (1997) Autoimmunity in myocarditis: Relevance of animal models. *Clin Immunol Immunopathol* 83: 93–102

7   Rose NR, Herskowitz A, Neumann DA, Neu N (1988) Autoimmune myocarditis: A paradigm of post-infection autoimmune disease. *Immunol Today* 9: 117–120

8   Neu N, Rose NR, Beisel KW, Herskowitz A, Gurri-Glass G, Craig SW (1987) Cardiac myosin induces myocarditis in genetically predisposed mice. *J Immunol* 139: 3630–3636

9   Smith SC, Allen PM (1991) Myosin-induced acute myocarditis is a T-cell-mediated disease. *J Immunol* 147: 2141–2147

10   Afanasyeva M, Wang Y, Kaya Z, Park S, Zilliox MJ, Schofield BH, Hill SL, Rose NR (2001) Experimental autoimmune myocarditis in A/J mice is an interleukin-4-dependent disease with a Th2 phenotype. *Am J Pathol* 159: 193–203

11   Penninger JM, Neu N, Timms E, Wallace VA, Koh DR, Kishihara K, Pummerer C, Mak

TW (1993) The induction of experimental autoimmune myocarditis in mice lacking CD4 or CD8 molecules. *J Exp Med* 178: 1837–1842

12   Opavsky MA, Penninger J, Aitken K, Wen WH, Dawood F, Mak T, Liu P (1999) Susceptibility to myocarditis is dependent on the response of alphabeta T lymphocytes to coxsackieviral infection. *Circ Res* 85: 551–558

13   Pummerer C, Berger P, Fruhwirth M, Ofner C, Neu N (1991) Cellular infiltrate, major histocompatibility antigen expression and immunopathogenic mechanisms in cardiac myosin-induced myocarditis. *Lab Invest* 65: 538–547

14   Neu N, Pummerer C, Rieker T, Berger P (1993) T-cells in cardiac myosin-induced myocarditis. *Clin Immunol Immunopathol* 68: 107–110

15   Wang Y, Afanasyeva M, Hill SL, Rose NR (1999) Characterization of murine autoimmune myocarditis induced by self and foreign cardiac myosin. *Autoimmunity* 31: 151–162

16   Lane JR, Neumann DA, Lafond-Walker A, Herskowitz A, Rose NR (1992) Interleukin 1 and tumor necrosis factor can promote coxsackie B3-induced myocarditis in resistant B10.A mice. *J Exp Med* 175: 1123–1129

17   Lane JR, Neumann DA, Lafond-Walker A, Herskowitz A, Rose NR (1993) Role of IL-1 and tumor necrosis factor in coxsackie virus-induced autoimmune myocarditis. *J Immunol* 151: 1682–1690

18   Neumann DA, Lane JR, Allen GS, Herskowitz A, Rose NR (1993) Viral myocarditis leading to cardiomyopathy: Do cytokines contribute to pathogenesis? *Clin Immunol Immunopathol* 68: 181–190

19   Smith SC, Allen PM (1992) Neutralization of endogenous tumor necrosis factor ameliorates the severity of myosin-induced myocarditis. *Circ Res* 70: 856–863

20   Bachmaier K, Pummerer C, Kozieradzki I, Pfeffer K, Mak TW, Neu N, Penninger JM (1997) Low-molecular-weight tumor necrosis factor receptor p55 controls induction of autoimmune heart disease. *Circulation* 95: 655–661

21   Cunningham MW (2001) Cardiac myosin and the TH1/TH2 paradigm in autoimmune myocarditis. *Am J Pathol* 159: 5–12

22   Afanasyeva M, Wang Y, Kaya Z, Stafford EA, Dohmen KM, Sadighi Akha AA, Rose NR (2001) Interleukin-12 receptor/STAT4 signaling is required for the development of autoimmune myocarditis in mice by an interferon-gamma-independent pathway. *Circulation* 104: 3145–3151

23   Okura Y, Takeda K, Honda S, Hanawa H, Watanabe H, Kodama M, Izumi T, Aizawa Y, Seki S, Abo T (1998) Recombinant murine interleukin-12 facilitates induction of cardiac myosin-specific Type 1 helper T-cells in rats. *Circ Res* 82: 1035–1042

24   Eriksson U, Kurrer MO, Sebald W, Brombacher F, Kopf M (2001) Dual role of the IL-12/IFN-gamma axis in the development of autoimmune myocarditis: Induction by IL-12 and protection by IFN-gamma. *J Immunol* 167: 5464–5469

25   Georgakopoulos D, Mitzner WA, Chen CH, Byrne BJ, Millar HD, Hare JM, Kass DA (1998) *In vivo* murine left ventricular pressure-volume relations by miniaturized conductance micromanometry. *Am J Physiol* 274: H1416–H1422

26 Afanasyeva M (2002) The role of T helper 1 and T helper 2 cytokines in murine experimental autoimmune myocarditis. Johns Hopkins University, PhD Dissertation

27 Kaya Z, Dohmen KM, Wang Y, Schlichting J, Afanasyeva M, Leuschner F, Rose NR
   (2002) Cutting edge: A critical role for IL-10 in induction of nasal tolerance in experimental autoimmune myocarditis. *J Immunol* 168: 1552–1556

28 Wang Y, Afanasyeva M, Hill SL, Kaya Z, Rose NR (2000) Nasal administration of cardiac myosin suppresses autoimmune myocarditis in mice. *J Am Coll Cardiol* 36:
   1992–1999

29 Watanabe K, Nakazawa M, Fuse K, Hanawa H, Kodama M, Aizawa Y, Ohnuki T,
   Gejyo F, Maruyama H, Miyazaki J (2001) Protection against autoimmune myocarditis
   by gene transfer of interleukin-10 by electroporation. *Circulation* 104: 1098–1100

30 Shioi T, Matsumori A, Nishio R, Ono K, Kakio T, Sasayama S (1997) Protective role of
   interleukin-12 in viral myocarditis. *J Mol Cell Cardiol* 29: 2327–2334

31 Yamamoto N, Shibamori M, Ogura M, Seko Y, Kikuchi M (1998) Effects of intranasal
   administration of recombinant murine interferon-gamma on murine acute myocarditis
   caused by encephalomyocarditis virus. *Circulation* 97: 1017–1023

32 Horwitz MS, La Cava A, Fine C, Rodriguez E, Ilic A, Sarvetnick N (2000) Pancreatic
   expression of interferon-gamma protects mice from lethal Coxsackie virus B3 infection
   and subsequent myocarditis. *Nat Med* 6: 693–697

33 Kaya Z, Afanasyeva M, Wang Y, Dohmen KM, Schlichting J, Tretter T, Fairweather D,
   Holers VM, Rose NR (2001) Contribution of the innate immune system to autoimmune
   myocarditis: a role for complement. *Nat Immunol* 2: 739–745

34 Afanasyeva M, Rose NR (2002) Cardiomyopathy is linked to complement activation.
   Am J Pathol 161: 351–357

35 Paupore EJ (2001) The role of CTLA-4 in autoimmune myocarditis. Baltimore, MD.
   Johns Hopkins University, MS Thesis

Nuclear factors in cardiac disease

Peroxisome proliferator activated receptors, inflammation, the vasculature and the heart

Quy N. Diep, Farhad Amiri and Ernesto L. Schiffrin

CIHR, Multidisciplinary Research Group on Hypertension, Clinical Research Institute of Montreal, 110 Avenue des Pins Ouest, Montreal, Quebec, Canada H2W 1R7

Introduction

Over the last dozen years since the discovery of the family of transcription factor termed peroxisome proliferator activated receptors (PPAR) [1], an impressive number of studies have investigated the characteristics, ligands and functional roles as well as molecular mechanisms of PPARs. Although PPARs were formerly believed to regulate genes involved only in lipid and glucose metabolism, a large number of more recent studies have explored the role of PPARs in cell growth, cell migration as well as in inflammation. The function of PPARs in inflammation was first demonstrated by Devchand et al. [2] who showed that pro-inflammatory eicosanoid leukotriene B4 binds to PPARα and induces transcription of genes involved in ω- and β-oxidation. In this chapter, we briefly summarize the role of PPARs in inflammation generally, and discuss in greater detail the role of PPARs in the heart. We will discuss molecular, biochemical, physiological and pharmacological roles of PPARα and PPARγ in the regulation of cardiac hypertrophy, inflammation and cardiac function, and introduce novel concepts relating to PPARs as transcription factors in the regulation of the expression of inflammatory response genes as mechanisms that participate in the pathophysiology of cardiac disease.

PPAR family

The first PPAR discovered was PPARα by Isseman and Green in 1990 [1]. These authors showed that PPARα was the receptor by which xenobiotics induce peroxisome proliferation in rodent liver. Shortly after, PPARδ (also called β or NUC-1) and PPARγ were identified [3]. All three PPAR isoforms share similar structure (reviewed in [4]) and differ in their ligand-binding domains. Basically, the PPAR structure consists of a N-terminal domain that plays an important role in regulating PPAR activity, a DNA binding domain that is responsible for the binding of PPAR to the PPAR response element (PPRE) in the promoter region of target genes, a docking domain for a cofactor, and a C-terminal ligand-binding domain that is responsible for ligand specificity and activation of PPAR binding to the PPRE to accelerate transcription of target genes [5]. A conformational change of these receptors occurs upon activation by PPAR ligands, allowing them to heterodimerize with retinoidX receptors (RXRα). The heterodimer then binds to PPRE in target genes and modulates gene transcription. PPRE consists of a direct repeat of the nuclear receptor hexameric AGGTCA recognition sequence separated by one or two nucleotides [6]. Although the PPAR-RXR heterodimer determines specific gene transcription on ligand activation, the differential recruitment of co-activators and co-repressors by PPAR-RXR heterodimers plays a crucial role. In the inactivated state, PPAR is believed to be present, binding to co-repressor proteins. Upon activation, PPAR dissociates from co-repressors and recruits co-activators, including a PPAR-binding protein and the steroid receptor coactivator-1, and binds to the cognate DNA response elements within the PPAR gene promoter [7].

PPARδ is expressed ubiquitously [8, 9] and its function remains unclear due to the unavailability of specific ligands. For this reason, only PPARα and PPARγ will be discussed in greater details in this chapter. PPARα is mainly expressed in tissues where fatty acid catabolism is important, such as liver, kidney, heart, and muscles. PPARγ is highly expressed in adipose tissue where it controls adipocyte differentiation and lipid storage and modulates the action of insulin. PPARα is activated by natural ligands such as fatty acids, eicosanoids and oxidized fatty acids. The synthetic ligands for PPARα are the lipid lowering fibrates. Selective activators of PPARγ are the insulin sensitizer's thiazolidinedione glitazones, such as troglitazone, pioglitazone and rosiglitazone.

PPAR and vascular inflammation

This subject has been well reviewed elsewhere [10–12] and will be summarized briefly. Until recently, PPAR was thought to regulate genes involved in lipid and glucose metabolism. During the last few years, there has been an exponential rise in the understanding of the role of PPAR in inflammation, particular in the vasculature and the heart. The anti-inflammatory effect of PPARα was first demonstrated by [2] who showed that the pro-inflammatory eicosanoid leukotriene B4 (LTB4) binds to PPARα and induces the transcription of genes involved in ω- and β-oxidation leading to its own catabolism.

The finding that PPARγ was highly expressed in the spleen [8, 9] lead to the discovery of high expression of PPARγ in monocytes/macrophages [13]. The same group demonstrated that PPARγ is markedly up-regulated in activated macrophages and inhibits the expression of inducible nitric oxide synthase (iNOS), gelatinase B (matrix metalloproteinase 9) and scavenger receptor A genes in response to 15d-PGJ2 and synthetic PPARγ ligands. PPARγ activation inhibits gene expression in part by antagonizing the activities of the transcription factors AP-1, STAT and NF-κB. Taken together, PPARs may function to protect the vascular system from injury by down-regulation of inflammatory mediators.

PPARα and vascular inflammation

Since both PPARα and PPARγ are expressed in vascular cells, such as endothelial cells [14, 15] vascular smooth muscle cells (VSMC) [16] and monocytes/macrophages [13], a number of studies have been carried out to elucidate the cellular and molecular mechanisms underlying inflammatory control by PPARs. In VSMC, PPARα ligands inhibit interleukin-1β-induced production of interleukin-6 and prostaglandin and expression of cyclooxygenase-2, as a result of PPARα repression of transcription factor NF-κB signaling [16]. From the clinical point of view, fenofibrate treatment decreases the plasma concentrations of interleukin-6, fibrinogen and C-reactive protein in hyperlipidemic patients [16]. Fenofibrate also significantly reduces plasma interferon-γ and tumor necrosis factor a (TNF-α) in hyperlipoproteinemia IIb patients [17], suggesting a potential role of PPARα in the treatment of chronic inflammatory diseases. Furthermore, PPARα activators down-regulate cytokine-induced genes, such as expression of vascular cell adhesion molecule (VCAM)-1 and tissue factor in endothelial cells [18]. *In vivo* studies have also demonstrated an anti-inflammatory action of PPARα. Indeed, PPARα-deficient mice displayed an exacerbated inflammatory response to lipopolysaccharide stimulation [19]. In addition, fibrates, which activate PPARα, did not affect LPS-induced IL-6 transcription in PPARα-deficient mice. Taken together, these data provide evidence that PPARα plays a role in the inflammatory response at the vascular level. The molecular mechanisms of this anti-inflammatory action of PPARα activators could be that PPARα negatively interferes with the inflammatory response by antagonizing the NF-κB signaling pathway, in which the anti-oxidant enzyme, catalase, might have a potential [18–20].

PPARγ and vascular inflammation

The mechanisms of the anti-inflammatory effects of PPARγ have been studied extensively. The underlying mechanisms for the anti-inflammatory effects of PPARγ have been reported in macrophage/monocytes and endothelial cells [10, 11]. In monocytes, PPARγ-dependent signaling suppresses the production of pro-inflammatory cytokines, whereas in vascular smooth muscle cells, PPARγ inhibits proliferation and migration. PPARγ was first demonstrated to be expressed in monocytes, where

PPARγ activators were shown to inhibit the expression of TNF-α, IL-6, IL-1β [21], iNOS, matrix metalloprotease-9 (MMP-9) and scavenger receptor A [22]. PPARγ is expressed in atherosclerotic plaques and in endothelial cells. The PPARγ activators, troglitazone and 15-deoxy-(delta12, 14)-prostaglandin J2 (15d-PGJ2), markedly attenuated TNF-induced VCAM-1 and intercellular adhesion molecule (ICAM)-1 expression in cultured endothelial cells. In addition, troglitazone significantly reduced monocyte/macrophage homing to atherosclerotic plaques in apoE-deficient mice [23]. Taken together, these findings suggest that PPARγ activators, currently used in treatment of Type II diabetes, may have beneficial effects in modulating inflammatory response in atherosclerosis. However, it should be pointed out that 15d-PGJ2 (a PPARγ agonist) induces synthesis of the inflammatory interleukin-8 in endothelial cells in a PPARγ-independent manner [24]. PPARγ also plays an anti-inflammatory role in hypertensive models, such as angiotensin (Ang) II-induced hypertension. We have recently demonstrated that the PPARγ activators rosiglita-zone and pioglitazone prevented hypertension in Ang II-infused rats, and abrogated the structural, functional and molecular changes induced by Ang II in blood vessels by exerting direct effects on the vascular wall, leading to inhibition of cell growth and inflammation [25].

Recently a mechanism for the anti-inflammatory action of PPARγ activators has been described. An interaction has been demonstrated between CCAAT/enhancer-binding protein (C/EBP)-δ that up-regulate transcription of various inflammatory cytokines and are present in tandem repeats in the PPARγ gene promoter, and are negatively auto-regulated by PPARγ in the vasculature [26]. PPARγ ligands troglita-zone, pioglitazone, and 15d-PGJ2, transcriptionally inhibited IL-1β-induced IL-6 expression in vascular smooth muscle cells. Thus C/EBP-δ may be negatively auto-regulated *via* transactivation of PPARγ, down-regulating inflammatory responses.

PPARα and cardiac inflammation

There is increasing evidence pointing to a potential role of PPARα in the patho-physiology of heart disease. PPARα appears to play a crucial role in mitochondrial fatty acid β-oxidation, a fuel generating mechanism in the heart [27]. Only two years after PPAR discovery, PPARα was identified as a new member of the steroid hormone receptor super-family that is activated by a peroxisome proliferator acti-vator WY 14643 and by fatty acids [28]. Since, it has been demonstrated that long-chain fatty acids regulate the transcription of a gene encoding a pivotal enzyme in the mitochondrial fatty acid uptake pathway in cardiac myocytes.

Even though PPARα is predominantly expressed in the heart, where the catabolic rate of fatty acids is high, it was only recently that the role of PPARα in the control of myocardial lipid metabolism was established through the activation of transcrip-tion of the muscle carnitine palmitoyltransferase I (CPT I) gene [27]. Moreover, in response to the metabolic stress induced by inhibition of translocation of mito-chondrial long-chain fatty acids with CPT I inhibitor etomoxir, PPARα serves as a molecular "lipostat" factor by inducing the expression of target genes involved in cardiac fatty acid metabolism [29].

Recent evidence has also linked PPARα to cardiac hypertrophy. PPARα is deac-tivated during cardiac hypertrophic growth [30], which suggests that PPARα is involved in the regulation of cardiac remodeling. Hypertrophied myocytes exhibit-ed reduced capacity for cellular lipid homeostasis, as evidenced by intracellular fat accumulation in response to oleate loading. These results indicate that during car-diac hypertrophic growth, PPARα is deactivated at several levels, leading to dimin-ished capacity for myocardial lipid and energy homeostasis. In addition to the role that PPARα might play in cardiac hypertrophy, PPARα also exerts direct anti-inflammatory action. PPARα and PPARγ activators inhibit cardiac expression of TNF-α and NF-κB induced by lipopolysaccharide [31], both of which have been reported to be elevated in the failing heart and have negative inotropic effects on cardiac myocytes. This data further suggests that PPARα may play a role in inflam-mation in the heart *via* specific signaling pathways and cytokines.

Using PPARα$^{-/-}$ mouse as a potentially useful model of inborn and acquired abnormalities of human fatty acid utilization, a critical role for PPARα in a tran-scriptional regulatory response to fasting has been demonstrated [32]. Indeed, the capacity for constitutive myocardial β-oxidation of the medium and long chain fatty acids octanoic acid and palmitic acid was markedly reduced in the PPARα-null mice compared to wild-type mice [33], indicating that mitochondrial fatty acid catabo-lism is impaired in the absence of PPARα. In contrast, constitutive β-oxidation of the very long chain fatty acid, lignoceric acid, did not differ between the PPARα-deficient mice and the wild-type, which suggests that the constitutive expression of enzymes involved in peroxisomal β-oxidation is independent of PPARα. It was implied that altered expression of fatty acid-metabolizing enzymes could lead to myocardial damage and fibrosis, *via* inflammation and abnormal cell growth.

Moreover, the PPARα activator fenofibrate decreased preproET-1 mRNA expression and attenuated collagen Type I and Type III mRNA, associated with reduced interstitial and perivascular fibrosis in hypertrophied rat hearts due to pres-sure-overload by abdominal aortic banding [34]. Since the ET-1 gene has AP-1 response elements in the 5'-flanking region, the authors suggested that myocardial fibrosis is effectively inhibited by fenofibrate through suppression of AP-1-mediat-ed ET-1 gene augmentation in the pressure-overloaded heart caused by aortic band-ing in rats. Thus the importance of PPARα as a regulator of the oxidative degrada-tion of fatty acids becomes more evident in pathophysiological states with high-energy demands that are associated with abnormal fatty acid metabolism, such as myocarditis and dilated cardiomyopathy.

Additionally, PPARα activator fenofibrate reduced cardiac hypertrophy and inflammatory lesion area associated with an increase in the anti-inflammatory

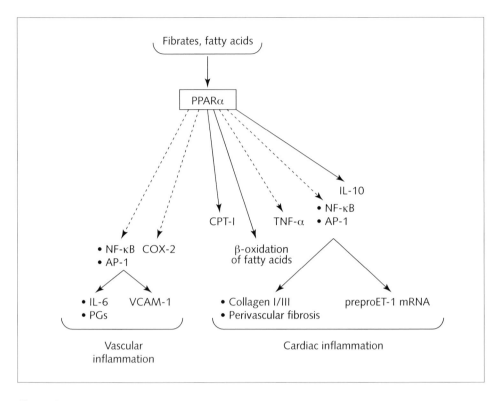

Figure 1
Some of the mechanisms activated by PPARα in the heart and in blood vessels leading to inflammation are depicted in this figure.
VCAM-1, vascular cell adhesion molecule-1; IL, interleukin; PGs, prostaglandins; NF-κB, nuclear factor kappa B; COX-2, cyclooxygenase-2; CPT-I, carnitine palmitoyltransferase I; TNF-α, tumor necrosis factor alpha; AP-1, activator protein-1; ET-1, endothelin-1;
——→, stimulation; ----→, inhibition.

cytokine IL-10 expression [35]. Furthermore, fenofibrate ameliorated changes in serum albumin and sialic acid, which are markers of inflammation. Supporting the role of PPARα in cardiac inflammation, we recently observed that fenofibrate had direct beneficial effects on inflammation and collagen deposition in the heart of Ang II-infused rats (unpublished data). This was associated with a decrease in NF-κB activity, VCAM-1, PECAM, ICAM-1 and ED-1 expression, and down-regulation of AT_1 and up-regulation of AT_2 receptors. Since PPARα activity was increased by fenofibrate treatment, these findings indicate that the favorable effects of fenofibrate on the heart of Ang II-infused rats were at least partly dependent on PPARα activation.

Pathways activated or inhibited by PPARα that participate in cardiac inflammation are summarized in Figure 1.

PPARγ and cardiac inflammation

In contrast to the clearer picture of PPARα function in the heart, the role of PPARγ in the heart has not been well explored. In addition, there is a discrepancy between clinical and experimental data. Recent *in vitro* and *in vivo* studies have suggested a role for PPARγ as an inhibitor of cardiac hypertrophy. Both troglitazone and the endogenous PPARγ ligand 15d-PGJ2 were able to block the hypertrophic phenotype and brain natriuretic peptide expression in cultured cardiomyocytes [36]. Moreover, PPARγ may function as a transducer of anti-hypertrophic signaling in the heart. In heterozygous PPARγ-deficient mice, an exaggerated hypertrophic response to pressure overload induced by aortic banding was noted [37]. In contrast, to the phenotype presented by PPARγ$^{-/-}$ mice in response to aortic banding, the PPARγ agonist pioglitazone significantly blunted myocardial hypertrophy in both wild-type and PPARγ$^{-/-}$ mice, although to various degrees. These findings are further supported by *in vitro* data indicating that angiotensin II-induced hypertrophic gene expression, as well as increased cardiomyocyte size, could also be attenuated by thiazolidinediones. Taken together, these data strongly suggest the involvement of PPARγ in a pathway for negative regulation of cardiac hypertrophy. In addition, PPARγ improved left ventricular diastolic function and decreased collagen accumulation in diabetic rats [38, 39], and protected myocardium from ischemic injury [40, 41]. However, clinical reports have recently warned that the PPARγ activator glitazones may lead to development or exacerbation of congestive heart failure [42]. Among molecular adaptations of the hypertrophic heart are the increase in glucose utilization and decreased fatty acid oxidation. Whether or not PPARγ has similar regulating effects on fatty acid metabolism as PPARa is unclear. Since both PPARα and PPARγ have a partially overlapping ligand profile, PPARγ could mediate to some degree similar signals as PPARα in cardiomyocytes. PPARγ signaling could attenuate cardiac remodeling *via* pathways not directly involved in controlling lipid and energy metabolism, such as inflammation. Inflammation is an important mechanism in the progression of cardiac remodeling and dysfunction. In macrophages, PPARγ is involved in regulation of inflammatory responses by antagonism of transcription factors NF-κB and AP-1 [13]. NF-κB is required for the hypertrophic response of neonatal rat cardiomyocytes *in vitro* [43]. Indeed, we recently observed that the PPARγ activator pioglitazone has beneficial long-term effects on cardiac hypertrophy, cardiac inflammation and cardiac function in spontaneously hypertensive rats (unpublished data).

Pathways activated or inhibited by PPARγ that participate in cardiac inflammation are shown in Figure 2.

343

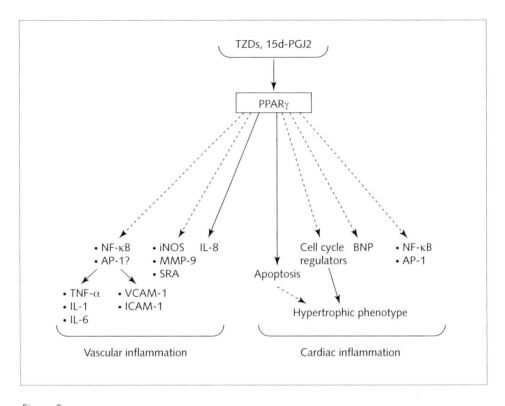

Figure 2
*PPARγ-activated mechanisms in heart and blood vessels leading to inflammation are depict-
ed in this figure.*
*Abbreviations as in Fig. 1. TZDs, thiazolidinediones; 15d-PGJ2, 15-deoxy-(delta12,14)-
prostaglandin J2; ICAM-1, intercellular adhesion molecule-1; iNOS, inducible nitric oxide
synthase; MMP-9, matrix metalloproteinase-9; SRA, scavenger receptor A; BNP, brain natriuretic peptide.*

Conclusions and future directions

Based on *in vivo* and *in vitro* studies with different cell types, it is clear that PPARα
and PPARγ play an important role in the regulation of inflammatory responses.
However, our knowledge of the regulatory mechanisms and signaling cascades
underlying the anti-inflammatory effect of PPARs, particularly in blood vessels and
the heart, is still limited. More research in this area is required. In addition, the discrepancy between the beneficial effect of PPARγ activators on the heart in experimental models and the clinical reports of heart failure that have occurred in a few
diabetic patients treated with PPARγ activators needs to be further clarified.

Acknowledgements

Work from our laboratory discussed in this chapter has been supported by grant 13570 and a Group grant to the Multidisciplinary Research Group on Hypertension (ELS) and a post-doctoral fellowship (QND), all from Canadian Institutes of Health Research (CIHR).

References

1   Issemann I, Green S (1990) Activation of a member of the steroid hormone receptor superfamily by peroxisome proliferators. *Nature* 347: 645–650

2   Devchand PR, Keller H, Peters JM, Vazquez M, Gonzalez FJ, Wahli W (1996) The PPA-Ralpha-leukotriene B4 pathway to inflammation control. *Nature* 384: 39–43

3   Dreyer C, Krey G, Keller H, Givel F, Helftenbein G, Wahli W (1992) Control of the peroxisomal beta-oxidation pathway by a novel family of nuclear hormone receptors. *Cell* 68: 879–87

4   Guan Y, Breyer MD (2001) Peroxisome proliferator-activated receptors (PPARs): Novel therapeutic targets in renal disease. *Kidney Int* 60: 14–30

5   Tugwood JD, Issemann I, Anderson RG, Bundell KR, McPheat WL, Green S (1992) The mouse peroxisome proliferator activated receptor recognizes a response element in the 5' flanking sequence of the rat acyl CoA oxidase gene. *EMBO J* 11: 433–439

6   Ijpenberg A, Jeannin E, Wahli W, Desvergne B (1997) Polarity and specific sequence requirements of peroxisome proliferator-activated receptor (PPAR)/retinoid X receptor heterodimer binding to DNA. A functional analysis of the malic enzyme gene PPAR response element. *J Biol Chem* 272: 20108–20117

7   Llopis J, Westin S, Ricote M, Wang Z, Cho CY, Kurokawa R, Mullen TM, Rose DW, Rosenfeld MG, Tsien RY et al (2000) Ligand-dependent interactions of coactivators steroid receptor coactivator-1 and peroxisome proliferator-activated receptor binding protein with nuclear hormone receptors can be imaged in live cells and are required for transcription. *Proc Natl Acad Sci USA* 97: 4363–4368

8   Kliewer SA, Forman BM, Blumberg B, Ong ES, Borgmeyer U, Mangelsdorf DJ, Umesono K, Evans RM (1994) Differential expression and activation of a family of murine peroxisome proliferator-activated receptors. *Proc Natl Acad Sci USA* 91: 7355–7359

9   Braissant O, Foufelle F, Scotto C, Dauca M, Wahli W (1996) Differential expression of peroxisome proliferator-activated receptors (PPARs): tissue distribution of PPAR-alpha, -beta, and -gamma in the adult rat. *Endocrinology* 137: 354–366

10 Delerive P, Fruchart C, Staels B (2001) Peroxisome proliferator-activated receptors in inflammation control. *J Endocrinol* 169: 453–459

11 Chinetti G, Fruchart JC, Staels B (2001) Peroxisome proliferator-activated receptors (PPARs): nuclear receptors with functions in the vascular wall. *Z Kardiol* 90 (Suppl 3): 125–132

12 Bishop-Bailey D (2000) Peroxisome proliferator-activated receptors in the cardiovascular system. *Br J Pharmacol* 129: 823–834

13 Ricote M, Li AC, Willson TM, Kelly CJ, Glass CK (1998) The peroxisome proliferator-activated receptor-gamma is a negative regulator of macrophage activation. *Nature* 391: 79–82

14 Inoue I, Shino K, Noji S, Awata T, Katayama S (1998) Expression of peroxisome proliferator-activated receptor alpha (PPAR alpha) in primary cultures of human vascular endothelial cells. *Biochem Biophys Res Commun* 246: 370–374

15 Satoh H, Tsukamoto K, Hashimoto Y, Hashimoto N, Togo M, Hara M, Maekawa H, Isoo N, Kimura S, Watanabe T (1999) Thiazolidinediones suppress endothelin-1 secretion from bovine vascular endothelial cells: a new possible role of PPARgamma on vascular endothelial function. *Biochem Biophys Res Commun* 254: 757–763

16 Staels B, Koenig W, Habib A, Merval R, Lebret M, Torra IP, Delerive P, Fadel A, Chinetti G, Fruchart JC et al (1998) Activation of human aortic smooth-muscle cells is inhibited by PPARalpha but not by PPARgamma activators. *Nature* 393: 790–793

17 Madej A, Okopien B, Kowalski J, Zielinski M, Wysocki J, Szygula B, Kalina Z, Herman ZS (1998) Effects of fenofibrate on plasma cytokine concentrations in patients with atherosclerosis and hyperlipoproteinemia IIb. *Int J Clin Pharmacol Ther* 36: 345–349

18 Marx N, Sukhova GK, Collins T, Libby P, Plutzky J (1999) PPARalpha activators inhibit cytokine-induced vascular cell adhesion molecule-1 expression in human endothelial cells. *Circulation* 99: 3125–3131

19 Delerive P, De Bosscher K, Besnard S, Vanden Berghe W, Peters JM, Gonzalez FJ, Fruchart JC, Tedgui A, Haegeman G, Staels B (1999) Peroxisome proliferator-activated receptor alpha negatively regulates the vascular inflammatory gene response by negative cross-talk with transcription factors NF-kappaB and AP-1. *J Biol Chem* 274: 32048–32054

20 Poynter ME, Daynes RA (1998) Peroxisome proliferator-activated receptor alpha activation modulates cellular redox status, represses nuclear factor-kappa-B signaling, and reduces inflammatory cytokine production in aging. *J Biol Chem* 273: 32833–32841

21 Jiang C, Ting AT, Seed B (1998) PPAR-gamma agonists inhibit production of monocyte inflammatory cytokines. *Nature* 391: 82–86

22 Ricote M, Huang JT, Welch JS, Glass CK (1999) The peroxisome proliferator-activated receptor (PPARgamma) as a regulator of monocyte/macrophage function. *J Leukoc Biol* 66: 733–739

23 Pasceri V, Wu HD, Willerson JT, Yeh ET (2000) Modulation of vascular inflammation *in vitro* and *in vivo* by peroxisome proliferator-activated receptor-gamma activators. *Circulation* 101: 235–238

24 Jozkowicz A, Dulak J, Prager M, Nanobashvili J, Nigisch A, Winter B, Weigel G, Huk I (2001) Prostaglandin-J2 induces synthesis of interleukin-8 by endothelial cells in a PPAR-gamma-independent manner. *Prostaglandins Other Lipid Mediat* 66: 165–177

25 Diep QN, El Mabrouk M, Cohn JS, Endemann D, Amiri F, Virdis A, Neves MF, Schiffrin EL (2002) Structure, endothelial function, cell growth, and inflammation in

blood vessels of angiotensin II-infused rats: Role of peroxisome proliferator-activated receptor-gamma. *Circulation* 105: 2296–2302

26   Takata Y, Kitami Y, Yang ZH, Nakamura M, Okura T, Hiwada K (2002) Vascular inflammation is negatively auto-regulated by interaction between CCAAT/enhancer-binding protein-δ and peroxisome proliferator-activated receptor-γ. *Circ Res* 91: 427–433

27   Brandt JM, Djouadi F, Kelly DP (1998) Fatty acids activate transcription of the muscle carnitine palmitoyltransferase I gene in cardiac myocytes *via* the peroxisome proliferator-activated receptor alpha. *J Biol Chem* 273: 23786–23792

28   Schmidt A, Endo N, Rutledge SJ, Vogel R, Shinar D, Rodan GA (1992) Identification of a new member of the steroid hormone receptor super-family that is activated by a peroxisome proliferator and fatty acids. *Mol Endocrinol* 6: 1634–1641

29   Djouadi F, Brandt JM, Weinheimer CJ, Leone TC, Gonzalez FJ, Kelly DP (1999) The role of the peroxisome proliferator-activated receptor alpha (PPAR alpha) in the control of cardiac lipid metabolism. *Prostaglandins Leukot Essent Fatty Acids* 60: 339–343

30   Barger PM, Brandt JM, Leone TC, Weinheimer CJ, Kelly DP (2000) Deactivation of peroxisome proliferator-activated receptor-alpha during cardiac hypertrophic growth. *J Clin Invest* 105: 1723–1730

31   Takano H, Nagai T, Asakawa M, Toyozaki T, Oka T, Komuro I, Saito T, Masuda Y (2000) Peroxisome proliferator-activated receptor activators inhibit lipopolysaccharide-induced tumor necrosis factor-alpha expression in neonatal rat cardiac myocytes. *Circ Res* 87: 596–602

32   Leone TC, Weinheimer CJ, Kelly DP (1999) A critical role for the peroxisome proliferator-activated receptor alpha (PPARalpha) in the cellular fasting response: The PPARalpha-null mouse as a model of fatty acid oxidation disorders. *Proc Natl Acad Sci USA* 96: 7473–7478

33   Watanabe K, Fujii H, Takahashi T, Kodama M, Aizawa Y, Ohta Y, Ono T, Hasegawa G, Naito M, Nakajima T et al (2000) Constitutive regulation of cardiac fatty acid metabolism through peroxisome proliferator-activated receptor alpha associated with age-dependent cardiac toxicity. *J Biol Chem* 275: 22293–22299

34   Ogata T, Miyauchi T, Sakai S, Irukayama-Tomobe Y, Goto K, Yamaguchi I (2002) Stimulation of peroxisome-proliferator-activated receptor alpha (PPARalpha) attenuates cardiac fibrosis and endothelin-1 production in pressure-overloaded rat hearts. *Clin Sci (Lond)* 103 (Suppl 1): 284S–288S

35   Maruyama S, Kato K, Kodama M, Hirono S, Fuse K, Nakagawa O, Nakazawa M, Miida T, Yamamoto T, Watanabe K et al (2002) Fenofibrate, a peroxisome proliferator-activated receptor alpha activator, suppresses experimental autoimmune myocarditis by stimulating the interleukin-10 pathway in rats. *J Atheroscler Thromb* 9:87–92

36   Yamamoto K, Ohki R, Lee RT, Ikeda U, Shimada K (2001) Peroxisome proliferator-activated receptor gamma activators inhibit cardiac hypertrophy in cardiac myocytes. *Circulation* 104: 1670–1675

37   Asakawa M, Takano H, Nagai T, Uozumi H, Hasegawa H, Kubota N, Saito T, Masu-

da Y, Kadowaki T, Komuro I F (2002) Peroxisome proliferator-activated receptor gamma plays a critical role in inhibition of cardiac hypertrophy *in vitro* and *in vivo*. *Circulation* 105: 1240–1246

38   Tsuji T, Mizushige K, Noma T, Murakami K, Ohmori K, Miyatake A, Kohno M (2001) Pioglitazone improves left ventricular diastolic function and decreases collagen accumulation in prediabetic stage of a type II diabetic rat. *J Cardiovasc Pharmacol* 38: 868–874

39   Zhu P, Lu L, Xu Y, Schwartz GG (2000) Troglitazone improves recovery of left ventricular function after regional ischemia in pigs. *Circulation* 101: 1165–1171

40   Sidell RJ, Cole MA, Draper NJ, Desrois M, Buckingham RE, Clarke K (2002) Thiazolidinedione treatment normalizes insulin resistance and ischemic injury in the zucker fatty rat heart. *Diabetes* 51: 1110–1117

41   Yue Tl TL, Chen J, Bao W, Narayanan PK, Bril A, Jiang W, Lysko PG, Gu JL, Boyce R, Zimmerman DM et al (2001) *In vivo* myocardial protection from ischemia/reperfusion injury by the peroxisome proliferator-activated receptor-gamma agonist rosiglitazone. *Circulation* 104: 2588–2594

42   Wooltorton E (2002) Rosiglitazone (Avandia) and pioglitazone (Actos) and heart failure. *CMAJ* 166: 219

43   Purcell NH, Tang G, Yu C, Mercurio F, DiDonato JA, Lin A (2001) Activation of NF-kappa-B is required for hypertrophic growth of primary rat neonatal ventricular cardiomyocytes. *Proc Natl Acad Sci USA* 98: 6668–6673

Chemokines and cardiac diseases

Role of chemokines in the pathogenesis of congestive heart failure

Joseph Winaver[1], Thomas M. Behr[2] and Zaid Abassi[1]

[1]Department of Physiology & Biophysics, Faculty of Medicine, Technion, P.O. Box 9649, Haifa 31096, Israel; [2]Department of Cardiology, Medizinische Poliklinik, University of Wuerzburg, Klinikstr. 6, 97084 Wuerzburg, Germany

Introduction

In 1990, Levin et al. [1] reported that high circulating levels of tumor necrosis factor (TNF-α) were found in patients with severe congestive heart failure (CHF), and suggested that this cytokine is involved in the pathogenesis of cardiac failure. Since then, increasing amounts of clinical and experimental data have accumulated to support a role of inflammatory mediators in the pathogenesis of myocardial dysfunction in CHF. The present chapter will review the current evidence on the involvement of chemokines, a subgroup of cytokines with chemo-attractant properties, in the mechanisms that lead to myocardial dysfunction and the development of CHF.

Chemokines (derived from chemotactic cytokines) are low-molecular-weight (8.0–12.0 kDa) proteins that have the ability to induce migration and attract circulating leukocytes into sites of inflammation in different tissues [2–5]. They are produced by a wide spectrum of cell types of both hematopoietic and non-hematopoietic origin, and are secreted in response to a variety of inflammatory and immunologic mediators. In addition to their important role in leukocyte trafficking, chemokines have biological effects on other cell types including, endothelial and vascular smooth muscle cells [6–8]. Currently, 40–50 human chemokines have been identified [4]. They are divided into four subgroups; CC, CXC, CX₃, and C, according to the position of the conserved cysteine residues in the N-terminal region of the peptide [2–4]. Of these, the first two groups, CC and CXC, contain the majority of the known chemokines at present. Monocyte chemo-attractant protein-1 (MCP-1), also known as CCL2 according to the newer nomenclature [4], is the prototype of the CC chemokines. Human MCP-1 is a 76 amino acid protein encoded by a gene that maps to the CC chemokine locus at 17q11.2 [4, 9]. The human and murine types differ in their molecular weight due to the high degree of glycosylation in the latter [10]. MCP-1 possesses potent chemo-attractant properties primarily for monocytes and was found to be involved in the pathogenesis of several cardiovascular disorders, including atherosclerosis and CHF [11, 12]. IL-8, the first pro-inflammatory chemokine discovered and the prototype of the CXC group, was initially identified in 1987 as a monocyte-derived neutrophil-activating/chemotactic factor [13]. As its name implies, it attracts primarily leukocytes, but not monocytes, and is also involved in the pathogenesis of several cardiovascular disorders [11].

Chemokines exert their biological actions by binding to chemokine receptors in target cells. According to the current nomenclature the receptors are defined as CXC, CC, XC, and CX3C followed by R and a number, whereas the chemokines are defined by the same structure-related acronyms followed by L (for ligand) [4, 14]. Unlike the classical cytokine and interleukin receptors, the chemokine receptors generally belong to the super-family of the G-protein-coupled- receptors [15]. Target cells can express more than one chemokine receptor, and apparently a single receptor can be activated by more than one ligand. This network arrangement provides a background for a complex interplay and crosstalk between intracellular transduction systems. Chemokine receptors may be linked to a number of intracellular transduction systems, depending on the type of cell and receptor activated. Several intracellular signaling pathways have been identified [16]. These include among other the activation of protein kinase C, JAK-STAT pathway, and Rho family of small G-protein which involve cell motility through the actin cytoskeleton [17, 18]. A detailed description of the cellular signaling of the chemokines network can be found in several recent reviews [16, 17, 19].

Chemokines and the cardiovascular system

A growing number of studies provide evidence for an important involvement of chemokines in the pathogenesis of cardiovascular disorders such as atherosclerosis [11, 20], CHF [12, 21], ischemic reperfusion injury [22, 23], neointimal hyperplasia following balloon injury [24] and vascular lesions induced by chronic nitric oxide (NO) blockade [25–27].

At present, there is compelling evidence for participation of chemokines, in particular MCP-1, in the mechanism of atherogenesis. This is based primarily on genetically modified, atherosclerosis-prone mice models in which the gene for MCP-1 or its receptor, CCR_2, were disrupted or over-expressed [11, 20]. The emerging view is that MCP-1 is induced in endothelial and vascular smooth muscle cells in response to atherogenic stimuli such as oxidized low density lipoproteins, cytokines and platelet derived growth factor. MCP-1 recruits monocytes into the sub-endothelial layer of the injured vessel wall, initiating an inflammatory response. Monocytes then differentiate into macrophages that express receptors for the oxidized lipids and are converted into foam cells within the fatty streak, providing a key element for atherosclerotic plaque formation. MCP-1 also induces the expression of tissue factor (TF) by vascular smooth muscle cells, which contributes to the pro-coagulatory nature of the atherosclerotic plaque [28]. Other chemokines, such as IL-8, stromal derived factor 1 (SDF-1), IP-10 and I-309 have been shown to be associated with atherogenic lesions in animal models of atherosclerosis [29–32]. However, additional studies are required to establish their exact role and relative contribution.

Role of MCP-1 and other chemokines in myocardial dysfunction and CHF

While the role of MCP-1 in atherogenesis is fairly established in experimental animal models, the involvement of chemokines in mediating myocardial injury and the development of CHF is less understood. In particular, the cause and effect relationship and the relative contribution of chemokines induction to myocardial dysfunction in CHF, appear to be less obvious. Currently, it is well established that other inflammatory mediators in addition to chemokines play an important role in the pathogenesis of CHF [33–36]. However, in the following sections we will limit ourselves only to chemokines and review the current knowledge, based on studies in patients and experimental models of CHF.

Role of chemokines in patients with CHF

The earliest study suggesting an involvement of chemokines in the pathogenesis of cardiac disorders in humans was reported by Seino and co-workers in 1995 [37]. They demonstrated by polymerase chain reaction (PCR) that IL-8 and MCP-1 mRNAs were expressed in endomyocardial specimen from seven patients with idiopathic dilated cardiomyopathy. In the same study, the authors demonstrated that exposure of cultured neonatal rat cardiac myocytes to human recombinant TNF-α resulted in increased expression of MCP-1 and IL-8 mRNAs. The findings that chemokines were synthesized by cardiomyocytes under stimulated conditions, and their abundant expression in the myocardium of patients with dilated cardiomyopathy led the authors to suggest that these chemokines may play an important signaling role in inflammatory heart muscle disorders. Three years later, Aukrust et al. [38] reported that circulating levels of the CC chemokines, MCP-1, MIP-1α and RANTES were increased in patients with chronic CHF, with the highest levels present in New York Heart Association Class IV patients. Moreover, MCP-1 and MIP-1α levels were inversely correlated with left ventricular ejection fraction, and elevated chemokine levels were found independent on the cause of heart failure, although MCP-1 was particularly high in patients with coronary artery disease [38]. The authors suggested that platelets, CD3[+] lymphocytes and monocytes were the origin of the elevated circulating chemokines, since cells obtained from patients with CHF released higher amounts of these chemokines than cells from healthy subjects. However, the possibility that the failing myocardium itself could be the source of the elevated chemokines was brought up as well. Subsequently, the cardiac origin of MCP-1 was verified in another study by Lehmann and co-workers [39]. This group reported that both mRNA expression and immunohistological staining of MCP-1 were higher in endomyocardial biopsy specimen of patients with dilated cardiomyopathy and severe left ventricular dysfunction than in patients with low to moderate impairment of left ventricular function. Using immunolocalization, they observed that MCP-1 was produced in the cardiac interstitium but did not identify positive staining of myocytes. Unfortunately, this study did not examine normal heart tissue or specimen from ischemic or valvular causes of heart failure. Thus, the authors were unable to conclude whether the increase in MCP-1 had a limited role only in dilated cardiomyopathy or was a more generalized phenomenon associated with heart failure.

The idea that increased chemokines levels in CHF is not limited only to the CC chemokines subgroup but is a more generalized phenomenon, was further advanced by Damas and co-workers [40]. Following their original report on the CC chemokines in CHF [38] this group demonstrated that the circulating levels of three chemokines of the CXC subgroup, namely IL-8, growth-regulated oncogene (GRO)α, and epithelial neutrophil activating peptide (ENA)-78, were also significantly elevated in patients with CHF [40]. In similarity to their findings with the CC chemokines, plasma levels of IL-8 and GROα correlated with the severity of heart failure according to the NYHA classification. Furthermore, at least for IL-8, there was an inverse correlation between plasma level of the chemokine and left ventricular ejection fraction. The authors also demonstrated that both unstimulated and lipopolysaccharide-stimulated monocytes from CHF patients released high amounts of all three chemokines, and that activated platelets stimulated the release of IL-8 from peripheral blood mononuclear cells. Based on the latter findings they suggested that activated monocytes and platelets could contribute to the enhanced CXC chemokine levels in CHF. Notwithstanding this, in a subsequent study the same group evaluated the expression (by RNAase protection assay) and immunolocalization (immunohistochemistry) of several CC and CXC chemokines and chemokine receptors in explanted heart tissues of patients with end-stage heart failure undergoing cardiac transplantation [41]. Interestingly, they found that the expression of MCP-1, IL-8, RANTES, and MIP-1α was significantly decreased in the failing hearts compared with non-failing control hearts. However, the chemokine receptors, CCR1, CCR2, and CXCR1 were rather up-regulated in failing hearts compared with the non-failing controls. By immunohistochemistry they were able to demonstrate that the chemokines MCP-1 and IL-8 and the CXCR4 chemokine receptor were localized to the cardiomyocytes and not only in "contaminating" leukocytes, endothelial cells and fibroblast. The finding of decreased myocardial expression of the major CC and CXC chemokines in CHF may appear difficult to reconcile with previous findings of the same group on elevated circulating levels of the same chemokines in patients with CHF. It is possible however, that the myocardial "chemokine system" is regulated in a different manner compared with circulating mononuclear cells. In addition, this may reflect the severe end-stage, cardiomyopathy in patients undergoing cardiac transplantation, or the possibility that the control hearts (taken from unused cardiac donation) were exposed to stressful or hypoxic conditions that caused artificial up-regulation of the chemokine in the non-failing control hearts. Nevertheless, this study provides evidence for the existence of a chemokine system containing both the ligands and their corresponding receptors in the myocardium itself, and that this system may be modulated in CHF. In an additional study by the same group, the expression of chemokines and their corresponding receptors was evaluated in peripheral mononuclear cells of patients with CHF [42]. This study revealed a significant increase in the expression of MIP-1α, MIP-1β, IL-8 and of the chemokine receptors CCR1, CCR2, CCR5, CXCR1, CXCR2, and CX_3CR. Furthermore, in response to treatment with intravenous immunoglobulins for 26 weeks there was a significant decrease in the mononuclear expression as well as in plasma protein levels of the chemokines [42]. At least for MIP-1α, a significant correlation was observed between the decrease in the chemokine levels and the increase in left ventricular ejection fraction.

Taken together, these data suggest that in human CHF the chemokine system (ligand and receptors) may be modulated in plasma, the myocardium itself and in mononuclear cells. Moreover, this modulation occurs at the transcription level (mRNA) as well as in the immunoreactive proteins themselves.

Role of chemokines in experimental models of CHF

The data on the involvement of chemokines in animal models of CHF are limited mainly to MCP-1. Although there were data indicating that chemokine synthesis may be experimentally induced in the isolated cardiomyocytes [37], the earliest study demonstrating an involvement of MCP-1 in an animal model of CHF was published in 1997 by Shioi et al. [43]. This study followed the expression of MCP-1 and IL-1β in Dahl salt-sensitive rats, a hypertensive model that develops cardiac hypertrophy and subsequently cardiac failure due to pressure overload. They were able to demonstrate a 3.6-fold increase inMCP-1 mRNA when left ventricular hypertrophy developed (11 weeks) and a further increase to 4.8-fold at the CHF stage, relative to age-matched Dahl salt-resistant control rats. The increase in the expression of the IL-1β cytokine was even more impressive (3.9- and 6.2-fold, respectively). This increase was associated with a diffuse macrophage infiltration throughout the left ventricle. MCP-1 immunoreactivity was localized to the endothelial cells and interstitial macrophages. Based on these findings, the authors suggested that the increase in the expression of chemokine and pro-inflammatory cytokine and in macrophage infiltration could play a role in the pathogenesis of cardiac hypertrophy and failure induced by chronic mechanical overload.

Perhaps the most convincing evidence that MCP-1 can cause significant myocardial injury was brought up by Kolattukudy and co-workers [44]. Using transgenic mice in which the murine MCP-1(JE) gene was expressed under the control of the α-cardiac myosin heavy chain promoter, they were able to target MCP-1 expression to the adult heart muscle. MCP-1 levels in the transgenic hearts increased up to 30–45 days after birth, and was detected in cardiac myocytes and also in the interstitium, with greater expression near the epicardium. Transgenic hearts were 65% heavier than normal controls, and histological analysis revealed signs of myocarditis, edema, macrophage infiltration and some fibrosis. Echocardiographic analysis of one-year-old transgenic mice revealed cardiac hypertrophy and dilatation, evidenced by increased left ventricular mass and systolic and diastolic diameters. Functionally, these signs were associated with a significant decline in the M-mode shortening fraction, indicating depressed contractile ability [44]. Admittedly, the method of targeted expression of MCP-1 gene may result in significantly higher myocardial levels of the chemokine compared with more "conventional" experimental models of CHF. Nevertheless, these findings clearly indicate that selective over-expression of MCP-1 in the myocardium may result in cardiac dysfunction characteristic of CHF and not only histological signs of an inflammatory reaction.

In support of the latter assumption, our group has studied the expression of MCP-1 in the myocardium of rats with aorto-caval fistula (ACF), an experimental model of volume-overload CHF [45]. This model is characterized by a marked degree of cardiac hypertrophy and dilatation, neurohumoral activation, and a tendency to avid sodium and water retention by the kidney and edema formation [46, 47]. Similar to patients with CHF, rats with ACF may be further subdivided into animals with compensated and decompensated heart failure, based on their daily urinary sodium excretion and the degree of neurohumoral activation [46, 47]. Using two independent methodologies, Northern blotting and real time PCR analysis (TaqMan), we were able to demonstrate increased MCP-1 mRNA expression in CHF rats, with significantly higher levels in rats with decompensated CHF than in the compensated CHF subgroup. MCP-1 immunoreactive protein was localized by immunohistochemistry to the vascular endothelium and smooth muscle cells, infiltrating leukocytes, and interstitial fibroblasts. Interestingly, as shown in Figure 1, in the more severe decompensated CHF animals positive staining was observed in cardiomyocytes, suggesting that these cells were an important source of the elevated MCP-1 [45].

In addition, a significant decrease in ^{125}I-labeled MCP-1 binding to myocardium-derived membrane preparations was observed in rats with compensated and decompensated CHF. The latter might be due to increased occupancy of the myocardial receptors by endogenous MCP-1 or, alternatively, due to down-regulation of the receptors.

Additional experimental models characterized by increased myocardial expression of MCP-1 have been reported. Tomita et al. [25] demonstrated that chronic

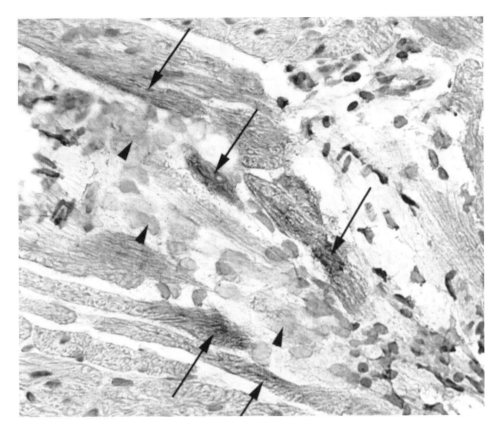

Figure 1
Immunohistological staining with anti-MCP-1 antibody of left ventricular tissue in a rat with decompensated CHF, induced by aorto-caval fistula. Positive staining for rat-MCP-1 is demonstrated in cardiomyocytes (arrows) and in adjacent infiltrative cells (arrowheads). Taken from [45] with permission.

nitric oxide (NO) inhibition by N^{ω}-nitro-L-arginine methyl ester (L-NAME) induces inflammatory changes in the heart and blood vessels. In this model, also characterized by the development of hypertension, the authors found a marked infiltration of mononuclear cells in the perivascular areas of the coronary vessels. This was associated with positive staining for MCP-1, by immunohistochemistry, in a major portion of the coronary arteries and veins in the visual field. In line with these findings, MCP-1 mRNA expression was similarly increased in animals with inhibition of NO synthesis. Furthermore, the infiltration of inflammatory cells into myocardial interstitial spaces was associated with myocytes necrosis and later (after 28 days of treatment) with signs of myocardial remodeling and fibrosis. Unfortunately, no data on cardiac function are available in this study and therefore, it is not clear whether these histological and immunological alterations were associated with myocardial dysfunction and/or development of CHF. Similarly, there is ample of evidence for the induction of MCP-1 and IL-8 in experimental models of myocardial ischemia and reperfusion injury [22, 23]. However, the relevance of these findings to the development of chronic cardiac failure is not clear at present.

Possible mechanisms of chemokines induction in CHF

Although there is evidence for increased circulating levels of chemokines in CHF as well as for up-regulation of the chemokine system in the failing myocardium, the mechanisms mediating these phenomena have not been thoroughly studied. Several potential mechanisms might be implicated; first, it has been shown that other inflammatory cytokines, in particular TNF-α, may induce MCP-1 and IL-8 generation in cultured neonatal rat cardiomyocytes [37], as well as MCP-1 expression in adult rat cardiomyocytes [48]. Second, in cultured endothelial cells, Okada et al.[49] demonstrated by Northern blotting that the mRNA levels of IL-8 and MCP-1 were up-regulated by cyclic stretch as a function of its intensity. They further demonstrated that phospholipase C, protein kinase C and tyrosine kinase, but not stretch-activated ion channels, were involved in the stretch-induced gene expression [49]. It is possible that a similar mechanism may be triggered in the myocardial wall and the endocardial layer when exposed to altered mechanical stretch in pressure overload CHF or in dilated cardiomyopathy. Finally, there is a possibility that the up-regulation of the chemokine system may be a consequence of neurohumoral activation in CHF. Thus, it has been reported that increased activity of angiotensin II (Ang II) is associated with the induction of MCP-1, in particular in the vascular wall of various hypertensive and atherosclerotic models [26, 50–52]. There is extensive evidence supporting the notion that Ang II, in addition to its action as a potent vasoconstrictor, also promotes vascular inflammation, proliferation and hypertrophy. The mechanisms mediating the latter phenomena are thought to act by activation of Ang II Type 1 receptor and through oxidative stress-related pathways [53]. Recently, it was reported that the Ang II-induced macrophage infiltration in arterial wall was virtually eliminated in CCR-2 deficient mice, suggesting a mandatory role of the MCP-1/CCR-2 pathway in the inflammatory response to Ang II [52].

Activation of the renin-angiotensin system (RAS) is thought to play a major role in the pathogenesis of CHF and to contribute significantly to myocardial dysfunction and neurohumoral disturbances characteristic of this syndrome [54]. It is also known that in CHF the RAS is activated within the failing myocardium, and that the local Ang II action is involved in the induction of cardiac hypertrophy as well as other manifestations of cardiac dysfunction [55, 56]. Thus, in view of the inflam-

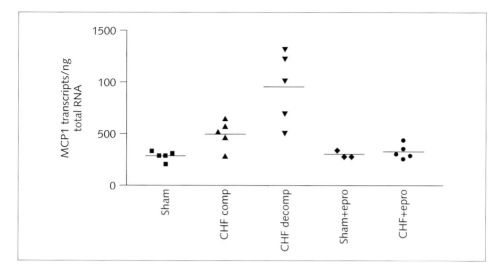

Figure 2
Number of MCP-1 mRNA transcripts in cardiac tissue samples obtained from control group (Sham), rats with compensated and decompensated CHF (CHF comp and CHF decomp, respectively), and in control and CHF rats treated for seven days with eprosartan (Sham + epro and CHF + epro, respectively). Data were obtained on the seventh day after surgical creation of aorto-caval fistula (CHF) or sham operation. Eprosartan was administered intraperitoneally via osmotic mini-pumps. For characterization of the compensated and decompensated CHF subgroups see [47].

matory effects of Ang II, it is possible that increased activity of the local RAS in the failing myocardium may also be involved in the induction of MCP-1. To test the latter hypothesis, we studied the effects of eprosartan, a selective Ang II Type 1 receptor antagonist, on the expression of MCP-1 mRNA in the myocardium of rats with volume overload CHF induced by aorto-caval fistula. As shown earlier, this experimental model of CHF is characterized by activation of the local cardiac RAS, as well as by a marked up-regulation of MCP-1 expression within the failing myocardium [45, 57]. Eprosartan was administered chronically, *via* osmotic mini-pumps inserted into the peritoneal cavity during the surgical creation of the aorto-caval fistula or in sham-operated control rats. MCP-1 mRNA expression in cardiac tissue samples was evaluated by the real time PCR analysis (TaqMan, Perkin-Elmer), as previously reported [45]. Figure 2 shows the number of MCP-1 mRNA transcripts normalized for ng of total RNA.

As depicted, on the seventh day after induction of CHF or sham operation, the highest number of MCP-1 transcripts was observed in the subgroup of rats with decompensated CHF. Furthermore, in the group of CHF rats treated with eprosartan the number of MCP-1 transcripts was similar to that observed in cardiac tissues of control animals. This finding demonstrate that blocking the actions of Ang II by a selective antagonist of its Type 1 receptor actually abolished the increase in myocardial MCP-1 expression in rats with CHF. Thus, activation of the RAS and elevated Ang II appear to be involved in the up-regulation of MCP-1 in the failing myocardium of this experimental model of CHF.

Effects of chemokines on cardiomyocytes

There are several potential mechanisms by which MCP-1 and other chemokines may exert their detrimental influence on the myocardium [12]. Chemokines play a crucial role in the induction of the inflammatory process by recruiting leukocytes into the affected tissue. MCP-1 and IL-8 have been also shown to trigger the firm adhesion of monocytes to vascular endothelium under flow conditions [58]. However, their role is not limited only to attraction and migration of mononuclear leukocytes, but also to their activation. The latter include release of lysozomal enzymes, generation of reactive oxygen species as well as induction of other inflammatory cytokines. Thus, chemokines may lead to myocardial damage by several secondary mechanisms. At least for MCP-1, there is evidence that sera from CHF patients stimulated oxygen free radicals generation in monocytes, which was inhibited by neutralizing antibodies against MCP-1 [38]. The oxidative stress may further induce the synthesis of chemokines and other cytokines in various cell types by activating the NF-κB transcription factor, thus creating a positive feedback loop that augments the inflammatory response. Recently, Damas et al. [48] demonstrated that exposure of cultured adult rat cardiomyocytes to incremental doses of MCP-1 resulted in a generation of IL-1β and IL-6 in a dose dependent manner. They further observed that IL-1β and IL-6 mRNAs were likewise elevated in MCP-1 stimulated cardiomyocytes. These finding indicate that MCP-1 is able to induce generation of other inflammatory cytokines in cardiomyocytes and that this effect is probably mediated by increased transcription. Moreover, oxidative stress and several cytokines such as TNF-α and IL-1 appear to be important mediators in the up-regulation of inducible NO synthase (iNOS). There is increasing evidence that myocardial iNOS may be up-regulated in patients and experimental models of CHF, and that induction of the latter isoform may be involved in the pathogenesis of contractile dysfunction [59]. Indeed, we have recently shown that the myocardial iNOS isoform was up-regulated in rats with volume-overload CHF [60]. Furthermore, treatment with W-1400, a selective inhibitor of iNOS, was associated with a significant improvement of beta-adrenergic receptor agonist mediated contractile responsiveness in isolated cardiomyocyte obtained from these animals. As mentioned earlier, this experimental model of CHF is also characterized by a marked up-regulation of MCP-1 in the failing myocardium [45]. Although it is tempting to speculate that the over-expression of iNOS in the myocardium is related to that of MCP-1, such an association remains to be established in future studies.

Finally, there is evidence that MCP-1 may modulate collagen synthesis by rat pulmonary fibroblasts and human skin fibroblasts [61, 62]. In rat lung fibroblasts, MCP-1 stimulates collagen gene expression by up-regulation of endogenous transforming growth factor (TGF)-β [61]. In addition, Yamamoto et al. [62] demonstrated that MCP-1 increased gene expression of matrix metalloproteinase-1 and 2 (MMP-1, 2) as well as that of tissue inhibitor of metalloproteinase-1 (TIMP-1) mRNAs in human fibroblasts. Interestingly, recent studies by Spinale and co-workers [63, 64] have underscored the importance of the MMP/TIMP system in the pathogenesis of myocardial remodeling and fibrosis in cardiac failure. Although purely speculative at present, it will be of interest to study if similar mechanisms may exist in cardiac fibroblasts, which could contribute to the development of CHF.

In summary, the overall effect of chemokines on myocardial function in CHF is complex and may be related to their effects on cardiomyocytes as well as on actions on infiltrating monocytes, endothelial cells, smooth muscle cells and fibroblasts. Moreover, these effects may be mediated indirectly, by activation of and interactions with secondary mechanisms such as other inflammatory cytokines, oxidative stress, and perhaps up-regulation of iNOS.

Summary and future perspectives

In the present review we analyzed the current literature on the involvement of chemokines, a selected subgroup of cytokines with chemo-attractant properties, in the pathogenesis of clinical and experimental CHF. Based on the published data it might be concluded that the chemokine system is modulated in CHF in three major domains; first, there is evidence for an increase in the circulating levels of several chemokines both of the CC and CXC subgroups in patients with CHF. Second, there is also compelling evidence that the expression of several chemokines and their receptors is altered in the myocardium of patients and in experimental models of CHF, and that these alterations are regulated at least in part at the transcriptional level. Furthermore, the altered expression of chemokines is followed by similar changes in their immunoreactive levels, and that their cellular site of induction appear to be the diseased cardiomyocytes and not only infiltrating leukocytes, fibroblasts or endothelial cells. Finally, in addition to changes in the plasma concentrations and in the myocardial levels, enhanced gene expression of chemokines and their corresponding receptors may be also found in mononuclear blood cells of patients with CHF. The induction of some chemokines, but not all, appears to correlate with the severity of cardiac dysfunction and the decrease in left ventricular ejection fraction. Among all the chemokines reported, MCP-1 seems to be dominant in its involvement both in clinical and experimental CHF, while the evidence for the others requires further support by additional studies. Although there are several potential mechanisms which might offer an explanation for the up-regulation of the chemokine system in CHF, in most of the studies reported the mechanisms mediating the altered expression of the chemokine remain unidentified. Similarly, a lot remains to be investigated about the mechanisms by which chemokines exert their deleterious effects on cardiac function and about their relative contribution compared with other mechanisms. Thus, the question whether the activation of the chemokine system takes an active part in the evolution of CHF or is merely an epiphenomenon, if not an "innocent bystander", remains largely unanswered in our opinion. One of the reasons for this uncertainty is the lack of effective and selective blockers of chemokines activity up till now. Most of the therapeutic maneuvers that are known to reduce chemokine levels such as angiotensin converting enzyme inhibitors [65] intravenous immunoglobulin infusion [42] and statins [66] are nonspecific and may exert their beneficial effects on cardiac function by other mechanisms, not related to their effects on chemokines. More specific therapies such as monoclonal anti-MCP-1 neutralizing antibodies and anti-MCP-1 gene therapy using 7ND, an amino-terminal deletion mutant of MCP-1, have not been studied in experimental models of CHF, although they have been documented to be highly beneficial in inhibiting cardiovascular remodeling induced by chronic blockade of NO synthesis [27, 67]. Finally, the possibility of finding an adequate therapy is further complicated by the redundancy of the chemokine system and the finding that several chemokines and/or their receptors may be activated simultaneously. Thus, targeting of one chemokine or its receptor by a selective blocker may be insufficient to block the induction of the inflammatory process.

Yet, despite these reservations, enormous progress has been made in recent years by the pharmaceutical industry in the field of anti-chemokine therapy. Understanding of the molecular interactions between chemokines and their G-protein-coupled receptors has led to the development of new classes of small molecules which demonstrate high selectivity against several chemokine receptors. As summarized in two recent reviews, there are now a large number of molecules that show nanomolar potency as selective antagonists of the chemokine receptors [15, 68]. In the future, it is anticipated that this class of molecules will produce clinically useful therapies. However, for the basic scientists and clinical investigators they may provide an excellent tool to study the specific role of chemokines in the pathogenesis of CHF.

References

1   Levine B, Kalman J, Mayer L, Fillit HM, Packer M (1990) Elevated circulating levels of tumor necrosis factor in severe chronic heart failure. *N Engl J Med* 323: 236–241

2   Adams DH, Lloyd A R (1997) Chemokines: leucocyte recruitment and activation cytokines. *Lancet* 349: 490–495

3   Luster AD (1998) Chemokines–chemotactic cytokines that mediate inflammation. *N Engl J Med* 338: 436–445

4   Baggiolini M (2001) Chemokines in pathology and medicine. *J Intern Med* 250: 91–104

5   Gerard C, Rollins BJ (2001) Chemokines and disease. *Nat Immunol* 2: 108–115

6   Krishnaswamy G, Kelley J, Yerra L, Smith JK., Chi DS (1999) Human endothelium as a source of multifunctional cytokines: Molecular regulation and possible role in human disease. *J Interferon Cytokine Res* 19: 91–104

7   Wang X, Yue TL, Ohlstein EH, Sung CP, Feuerstein GZ (1996) Interferon-inducible protein-10 involves vascular smooth muscle cell migration, proliferation, and inflammatory response. *J Biol Chem* 271: 24286–24293

8   Yue TL, Wang X, Sung CP, Olson B, McKenna PJ, Gu JL, Feuerstein GZ (1994) Interleukin-8. A mitogen and chemo-attractant for vascular smooth muscle cells. *Circ Res* 75: 1–7

9   Gu L, Tseng SC, Rollins BJ (1999) Monocyte chemo-attractant protein-1. *Chem Immunol* 72: 7–29

10   Zhang Y, Ernst CA, Rollins BJ (1996) MCP-1: Structure/activity analysis. *Methods* 10: 93–103

11   Shin WS, Szuba A, Rockson SG (2002) The role of chemokines in human cardiovascular pathology: enhanced biological insights. *Atherosclerosis* 160: 91–102

12   Aukrust P, Damas JK, Gullestad L, Froland SS (2001) Chemokines in myocardial failure – pathogenic importance and potential therapeutic targets. *Clin Exp Immunol* 124: 343–345

13   Walz A, Peveri P, Aschauer H, Baggiolini M (1987) Purification and amino acid sequencing of NAF, a novel neutrophil-activating factor produced by monocytes. *Biochem Biophys Res Commun* 149: 755–761

14   Zlotnik A, Yoshie O (2000) Chemokines: A new classification system and their role in immunity. *Immunity* 12: 121–127

15   Schwarz MK, Wells TN (2002) New therapeutics that modulate chemokine networks. *Nat RevDrug Discov* 1: 347–358

16   Thelen M (2001) Dancing to the tune of chemokines. *Nat Immunol* 2: 129–134

17   Rodriguez-Frade JM, Mellado M, Martinez A (2001) Chemokine receptor dimerization: Two are better than one. *Trends Immunol* 22: 612–617

18   Laudanna C, Campbell JJ, Butcher EC (1996) Role of Rho in chemo-attractant-activated leukocyte adhesion through integrins. *Science* 271: 981–983

19   Premack BA, Schall TJ (1996) Chemokine receptors: Gateways to inflammation and infection. *Nat Med* 2: 1174–1178

20   Peters W, Charo IF (2001) Involvement of chemokine receptor 2 and its ligand, monocyte chemo-attractant protein-1, in the development of atherosclerosis: Lessons from knockout mice. *Curr Opin Lipidol* 12: 175–180

21   Sasayama S, Okada M, Matsumori A (2000) Chemokines and cardiovascular diseases. *Cardiovasc Res* 45: 267–269

22 Kukielka GL, Smith CW, LaRosa GJ, Manning AM, Mendoza LH, Daly TJ, Hughes BJ, Youker KA, Hawkins HK, Michael LH (1995) Interleukin-8 gene induction in the myocardium after ischemia and reperfusion *in vivo*. *J Clin Invest* 95: 89–103

23 Kakio T, Matsumori A, Ono K, Ito H, Matsushima K, Sasayama S (2000) Roles and relationship of macrophages and monocyte chemotactic and activating factor/monocyte chemo-attractant protein-1 in the ischemic and reperfused rat heart. *Lab Invest* 80: 1127–1136

24 Furukawa Y, Matsumori A, Ohashi N, Shioi T, Ono K, Harada A, Matsushima K, Sasayama S (1999) Anti-monocyte chemo-attractant protein-1/monocyte chemotactic and activating factor antibody inhibits neointimal hyperplasia in injured rat carotid arteries. *Circ Res* 84: 306–314

25 Tomita H, Egashira K, Kubo-Inoue M, Usui M, Koyanagi M, Shimokawa H, Takeya M, Yoshimura T, Takeshita A (1998) Inhibition of NO synthesis induces inflammatory changes and monocyte chemo-attractant protein-1 expression in rat hearts and vessels. *Arterioscler Thromb Vasc Biol* 18: 1456–1464

26 Usui M, Egashira K, Tomita H, Koyanagi M, Katoh M, Shimokawa H, Takeya M, Yoshimura T, Matsushima K, Takeshita A (2000) Important role of local angiotensin II activity mediated *via* Type 1 receptor in the pathogenesis of cardiovascular inflammatory changes induced by chronic blockade of nitric oxide synthesis in rats. *Circulation* 101: 305–310

27 Egashira K, Koyanagi M, Kitamoto S, Ni W, Kataoka C, Morishita R, Kaneda Y, Akiyama C, Nishida KI, Sueishi K et al (2000) Anti-monocyte chemoattractant protein-1 gene therapy inhibits vascular remodeling in rats: Blockade of MCP-1 activity after intramuscular transfer of a mutant gene inhibits vascular remodeling induced by chronic blockade of NO synthesis. *FASEB J* 14: 1974–1978

28 Schecter AD, Rollins BJ, Zhang YJ, Charo IF, Fallon JT, Rossikhina M, Giesen PL, Nemerson Y, Taubman MB (1997) Tissue factor is induced by monocyte chemo-attractant protein-1 in human aortic smooth muscle and THP-1 cells. *J Biol Chem* 272: 28568–28573

29 Boisvert WA, Curtiss LK, Terkeltaub RA (2000) Interleukin-8 and its receptor CXCR2 in atherosclerosis. *Immunol Res* 21: 129–137

30 Abi-Younes S, Sauty A, Mach F, Sukhova GK, Libby P, Luster AD (2000) The stromal cell-derived factor-1 chemokine is a potent platelet agonist highly expressed in atherosclerotic plaques. *Circ Res* 86: 131–138

31 Mach F, Sauty A, Iarossi AS, Sukhova GK, Neote K, Libby P, Luster AD (1999) Differential expression of three T lymphocyte-activating CXC chemokines by human atheroma-associated cells. *J Clin Invest* 104: 1041–1050

32 Haque NS, Zhang X, French DL, Li J, Poon M, Fallon JT, Gabel BR, Taubman MB, Koschinsky M, Harpel PC (2000) CC chemokine I-309 is the principal monocyte chemoattractant induced by apolipoprotein(a) in human vascular endothelial cells. *Circulation* 102: 786–792

33 Sasayama S, Matsumori A, Kihara Y (1999) New insights into the pathophysiological role for cytokines in heart failure. *Cardiovasc Res* 42: 557–564

34 Aukrust P, Ueland T, Lien E, Bendtzen K, Muller F, Andreassen, A K, Nordoy I, Aass H, Espevik T, Simonsen S et al (1999) Cytokine network in congestive heart failure secondary to ischemic or idiopathic dilated cardiomyopathy. *Am J Cardiol* 83: 376–382

35 Blum A, Miller H (2001) Pathophysiological role of cytokines in congestive heart failure. *Annu Rev Med* 52: 15–27

36 Dinarello CA, Pomerantz BJ (2001) Proinflammatory cytokines in heart disease. *Blood Purif* 19: 314–321

37 Seino Y, Ikeda U, Sekiguchi H, Morita M, Konishi K, Kasahara T, Shimada K. (1995) Expression of leukocyte chemotactic cytokines in myocardial tissue. *Cytokine* 7: 301–304

38 Aukrust P, Ueland T, Muller F, Andreassen A K, Nordo I, Aass H, Kjekshus J, Simonsen S, Froland SS, Gullestad L (1998) Elevated circulating levels of C-C chemokines in patients with congestive heart failure. *Circulation* 97: 1136–1143

39 Lehmann MH, Kuhnert H, Muller S, Sigusch HH (1998) Monocyte chemoattractant protein 1 (MCP-1) gene expression in dilated cardiomyopathy. *Cytokine* 10: 739–746

40 Damas JK, Gullestad L, Ueland T, Solum NO, Simonsen S, Froland SS, Aukrust P (2000) CXC-chemokines, a new group of cytokines in congestive heart failure–possible role of platelets and monocytes. *Cardiovasc Res* 45: 428–436

41 Damas JK, Eiken HG, Oie E, Bjerkeli V, Yndestad A, Ueland T, Tonnessen T, Geiran OR, Aass H, Simonsen S et al (2000) Myocardial expression of CC- and CXC-chemokines and their receptors in human end-stage heart failure. *Cardiovasc Res* 47: 778–787

42 Damas JK, Gullestad L, Aass H, Simonsen S, Fjeld JG, Wikeby L, Ueland T, Eiken HG, Froland SS, Aukrust P (2001) Enhanced gene expression of chemokines and their corresponding receptors in mononuclear blood cells in chronic heart failure–modulatory effect of intravenous immunoglobulin. *J Am Coll Cardiol* 38: 187–193

43 Shioi T, Matsumori A, Kihara Y, Inoko M, Ono K, Iwanaga Y, Yamada T, Iwasaki A, Matsushima K, Sasayama S (1997) Increased expression of interleukin-1 beta and monocyte chemotactic and activating factor/monocyte chemo-attractant protein-1 in the hypertrophied and failing heart with pressure overload. *Circ Res* 81: 664–671

44 Kolattukudy PE, Quach T, Bergese S, Breckenridge S, Hensley J, Altschuld R, Gordillo G, Klenotic S, Orosz C, Parker-Thornburg J (1998) Myocarditis induced by targeted expression of the MCP-1 gene in murine cardiac muscle. *Am J Pathol* 152: 101–111

45 Behr TM, Wang X, Aiyar N, Coatney RW, Li X, Koster P, Angermann CE, Ohlstein E, Feuerstein GZ, Winaver J (2000) Monocyte chemo-attractant protein-1 is upregulated in rats with volume-overload congestive heart failure. *Circulation* 102: 1315–1322

46 Winaver J, Hoffman A, Burnett JCJ, Haramati A (1988) Hormonal determinants of sodium excretion in rats with experimental high-output heart failure. *Am J Physiol* 254: R776–R784

47 Abassi ZA, Brodsky S, Karram T, Dobkin I, Winaver J, Hoffman A (2001) Temporal

changes in natriuretic and antinatriuretic systems after closure of a large arteriovenous fistula. *Cardiovasc Res* 51: 567–576

48   Damas JK, Aukrust P, Ueland T, Odegaard A, Eiken HG., Gullestad L, Sejersted OM, Christensen G (2001) Monocyte chemoattractant protein-1 enhances and interleukin-10 suppresses the production of inflammatory cytokines in adult rat cardiomyocytes. *Basic Res Cardiol* 96: 345–352

49   Okada M, Matsumori A, Ono K, Furukawa Y, Shioi T, Iwasaki A, Matsushima K, Sasayama S (1998) Cyclic stretch upregulates production of interleukin-8 and monocyte chemotactic and activating factor/monocyte chemo-attractant protein-1 in human endothelial cells. *Arterioscler Thromb Vasc Biol* 18: 894–901

50   Capers Q, Alexander RW, Lou P, De Leon H, Wilcox JN, Ishizaka N, Howard AB, Taylor WR (1997) Monocyte chemo-attractant protein-1 expression in aortic tissues of hypertensive rats. *Hypertension* 30: 1397–1402

51   Hernandez-Presa M, Bustos C, Ortego M, Tunon J, Renedo G, Ruiz-Ortega M, Egido J (1997) Angiotensin-converting enzyme inhibition prevents arterial nuclear factor-kappa-B activation, monocyte chemo-attractant protein-1 expression, and macrophage infiltration in a rabbit model of early accelerated atherosclerosis. *Circulation* 95: 1532–1541

52   Bush E, Maeda N, Kuziel WA, Dawson TC, Wilcox JN, DeLeon H, Taylor W R (2000) CC chemokine receptor 2 is required for macrophage infiltration and vascular hypertrophy in angiotensin II-induced hypertension. *Hypertension* 36: 360–363

53   Griendling KK, Ushio-Fukai M, Lassegue B, Alexander RW (1997) Angiotensin II signaling in vascular smooth muscle. New concepts. *Hypertension* 29: 366–373

54   Dzau VJ (1987) Renal and circulatory mechanisms in congestive heart failure. *Kidney Int* 31: 1402–1415

55   Dzau VJ (1993) Tissue renin-angiotensin system in myocardial hypertrophy and failure. *Arch Intern Med* 153: 937–942

56   Yamazaki T, Komuro I, Yazaki Y (1999) Role of the renin-angiotensin system in cardiac hypertrophy. *Am J Cardiol* 83: 53H–57H

57   Pieruzzi F, Abassi ZA, Keiser HR (1995) Expression of renin-angiotensin system components in the heart, kidneys, and lungs of rats with experimental heart failure. *Circulation* 92: 3105–3112

58   Gerszten RE, Garcia-Zepeda EA, Lim YC, Yoshida M, Ding HA, Gimbrone M A Jr., Luster AD, Luscinskas FW, Rosenzweig A (1999) MCP-1 and IL-8 trigger firm adhesion of monocytes to vascular endothelium under flow conditions. *Nature* 398: 718–723

59   Balligand JL, Cannon PJ (1997) Nitric oxide synthases and cardiac muscle. Autocrine and paracrine influences. *Arterioscler Thromb Vasc Biol* 17: 1846–1858

60   Gealekman O, Abassi Z, Rubinstein I, Winaver J, Binah O (2002) Role of myocardial inducible nitric oxide synthase in contractile dysfunction and beta-adrenergic hyporesponsiveness in rats with experimental volume-overload heart failure. *Circulation* 105: 236–243

61   Gharaee-Kermani M, Denholm EM, Phan SH (1996) Costimulation of fibroblast colla-

gen and transforming growth factor beta1 gene expression by monocyte chemo-attractant protein-1 *via* specific receptors. *J Biol Chem* 271: 17779–17784

62 Yamamoto T, Eckes B, Mauch C, Hartmann K, Krieg T (2000) Monocyte chemo-attractant protein-1 enhances gene expression and synthesis of matrix metalloproteinase-1 in human fibroblasts by an autocrine IL-1 alpha loop. *J Immunol* 164: 6174–6179

63 Spinale FG (2002) Matrix metalloproteinases: regulation and dysregulation in the failing heart. *Circ Res* 90: 520–530

64 Bradham WS, Moe G, Wendt KA, Scott AA, Konig A, Romanova M, Naik G, Spinale FG (2002) TNF-alpha and myocardial matrix metalloproteinases in heart failure: relationship to LV remodeling. *Am J Physiol Heart Circ Physiol* 282: H1288–H1295

65 Soejima H, Ogawa H, Yasue H, Kaikita K, Takazoe K, Nishiyama K, Misumi, K, Miyamoto S, Yoshimura M, Kugiyama K, Nakamura S, Tsuji I (1999) Angiotensin-converting enzyme inhibition reduces monocyte chemo-attractant protein-1 and tissue factor levels in patients with myocardial infarction. *J Am Coll Cardiol* 34: 983–988

66 Romano M, Diomede L, Sironi M, Massimiliano L, Sottocorno M, Polentarutti N, Guglielmotti A, Albani D, Bruno A, Fruscella P et al (2000) Inhibition of monocyte chemotactic protein-1 synthesis by statins. *Lab Invest* 80: 1095–1100

67 Koyanagi M, Egashira K, Kitamoto S, Ni W, Shimokawa H, Takeya M, Yoshimura T, Takeshita A (2000) Role of monocyte chemoattractant protein-1 in cardiovascular remodeling induced by chronic blockade of nitric oxide synthesis. *Circulation* 102: 2243–2248

68 Carter PH (2002) Chemokine receptor antagonism as an approach to anti-inflammatory therapy: "just right" or plain wrong? *Curr Opin Chem Biol* 6: 510–525

Neurohormonal mediators
and cardiac inflammation

The role of endothelin-1 in myocardial inflammation and fibrosis

Li L. Yang[1,2,4], Mansoor Husain[1,2,3,4] and Duncan J. Stewart[1,2,3,5]

[1]Heart and Stroke Richard Lewar Centre of Excellence, University of Toronto, Ontario, Canada; [2]The Department of Laboratory Medicine and Pathobiology, and [3]The Department of Medicine, University of Toronto, Ontario, Canada; [4]Division of Cellular and Molecular Biology, Toronto General Hospital Research Institute, Ontario, Canada; [5]Terrence Donnelley Heart Center, St. Michael's Hospital, Q7-810, 30 Bond Street, Toronto, Ontario M5G 2C4, Canada

Introduction

The endothelins are a family of endothelium-derived peptides that possess vasoconstrictor properties [1]. The three isoforms identified, namely endothelin-1 (ET-1), endothelin-2 (ET-2) and endothelin-3 (ET-3), are encoded by three different genes. Each isoform contains two intra-chain disulphide bridges between paired cysteine amino-acid residues, producing an unusual semi-conical structure [2]. ET-1 is the isoform predominantly responsible for cardiovascular effects, while ET-2 may function as a mediator in the intestinal tract, and ET-3 may play a role in the central nervous system and intestinal tract [3].

The initial product of the human ET-1 gene is preproendothelin-1, a 212 amino acid peptide. Proendothelin-1 is formed after removal of a short secretory sequence, and is further cleaved by a furin-like enzyme to generate the 38 amino acid peptide, big ET-1. Formation of the mature 21-amino-acid-peptide ET-1 requires cleavage of big ET-1 by endothelin converting enzymes (ECE), which are membrane-bound zinc metalloproteases [4].

In mammals, two G-protein-coupled endothelin receptors (ET_A and ET_B) have been identified [5, 6]. Under basal conditions, endogenous generation of ET-1 contributes to maintenance of vascular tone and blood pressure through activation of ET_A and ET_B receptors. The activation of both of these receptors in vascular smooth cells leads to activation of Gq-coupled signaling and vasoconstriction [1, 7]. In contrast, activation of ET_B receptor in endothelial cells leads to vasodilation through the endothelial cell release of nitric oxide and prostacyclin [2, 4].

The role of ET-1 and its receptors in cardiac diseases

ET-1 can be secreted by cardiomyocytes, cardiac endothelial cells, and cardiac fibroblasts [1, 8, 9]. Both ET_A and ET_B are found on cardiomyocytes and cardiac

Inflammation and Cardiac Diseases, edited by Giora Z. Feuerstein, Peter Libby and Douglas L. Mann
© 2003 Birkhäuser Verlag Basel/Switzerland

fibroblasts, with ET_A representing 90% of the endothelin receptors found on cardiomyocytes [10, 11]. ET_A and ET_B receptors are also found on the smooth muscle and endothelial cells of coronary vessels. With robust expression of ET-1 and its receptors in the heart, it is perhaps not surprising that the ET-1 system has been implicated in many cardiac diseases.

Severe cardiac ischemia causes plasma ET-1 concentrations to increase >5-fold within a few hours [12]. Plasma ET-1 concentrations are also elevated in patients with modest to severe heart failure (NYHA Class II-IV) [13–16]. Indeed, a high plasma level of ET-1 is a marker of poor prognosis, correlating with the extent of cardiac hemodynamic impairment [13–16]. Additionally, local production of ET-1 is increased in the failing myocardium of patients with idiopathic and ischemic dilated cardiomyopathy [17, 18]. Similar results are found in experimental animal models of heart failure [8, 11]. ET-1 may also be involved in the pathophysiology of viral and parasitic myocarditis, as suggested by studies showing increased plasma levels and local production of ET-1 in these diseases [19, 20].

It is still unclear which of the two distinct ET-1 receptors is more involved in ET-1-mediated cardiac diseases. Studies on expression levels of ET_A and ET_B in failing hearts reveal inconsistent results. The levels of ET_A and ET_B expression in failing hearts in patients with idiopathic dilated cardiomyopathy (DCM) or ischemic dilated cardiomyopathy (ICM) have been found to increase, not change, or decrease [17, 18, 21–24]. These discrepant results may partly reflect differences in experimental conditions (i.e., different portion of the heart were examined at various stages of the disease), and the diverse expression patterns of ET-1 and its receptors in the heart. Further investigations aimed at identifying receptor subtypes expressed on different cell types (i.e., cardiomyocytes, fibroblasts, endothelial cells and smooth muscle cells) instead of in homogenized heart tissues may clarify this question.

Controversy also exists with regards to the benefit of endothelin receptor antagonists in heart failure. While use of the combined ET_A/ET_B antagonist Bosentan has been reported to improve hemodynamic parameters and survival in experimental models of CHF [25], it has not reduced mortality in heart failure patients [26]. Studies employing selective ET_A antagonists have also demonstrated both beneficial [27] and deleterious effects in experimental models [28].

Myocardial inflammation and fibrosis in the cardiac pathophysiology

Studies over the past two decades have led to a profound shift in the conceptual paradigm of heart failure. Heart failure is now considered to be a complex syndrome encompassing not only hemodynamic dysfunction, but also a state of immune activation triggered by pro-inflammatory cytokines [29]. Monocyte invasion, adherence, and *in situ* proliferation during the inflammatory phase result in the activation and release of a variety of bioactive substances including cytokines [30]. Pro-inflammatory cytokines, at sufficient concentrations, are able to mimic some aspects of the so-called heart failure phenotype, including progressive left ventricular dysfunction, pulmonary edema, LV remodeling, fetal gene expression, and cardiomyopathy [29]. Thus heart failure results, at least in part, from the toxic effects exerted by endogenous cytokine cascades on the heart and the peripheral circulation.

The fibrotic repair process following damage and inflammation may also contribute to the progression of heart failure. Interstitial fibrosis impairs ventricular systolic and diastolic function [31, 32]. It also leads to an increase in the distance that oxygen must diffuse, thus potentially lowering the oxygen tension of working myocytes [33]. Furthermore, electrical coupling of the cardiomyocytes may be impaired by the accumulation of extracellular matrix (ECM) proteins and fibroblasts and the resulting increase in myocyte separation [34].

The role of ET-1 in myocardial inflammation and fibrosis

It is well determined that ET-1 exerts trophic effects in cardiomyocytes, leading to LV remodeling and dysfunction [35, 36]. However, there is also accumulating evidence supporting a role for ET-1 as a pro-inflammatory cytokine and fibrotic factor [30]. In this review, we will discuss the role of ET-1 in the pathogenesis of cardiac diseases from the perspective of myocardial inflammation and fibrosis.

ET-1 has been implicated in many disease states characterized by inflammation and/or fibrotic remodeling, such as atherosclerosis [37, 38], ischemia-reperfusion-induced cystitis [39], airway inflammation [40, 41], cutaneous inflammation [42], Crohn's disease and ulcerative colitis [43, 44], liver cirrhosis [45], and kidney fibrosis [46].

ET-1 may also be involved in inflammation and fibrosis of the heart. Ono et al. documented that myocardial and plasma ET-1 levels increase in mice with encephalomyocarditis (EMC) virus-induced myocarditis, in parallel with the progression of myocardial injury [19]. The fact that the local ET-1 level in myocardium was higher than that in plasma suggested that the heart is a major source of endogenous ET-1 in myocarditis [19]. The combined ET_A/ET_B antagonist Bosentan improved survival in these mice and reduced cellular infiltration and myocardial necrosis [19].

Recently, Ammarguellat et al. reported that the myocardial inflammation and fibrosis in hearts of deoxycorticosterone acetate (DOCA) hypertensive rats were, at least in part, mediated by ET-1 [47, 48]. In this model, the selective ET_A antagonist A-127722 prevented cardiac fibrosis in hearts by normalizing the level of procollagen I and III and fibrotic factor TGF-β1. A-127722 also abrogated activation of the inflammatory mediator NF-κB and expression of the platelet-endothelial cell adhesion molecule (PECAM-1) and the vascular cell adhesion molecule (VCAM-1). Hocher et al. also demonstrated that ET-1 played an important role in the development of cardiac fibrosis in a 2-kidney 1-clip rat model of renovascular hypertension [49]. In this model, use of the selective ET_B antagonist IRL1038, but not the selective ET_A antagonist BQ123, attenuated cardiac fibrosis. Further study is needed to distinguish between ET_A- and ET_B-mediated effects on cardiac remodeling.

Lessons learned from knock-out and transgenic models

Although a number of studies have suggested an important role for ET-1 in the pathophysiology of cardiac diseases, there has been no direct demonstration that ET-1 induces myocardial inflammation and/or fibrosis *in vivo*.

Unfortunately, homozygous ET-1$^{-/-}$, $ET_A^{-/-}$, ECE1$^{-/-}$ knock out mice develop lethal defects in the development of cephalic and cardiac neural crest derivatives [50–52]. These mice die either *in utero* or soon after birth, thus limiting the use of these models to extend our knowledge of the role of ET-1 in inflammation and fibrosis.

Recently, Huang et al. were able to study the role of ET-1 in a murine model of myocarditis in which ET-1 was deleted only from cardiac myocytes [53]. The cardiac-specific ET-1 knock-out mice and their controls were subject to inoculation of *Trypanosoma cruzi*, an etiological agent of Chagas's disease. Chagas's disease is characterized by acute myocarditis and chronic cardiomyopathy. In this study, cardiac-specific ET-1 knock-out mice showed reduced left ventricular end diastolic diameter (LVEDD) and improved fractional shortening as compared to controls [53]. These data suggested that the absence of ET-1 gene expression in cardiac myocytes markedly attenuated the functional and structural cardiac abnormalities induced by *T. cruzi* infection [53]. However, whether ET-1 exerted direct effects on inflammation and necrosis was not tested in this model.

Griswold et al. also suggested that ET_B might be involved in inflammation [42]. ET_B knock-out mice were subjected to topical arachidonic acid (AA) challenge to induce cutaneous inflammation [42]. Herozygous (+/–) and homozygous (–/–) knock-out mice demonstrated significantly decreased cutaneous inflammation and neutrophil infiltration [42]. Moreover, the selective ET_B receptor antagonist A192621, but not the selective ET_A receptor antagonist SB234551, inhibited topical AA-induced inflammatory responses in wild type animals [42].

Previous attempts to develop transgenic models over-expressing ET-1 have failed to demonstrate any cardiac phenotype [46, 54]. This may be due to a lack of efficient expression of ET-1 in the heart, embryonic lethality of lines with high levels of cardiac ET-1 production, and/or selection bias for lines exhibiting low levels of ET-1 expression within the heart. Indeed, as discussed above, ET-1 plays a pivotal role in cardiac development [50–52]. In transgenic mice in which preproET-1 was driven by its own promoter, chronic inflammation of the kidney leading to nephrosclerosis and polycystic renal disease has been reported [46, 54]. It is likely that this pathology resulted from enhanced ET-1 expression by inflammatory cells, specifically macrophages, which perpetuated a low-grade inflammatory response in the renal parenchyma, ultimately leading to glomerular damage [46, 54]. Hocher et al. also reported that ET-1 over-expression resulted in the development of pulmonary fibrosis by increasing collagen synthesis and a chronic inflammatory lung disease characterized by an increased infiltration of CD4-positive cells [55]. The lack of an obvious pathology in the cardiovascular system of these models may reflect the relatively low level of gene expression, and the lack of relevant environmental triggers for cardiac pathology.

To overcome this limitation, we have generated transgenic mice restricting ET-1 over-expression to the heart by utilizing the α-myosin heavy chain (α-MHC) promoter-dependent cardiac-specific tetracycline-regulated gene expression system (Tet-OFF) [56]. This method allows temporal control of transgene expression and thus avoids negative selection bias against mice with high levels of ET-1 expression during development. Our data suggest that conditional cardiac-restricted over-expression of ET-1 is sufficient to cause a chronic inflammatory infiltration and mild cardiac fibrosis, associated with the elevated expression of cytokines, which ultimately leads to progressive dilated cardiomyopathy, heart failure and death [57]. Interestingly, a combined ET_A/ET_B antagonist but not a selective ET_A antagonist prolonged survival in ET-1 over-expressing mice, suggesting a potentially important role of ET_B in the pathogenesis of ET-1-induced cardiomyopathy [57].

Cellular and molecular mechanisms involved in ET-1-mediated myocardial inflammation

ET-1 can be secreted by macrophage/monocytes [58] and polymorphonuclear leukocytes [59], suggesting a role for ET-1 in inflammation. Indeed, many studies have indicated that ET-1 may act as a chemo-attractant for leukocytes in an autocrine/paracrine manner, stimulate the expression of adhesion molecules, and induce the expression of pro-inflammatory cytokines. Lopez-Farre et al. demonstrated that ET-1 enhanced neutrophil accumulation in the isolated rabbit heart, suggesting a direct link between ET-1 and myocardial inflammation [60]. In cultured bovine endothelial cells, ET-1 promotes neutrophil aggregation [61, 62], stimulates surface expression of CD11b/CD1 on human neutrophils and augments their adhesion to endothelial cells [60] and cardiac myocytes [63]. Additionally, ET-1 is a chemo-attractant for monocytes [64, 65] and is able to activate mast cells [66]. Furthermore, ET-1 increases vascular permeability [67], and causes a time- and dose-dependent entrapment of circulating platelets [68]. Finally, ET-1 increases the release of elastase by activating neutrophils, contributing to tissue damage [69].

In addition to its chemo-attractant ability, ET-1 stimulates the expression of adhesion molecules that are key players in leukocyte-endothelial cell interaction

[70]. Hayasaki et al. documented that ET-1 induced intercellular adhesion molecule (ICAM)-1 expression on cultured cardiomyocytes and aortic endothelial cells. Similarly, Zouki et al. reported that ET-1 increased the expression of E-selectin and ICAM-1 on cultured human coronary artery endothelial cells in a concentration-dependent fashion [24]. Furthermore, the production of monocyte chemo-attractant protein (MCP)-1, a potent chemo-attractant for monocytes, can be induced by ET-1 through ET_A receptor activation in human brain-derived endothelial cells [71]. This effect is augmented by the pro-inflammatory cytokines, tumor necrosis factor (TNF)-α and interleukin (IL)-1β [71].

Moreover, ET-1 induces the release a variety of inflammatory cytokines such as TNF-α [41, 72], IL-1β [41], IL-6 [73-75], and IL-8 [76]. These cytokines are known to be expressed by all nucleated cell types in the myocardium. Elaboration of these cytokines can produce maladaptive effects in the heart, contributing to the disease progression in heart failure [29]. Interestingly, TNF-α and IL-1 also induce the expression of ET-1 [77, 78], which may further amplify deleterious effects.

Both ET_A and ET_B may be involved in ET-1-mediated inflammation. Macrophages express predominantly ETB receptor [38, 79]. Both neutrophil-endothelial cell adhesion and increased ICAM-1 expression on endothelial cells are inhibited by the selective ET_B receptor antagonist BQ788 [24, 63], whereas neutrophil-cardiac myocyte adhesion and increased ICAM-1 production on cardiac myocytes are attenuated by selective ET_A receptor antagonist S-0139 [63]. This may be related to the differences in receptor density on various cell types. For example, ET_A represents 90% of receptors on the surface of cardiac myocytes while ET_B is the dominant receptor on endothelial cells. However, different groups have reported varying results. Zouki et al. reported that a selective ET_A antagonist FR 139317 markedly attenuated the ET-1 stimulated neutrophil adherence, suggesting the role of ET_A in netrophil-endothelial attachment [24]. This discrepancy may be due to the use of different antagonists. It remains also possible that short- *versus* long-term exposure of endothelial cells to ET-1 may affect endothelial adhesiveness differently. The fact that the selective ET_A antagonist BQ610 but not ET_B antagonist BQ788 decreases ET-1-induced MCP-1 expression [71] further implicates the role of ET_A receptor in ET-1-mediated inflammation. The controversy underlying signaling pathways mediating ET-1-induced inflammation requires further investigation, particularly, in intact organs in which many cell types reside.

Cellular and molecular mechanisms involved in ET-1-mediated myocardial fibrosis

During the fibrotic repair phase, ET-1 induces expression of the fibrotic cytokine TGF-β [80] which plays an important role in extracellular matrix remodeling by stimulating collagen synthesis and increasing turnover and degradation of collagen

[81]. In addition, ET-1 has been shown to induce the expression and release of fibronectin, a key extracellular matrix component, as well as act as a chemotactic factor for fibroblasts. Moreover, ET-1 stimulates cardiac fibroblast proliferation [82, 83] and induces collagen Type-I and -III synthesis in vascular smooth muscle cells [84, 85]. Taken together, ET-1 is able to induce interstitial fibrosis *via* different mechanisms, leading to cardiac remodeling, ventricular stiffness, and ultimately compromising the function of the heart.

It is also worth mentioning that ET-1 may, in the short term, exert salutary effects on cardiac muscle healing following myocardial infarction (MI). This effect may depend on it ability to promote inflammation and fibrotic repair. Our group has shown that administration of an ET antagonist within the first few days following MI can interfere with infarct healing and result in scar dilatation, compromise contractility and worsen heart failure [28, 86]. This finding has now been confirmed by other groups [80, 87], and underlines the importance of this multifaceted biological mediator in diverse physiological and pathophysiological mechanisms related to the regulation of cardiac structure and function.

Summary

There is growing evidence to suggest that ET-1 may act as a pro-inflammatory molecule and fibrotic factor in various tissues. In the heart, ET-1 may induce myocardial inflammation by recruitment of leukocytes, stimulating production of adhesion molecules, and inducing cytokine expression. It may also induce cardiac fibrosis by activating fibrotic factor TGF-β, increasing collagen synthesis, and stimulating fibroblast proliferation. While it remains unclear which mechanisms underlie ET_A and/or ET_B receptor-mediated contributions to these processes, both receptors appear to be involved.

Comparison of treatments of different ET receptor antagonists in conditional cardiac specific transgenic and/or knock-out model will further dissect out these mechanisms. The less than optimal results of ET receptor antagonist in clinical trials of heart failure may be partially due to the lack of recognition of the importance of ET-1-mediated myocardial inflammation and fibrosis contributing to ventricular remodeling and dysfunction. The further understanding of the role of ET-1 in the pathogenesis of cardiac diseases will provide new insights into the potential therapeutic importance of blocking ET-1 signaling pathways in these diseases.

Acknowledgements
LLY is supported by a Heart & Stroke Richard Lewar Centre of Excellence/OGSST Studentship and Heart & Stroke Foundation of Ontario (HSFO) Doctoral Research Award. MH is a recipient of a Clinician Scientist Award from the Canadian Insti-

tute of Health Research (CIHR). This study referenced in this review were from our laboratory supported in part by CIHR operating grant 11620 (DJS and MH).

Reference

1   Yanagisawa M, Kurihara H, Kimura S, Tomobe Y, Kobayashi M, Mitsui Y, Yazaki Y, Goto K, Masaki T (1988) A novel potent vasoconstrictor peptide produced by vascular endothelial cells. *Nature* 332: 411–415

2   Inoue A, Yanagisawa M, Kimura S, Kasuya Y, Miyauchi T, Goto K, Masaki T (1989) The human endothelin family: three structurally and pharmacologically distinct isopeptides predicted by three separate genes. *Proc Natl Acad Sci USA* 86: 2863–2867

3   Kedzierski RM, Yanagisawa M (2001) Endothelin system: The double-edged sword in health and disease. *Annu Rev Pharmacol Toxicol* 41: 851–876

4   Xu D, Emoto N, Giaid A, Slaughter C, Kaw S, deWit D, Yanagisawa M (1994) ECE-1: A membrane-bound metalloprotease that catalyzes the proteolytic activation of big endothelin-1. *Cell* 78: 473–485

5   Arai H, Hori S, Aramori I, Ohkubo H, Nakanishi S (1990) Cloning and expression of a cDNA encoding an endothelin receptor. *Nature* 348: 730–732

6   Sakurai T, Yanagisawa M, Takuwa Y, Miyazaki H, Kimura S, Goto K, Masaki T (1990) Cloning of a cDNA encoding a non-isopeptide-selective subtype of the endothelin receptor. *Nature* 348: 732–735

7   Haynes WG, Ferro CJ, O'Kane KP, Somerville D, Lomax CC, Webb DJ (1996) Systemic endothelin receptor blockade decreases peripheral vascular resistance and blood pressure in humans. *Circulation* 93: 1860–1870

8   Sakai S, Miyauchi T, Sakurai T, Kasuya Y, Ihara M, Yamaguchi I, Goto K, Sugishita Y (1996) Endogenous endothelin-1 participates in the maintenance of cardiac function in rats with congestive heart failure. Marked increase in endothelin-1 production in the failing heart. *Circulation* 93: 1214–1222

9   Gray MO, Long CS, Kalinyak JE, Li HT, Karliner JS (1998) Angiotensin II stimulates cardiac myocyte hypertrophy *via* paracrine release of TGF-beta 1 and endothelin-1 from fibroblasts. *Cardiovasc Res* 40: 352–363

10 Fareh J, Touyz RM, Schiffrin EL, Thibault G (1996) Endothelin-1 and angiotensin II receptors in cells from rat hypertrophied heart. Receptor regulation and intracellular Ca^{2+} modulation. *Circ Res* 78: 302–311

11 Sakai S, Miyauchi T, Kobayashi M, Yamaguchi I, Goto K, Sugishita Y (1996) Inhibition of myocardial endothelin pathway improves long-term survival in heart failure. *Nature* 384: 353–355

12 Stewart DJ, Kubac G, Costello KB, Cernacek P (1991) Increased plasma endothelin-1 in the early hours of acute myocardial infarction. *J Am Coll Cardiol* 18: 38–43

13 Stewart DJ, Cernacek P, Costello KB, Rouleau JL (1992) Elevated endothelin-1 in heart failure and loss of normal response to postural change. *Circulation* 85: 510–517

14   McMurray JJ, Ray SG, Abdullah I, Dargie HJ, Morton JJ (1992) Plasma endothelin in chronic heart failure. *Circulation* 85: 1374–1379

15   Pousset F, Isnard R, Lechat P, Kalotka H, Carayon A, Maistre G, Escolano S, Thomas D, Komajda M (1997) Prognostic value of plasma endothelin-1 in patients with chronic heart failure. *Eur Heart J* 18: 254

16   Wei CM, Lerman A, Rodeheffer RJ, McGregor CG, Brandt RR, Wright S, Heublein DM, Kao PC, Edwards WD, Burnett JC Jr. (1994) Endothelin in human congestive heart failure. *Circulation* 89: 1580–1586

17   Pieske B, Beyermann B, Breu V, Loffler BM, Schlotthauer K, Maier LS, Schmidt-Schweda S, Just H, Hasenfuss G (1999) Functional effects of endothelin and regulation of endothelin receptors in isolated human nonfailing and failing myocardium. *Circulation* 99: 1802–1809

18   Serneri GG, Cecioni I, Vanni S, Paniccia R, Bandinelli B, Vetere A, Janming X, Bertolozzi I, Boddi M, Lisi GF et al (2000) Selective upregulation of cardiac endothelin system in patients with ischemic but not idiopathic dilated cardiomyopathy: Endothelin-1 system in the human failing heart. *Circ Res* 86: 377–385

19   Ono K, Matsumori A, Shioi T, Furukawa Y, Sasayama S (1999) Contribution of endothelin-1 to myocardial injury in a murine model of myocarditis: Acute effects of bosentan, an endothelin receptor antagonist. *Circulation* 100: 1823–1829

20   Petkova SB, Tanowitz HB, Magazine HI, Factor SM, Chan J, Pestell RG, Bouzahzah B, Douglas SA, Shtutin V, Morris SA et al (2000) Myocardial expression of endothelin-1 in murine Trypanosoma cruzi infection. *Cardiovasc Pathol* 9: 257–265

21   Ponicke K, Vogelsang M, Heinroth M, Becker K, Zolk O, Bohm M, Zerkowski HR, and Brodde OE (1998) Endothelin receptors in the failing and nonfailing human heart. *Circulation* 97: 744–751

22   Zolk O, Quattek J, Sitzler G, Schrader T, Nickenig G, Schnabel P, Shimada K, Takahashi M, and Bohm M (1999) Expression of endothelin-1, endothelin-converting enzyme, and endothelin receptors in chronic heart failure. *Circulation* 99: 2118–2123

23   Walker CA, Ergul A, Grubbs A, Zile MR, Zellner JL, Crumbley AJ, Spinale FG (2001) beta-Adrenergic and endothelin receptor interaction in dilated human cardiomyopathic myocardium. *J Card Fail* 7: 129–137

24   Zouki C, Baron C, Fournier A, Filep JG (1999) Endothelin-1 enhances neutrophil adhesion to human coronary artery endothelial cells: Role of ET(A) receptors and platelet-activating factor. *Br J Pharmacol* 127: 969–979

25   Fraccarollo D, Hu K, Galuppo P, Gaudron P, Ertl G (1997) Chronic endothelin receptor blockade attenuates progressive ventricular dilation and improves cardiac function in rats with myocardial infarction: Possible involvement of myocardial endothelin system in ventricular remodeling. *Circulation* 96: 3963–3973

26   Mylona P, Cleland JG (1999) Update of REACH-1 and MERIT-HF clinical trials in heart failure. Cardio.net Editorial Team. *Eur J Heart Fail* 1: 197–200

27   Yamauchi-Kohno R, Miyauchi T, Hoshino T, Kobayashi T, Aihara H, Sakai S, Yabana H, Goto K, Sugishita Y, and Murata S (1999) Role of endothelin in deterioration of

heart failure due to cardiomyopathy in hamsters: Increase in endothelin-1 production in the heart and beneficial effect of endothelin-A receptor antagonist on survival and cardiac function. *Circulation* 99: 2171–2176

28 Nguyen QT, Cernacek P, Calderoni A, Stewart DJ, Picard P, Sirois P, White M, Rouleau JL (1998) Endothelin A receptor blockade causes adverse left ventricular remodeling but improves pulmonary artery pressure after infarction in the rat. *Circulation* 98: 2323–2330

29 Mann DL (2002) Inflammatory mediators and the failing heart: Past, present, and the foreseeable future. *Circ Res* 91: 988–998

30 Teder P, Noble PW (2000) A cytokine reborn? Endothelin-1 in pulmonary inflammation and fibrosis. *Am J Respir Cell Mol Biol* 23: 7–10

31 Doering CW, Jalil JE, Janicki JS, Pick R, Aghili S, Abrahams C, and Weber KT (1988) Collagen network remodelling and diastolic stiffness of the rat left ventricle with pressure overload hypertrophy. *Cardiovasc Res* 22: 686–695

32 Jalil JE, Doering CW, Janicki JS, Pick R, Shroff SG, Weber KT (1989) Fibrillar collagen and myocardial stiffness in the intact hypertrophied rat left ventricle. *Circ Res* 64: 1041–1050

33 Sabbah HN, Sharov VG, Lesch M, Goldstein S (1995) Progression of heart failure: A role for interstitial fibrosis. *Mol Cell Biochem* 147: 29–34

34 Weber KT, Brilla CG (1991) Pathological hypertrophy and cardiac interstitium. Fibrosis and renin- angiotensin-aldosterone system. *Circulation* 83: 1849–1865

35 Ito H, Hirata Y, Hiroe M, Tsujino M, Adachi S, Takamoto T, Nitta M, Taniguchi K, Marumo F (1991) Endothelin-1 induces hypertrophy with enhanced expression of muscle- specific genes in cultured neonatal rat cardiomyocytes. *Circ Res* 69: 209–215

36 Eble DM, Strait JB, Govindarajan G, Lou J, Byron KL, Samarel AM (2000) Endothelin-induced cardiac myocyte hypertrophy: role for focal adhesion kinase. *Am J Physiol Heart Circ Physiol* 278: H1695–1707

37 Barton M, Haudenschild CC, d'Uscio LV, Shaw S, Munter K, Luscher TF (1998) Endothelin ETA receptor blockade restores NO-mediated endothelial function and inhibits atherosclerosis in apolipoprotein E-deficient mice. *Proc Natl Acad Sci USA* 95: 14367–14372

38 Babaei S, Picard P, Ravandi A, Monge JC, Lee TC, Cernacek P, Stewart DJ (2000) Blockade of endothelin receptors markedly reduces atherosclerosis in LDL receptor deficient mice: Role of endothelin in macrophage foam cell formation. *Cardiovasc Res* 48: 158–167

39 Bajory Z, Hutter J, Krombach F, Messmer K (2002) The role of endothelin-1 in ischemia-reperfusion induced acute inflammation of the bladder in rats. *J Urol* 168: 1222–1225

40 Kraft M, Beam WR, Wenzel SE, Zamora MR, O'Brien RF, Martin RJ (1994) Blood and bronchoalveolar lavage endothelin-1 levels in nocturnal asthma. *Am J Respir Crit Care Med* 149: 946–952

41 Finsnes F, Lyberg T, Christensen G, Skjonsberg OH (2001) Effect of endothelin antago-

nism on the production of cytokines in eosinophilic airway inflammation. *Am J Physiol Lung Cell Mol Physiol* 280: L659–665

42   Griswold DE, Douglas SA, Martin LD, Davis TG, Davis L, Ao Z, Luttmann MA, Pullen M, Nambi P, Hay DW et al (1999) Endothelin B receptor modulates inflammatory pain and cutaneous inflammation. *Mol Pharmacol* 56: 807–812

43   Murch SH, Braegger CP, Sessa WC, MacDonald TT (1992) High endothelin-1 immunoreactivity in Crohn's disease and ulcerative colitis. *Lancet* 339: 381–385

44   McCartney SA, Ballinger AB, Vojnovic I, Farthing MJ, Warner TD (2002) Endothelin in human inflammatory bowel disease: Comparison to rat trinitrobenzenesulphonic acid-induced colitis. *Life Sci* 71: 1893–1904

45   Rockey DC, Chung JJ (1996) Endothelin antagonism in experimental hepatic fibrosis. Implications for endothelin in the pathogenesis of wound healing. *J Clin Invest* 98: 1381–1388

46   Hocher B, Thone-Reineke C, Rohmeiss P, Schmager F, Slowinski T, Burst V, Siegmund F, Quertermous T, Bauer C, Neumayer HH et al (1997) Endothelin-1 transgenic mice develop glomerulosclerosis, interstitial fibrosis, and renal cysts but not hypertension. *J Clin Invest* 99: 1380–9

47   Ammarguellat F, Larouche II, Schiffrin EL (2001) Myocardial fibrosis in DOCA-salt hypertensive rats: Effect of endothelin ET(A) receptor antagonism. *Circulation* 103: 319–324

48   Ammarguellat FZ, Gannon PO, Amiri F, Schiffrin EL (2002) Fibrosis, matrix metalloproteinases, and inflammation in the heart of DOCA-salt hypertensive rats: role of ET(A) receptors. *Hypertension* 39: 679–684

49   Hocher B, George I, Rebstock J, Bauch A, Schwarz A, Neumayer HH, Bauer C (1999) Endothelin system-dependent cardiac remodeling in renovascular hypertension. *Hypertension* 33: 816–822

50   Kurihara Y, Kurihara H, Suzuki H, Kodama T, Maemura K, Nagai R, Oda H, Kuwaki T, Cao WH, Kamada N et al (1994) Elevated blood pressure and craniofacial abnormalities in mice deficient in endothelin-1. *Nature* 368: 703–710

51   Clouthier DE, Hosoda K, Richardson JA, Williams SC, Yanagisawa H, Kuwaki T, Kumada M, Hammer RE, Yanagisawa M (1998) Cranial and cardiac neural crest defects in endothelin-A receptor- deficient mice. *Development* 125: 813–824

52   Yanagisawa H, Yanagisawa M, Kapur RP, Richardson JA, Williams SC, Clouthier DE, de Wit D, Emoto N, Hammer RE (1998) Dual genetic pathways of endothelin-mediated intercellular signaling revealed by targeted disruption of endothelin converting enzyme-1 gene. *Development* 125: 825–836

53   Huang H, Yanagisawa M, Kisanuki YY, Jelicks LA, Chandra M, Factor SM, Wittner M, Weiss LM, Pestell RG, Shtutin V et al (2002) Role of cardiac myocyte-derived endothelin-1 in chagasic cardiomyopathy: Molecular genetic evidence. *Clin Sci (Lond)* 103 Suppl 48: 263S–266S

54   Shindo T, Kurihara H, Maemura K, Kurihara Y, Ueda O, Suzuki H, Kuwaki T, Ju KH,

Wang Y, Ebihara A et al (2002) Renal damage and salt-dependent hypertension in aged transgenic mice overexpressing endothelin-1. *J Mol Med* 80: 105–116

55 Hocher B, Schwarz A, Fagan KA, Thone-Reineke C, El-Hag K, Kusserow H, Elitok S, Bauer C, Neumayer HH, Rodman DM et al (2000) Pulmonary fibrosis and chronic lung inflammation in ET-1 transgenic mice. *Am J Respir Cell Mol Biol* 23: 19–26

56 Yu Z, Redfern CS, Fishman GI (1996) Conditional transgene expression in the heart. *Circ Res* 79: 691–697

57 Yang LL, Gros R, Golam K, Gotlieb AI, Husain M, and Stewart DJ (2002) Conditional cardiac-overexpression of endothelin-1 in transgenic mice causes a fatal inflammatory cardiomyopathy. *Circulation* 106 (Suppl) II–160

58 Ehrenreich H, Anderson RW, Fox CH, Rieckmann P, Hoffman GS, Travis WD, Coligan JE, Kehrl JH, Fauci AS (1990) Endothelins, peptides with potent vasoactive properties, are produced by human macrophages. *J Exp Med* 172: 1741–1748

59 Sessa WC, Kaw S, Zembowicz A, Anggard E, Hecker M, Vane JR (1991) Human polymorphonuclear leukocytes generate and degrade endothelin-1 by two distinct neutral proteases. *J Cardiovasc Pharmacol* 17: S34–38

60 Lopez Farre A, Riesco A, Espinosa G, Digiuni E, Cernadas MR, Alvarez V, Monton M, Rivas F, Gallego MJ, Egido J et al (1993) Effect of endothelin-1 on neutrophil adhesion to endothelial cells and perfused heart. *Circulation* 88: 1166–1171

61 Gomez-Garre D, Guerra M, Gonzalez E, Lopez-Farre A, Riesco A, Caramelo C, Escanero J, and Egido J (1992) Aggregation of human polymorphonuclear leukocytes by endothelin: Role of platelet-activating factor. *Eur J Pharmacol* 224: 167–172

62 Lopez-Farre A, Caramelo C, Esteban A, Alberola ML, Millas I, Monton M, and Casado S (1995) Effects of aspirin on platelet-neutrophil interactions. Role of nitric oxide and endothelin-1. *Circulation* 91: 2080–2088

63 Hayasaki Y, Nakajima M, Kitano Y, Iwasaki T, Shimamura T, Iwaki K (1996) ICAM-1 expression on cardiac myocytes and aortic endothelial cells *via* their specific endothelin receptor subtype. *Biochem Biophys Res Commun* 229: 817–824

64 Achmad TH, Rao GS (1992) Chemotaxis of human blood monocytes toward endothelin-1 and the influence of calcium channel blockers. *Biochem Biophys Res Commun* 189: 994–1000

65 Langenfeld MR, Nakhla S, Death AK, Jessup W, Celermajer DS (2001) Endothelin-1 plus oxidized low-density lipoprotein, but neither alone, increase human monocyte adhesion to endothelial cells. *Clin Sci (Lond)* 101: 731–738

66 Uchida Y, Ninomiya H, Sakamoto T, Lee JY, Endo T, Nomura A, Hasegawa S, Hirata F (1992) ET-1 released histamine from guinea pig pulmonary but not peritoneal mast cells. *Biochem Biophys Res Commun* 189: 1196–1201

67 Helset E, Kjaeve J, Hauge A (1993) Endothelin-1-induced increases in microvascular permeability in isolated, perfused rat lungs requires leukocytes and plasma. *Circ Shock* 39: 15–20

68 Helset E, Lindal S, Olsen R, Myklebust R, Jorgensen L (1996) Endothelin-1 causes

sequential trapping of platelets and neutrophils in pulmonary microcirculation in rats *Am J Physiol* 271: L538–546

69 Halim A, Kanayama N, el Maradny E, Maehara K, Terao T (1995) Activated neutrophil by endothelin-1 caused tissue damage in human umbilical cord. *Thromb Res* 77: 321–327

70 Springer TA (1994) Traffic signals for lymphocyte recirculation and leukocyte emigration: the multistep paradigm. *Cell* 76: 301–314

71 Chen P, Shibata M, Zidovetzki R, Fisher M, Zlokovic BV, Hofman FM (2001) Endothelin-1 and monocyte chemo-attractant protein-1 modulation in ischemia and human brain-derived endothelial cell cultures. *J Neuroimmunol* 116: 62–73

72 Ruetten H, Thiemermann C (1997) Endothelin-1 stimulates the biosynthesis of tumour necrosis factor in macrophages: ET-receptors, signal transduction and inhibition by dexamethasone. *J Physiol Pharmacol* 48: 675–688

73 Stankova J, D'Orleans-Juste P, Rola-Pleszczynski M (1996) ET-1 induces IL-6 gene expression in human umbilical vein endothelial cells: synergistic effect of IL-1. *Am J Physiol* 271: C1073–1078

74 Saito S, Aikawa R, Shiojima I, Nagai R, Yazaki Y, Komuro I (1999) Endothelin-1 induces expression of fetal genes through the interleukin-6 family of cytokines in cardiac myocytes. *FEBS Lett* 456: 103–107

75 McMillen MA, Huribal M, Cunningham ME, Kumar R, Sumpio BE (1995) Endothelin-1 increases intracellular calcium in human monocytes and causes production of interleukin-6. *Crit Care Med* 23: 34–40

76 Zidovetzki R, Chen P, Chen M, Hofman FM (1999) Endothelin-1-induced interleukin-8 production in human brain-derived endothelial cells is mediated by the protein kinase C and protein tyrosine kinase pathways. *Blood* 94: 1291–1299

77 Maemura K, Kurihara H, Morita T, Oh-hashi Y, Yazaki Y (1992) Production of endothelin-1 in vascular endothelial cells is regulated by factors associated with vascular injury. *Gerontology* 38: 29–35

78 Klemm P, Warner TD, Hohlfeld T, Corder R, Vane JR (1995) Endothelin 1 mediates ex vivo coronary vasoconstriction caused by exogenous and endogenous cytokines. *Proc Natl Acad Sci USA* 92: 2691–2695

79 Sakurai-Yamashita Y, Yamashita K, Yoshida A, Obana M, Takada K, Shibaguchi H, Shigematsu K, Niwa M, Taniyama K (1997) Rat peritoneal macrophages express endothelin ET(B) but not endothelin ET(A) receptors. *Eur J Pharmacol* 338: 199–203

80 Fraccarollo D, Galuppo P, Bauersachs J, Ertl G (2002) Collagen accumulation after myocardial infarction: effects of ETA receptor blockade and implications for early remodeling. *Cardiovasc Res* 54: 559–567

81 Nicoletti A, Michel JB (1999) Cardiac fibrosis and inflammation: interaction with hemodynamic and hormonal factors. *Cardiovasc Res* 41: 532–543

82 Fujisaki H, Ito H, Hirata Y, Tanaka M, Hata M, Lin M, Adachi S, Akimoto H, Marumo F, Hiroe M (1995) Natriuretic peptides inhibit angiotensin II-induced proliferation

of rat cardiac fibroblasts by blocking endothelin-1 gene expression. *J Clin Invest* 96: 1059–1065

83 Piacentini L, Gray M, Honbo NY, Chentoufi J, Bergman M, Karliner JS (2000) Endothelin-1 stimulates cardiac fibroblast proliferation through activation of protein kinase C. *J Mol Cell Cardiol* 32: 565–576

84 Rizvi MA, Katwa L, Spadone DP, Myers PR (1996) The effects of endothelin-1 on collagen Type I and Type III synthesis in cultured porcine coronary artery vascular smooth muscle cells. *J Mol Cell Cardiol* 28: 243–252

85 Hirata Y, Yoshimi H, Takaichi S, Yanagisawa M, Masaki T (1988) Binding and receptor down-regulation of a novel vasoconstrictor endothelin in cultured rat vascular smooth muscle cells. *FEBS Lett* 239: 13–17

86 Nguyen QT, Cernacek P, Sirois MG, Calderone A, Lapointe N, Stewart DJ, Rouleau JL (2001) Long-term effects of nonselective endothelin A and B receptor antagonism in postinfarction rat: importance of timing. *Circulation* 104: 2075–2081

87 Pfeffer JM, Finn PV, Zornoff LA, and Pfeffer MA (2000) Endothelin-A receptor antagonism during acute myocardial infarction in rats. *Cardiovasc Drugs Ther* 14: 579–587

Cyclooxygenases and
cardiac diseases

Cyclooxygenase-2 and myocardial ischemia

Gary F. Baxter and Caroline P. D. Wheeler-Jones

Infection, Inflammation and Vascular Biology Research Group, Department of Basic Sciences, The Royal Veterinary College, University of London, Royal College Street, London NW1 0TU, UK

Introduction

Acute myocardial ischemia, usually as a result of thrombotic occlusion of one or more epicardial coronary arteries, is predicted to become the leading cause of death worldwide by 2020 [1]. Following myocardial infarction, tissue remodelling plays a major role in determining the chronic haemodynamic competency of the infarcted heart but may contribute ultimately to the development of chronic cardiac failure in patients who survive the acute ischaemic episode. Co-ordinated activation and interaction of a host of mediators is therefore critical in determining both early salvage of myocardium during and immediately following ischemia, and also in the later development of remodelling in the surviving myocardium. Among the numerous mediators that have been proposed to play roles in the ischaemic myocardium are the prostaglandins (PGs). PGs exert a diverse range of physiological and pathological roles throughout the cardiovascular system [2, 3]. Although synthetic PG derivatives have been extensively studied with regard to their ability to modify acute ischaemic injury and to influence coronary vascular reactivity, little is known about the endogenous roles of PGs, or the regulation of their synthesis, in the heart following ischemia.

Cyclooxygenase-2 and prostaglandin synthesis

Cleavage of arachidonic acid from the sn-2 position of phospholipids is the first step in the formation of PGs from membrane phospholipids and is catalysed by phospholipases A_2 (PLA_2), principally $cPLA_2\alpha$. Arachidonic acid is converted into PGH_2 by the action of cyclooxygenases (COXs). Terminal PG synthases subsequently catalyse the conversion of the unstable intermediate PGH_2 into the various PGs [4]. COX activity is thus a rate-limiting step for PG synthesis and the precise range of PGs produced in any cell type will depend on the pathophysiological milieu and the inherent terminal synthase capacity of the cells. Presently, there are two known

Inflammation and Cardiac Diseases, edited by Giora Z. Feuerstein, Peter Libby and Douglas L. Mann
© 2003 Birkhäuser Verlag Basel/Switzerland

forms of COX [5]. These iso-enzymes are the products of distinct genes and they sub-serve distinct physiological roles within the body. Thus, COX-1 is constitutively expressed in most tissues and is thought to be necessary for PG production relating to normal homeostasis. In contrast, COX-2 is expressed at very low levels or is absent in most normal tissues but is induced by a number of stimuli including cytokines, oxidative stress, tumour promoters and growth factors [6]. Regulation of COX-2 occurs at transcriptional, post-transcriptional and post-translational levels, and its activity plays a central role in the exaggerated production of PGs during inflammatory responses. This prevailing view of COX-1 being a constitutive enzyme accounting for PG formation under physiological conditions and COX-2 being an inducible enzyme, promoting increased PG formation during disease, may be questionable since there is accumulating evidence that COX-2 plays important roles in normal physiological regulation [7, 8].

Therapeutic COX-2 inhibition and cardiovascular risk

Selective COX-2 inhibitors have been introduced for the symptomatic treatment of inflammatory conditions, particularly the arthritides. The effect of chronic COX-2 inhibition on the risk of coronary vascular events is an area of current controversy. Large clinical studies assessing the safety of COX-2 inhibition in rheumatoid arthritis and osteoarthritis have reported conflicting data on the incidence of thrombotic events in patients treated with COX-2 inhibitors. Meta-analysis including more than 16,000 patients from the CLASS and VIGOR studies has suggested that the rate of myocardial infarction in patients taking COX-2 inhibitors is increased [9]. However, analysis of eight Phase IIB and Phase III trials involving more than 5,000 patients concluded that there was no increase in the risk of cardiovascular events [10]. At present it is impossible to conclude if, and how, selective COX-2 inhibition is associated with increased cardiovascular mortality and there is a need for prospective studies of COX-2 inhibition in patients with documented cardiovascular risk. A plausible mechanism is increased platelet responsiveness as a result of inhibition of vascular PGI_2 synthesis (a physiological action thought to be under the control of COX-2) in the face of unopposed platelet thromboxane A_2, primarily synthesised through COX-1. However, alternative or additional pathological mechanisms, might include the abrogation of any potentially beneficial effects of COX-2 in ischaemic and infarcted myocardium.

Regulation of cyclooxygenase-2 in myocardium

Few studies to date have described the expression of COX-2 in myocardium. Immunoblotting studies in rat and rabbit myocardium reported low constitutive

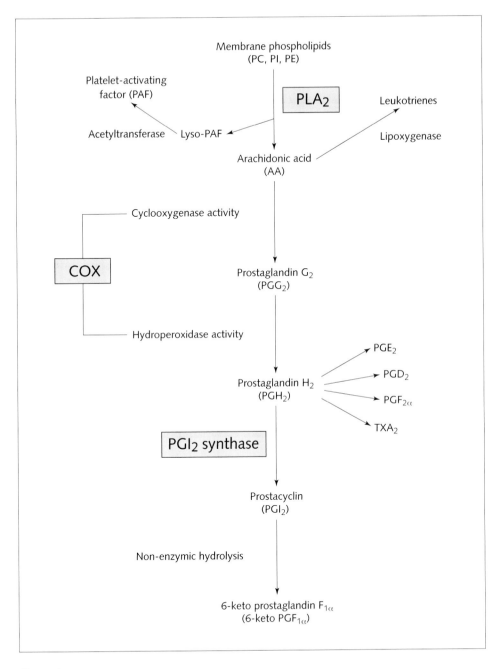

Figure 1
Major enzymatic pathways of prostanoid formation illustrating the central role of cyclo-oxygenases-1 and -2 (COX).

expression of COX-2 [11–13] whereas immunoblotting failed to detect COX-2 expression in mouse myocardium [14]. Similarly, immunohistochemical analysis of intact human myocardium showed either undetectable or low-level COX-2 expression [15, 16]. Studies in Wheeler-Jones's laboratory have shown that endothelial cells express both COX-1 and COX-2 in the absence of inflammatory stimuli. Basal PGI2 synthesis by human umbilical vein endothelial cells was partially inhibited by selective COX-2 inhibition, suggesting that both isoforms contribute to PGI2 synthesis in normal, unperturbed endothelium. In contrast, COX-2 expression in myocardial arteriolar endothelial and smooth muscle cells is barely detectable by immunohistochemistry under basal conditions [16]. Thus, the available evidence suggests that COX-2 may be expressed constitutively in myocardium at low levels but definitive evidence for this is lacking.

Under hypoxic conditions, expression of COX-2 increases markedly in myocardium. For example, during low-flow ischemia in the rat isolated heart, COX-2 mRNA and protein increased whereas COX-1 was unaffected [17]. Following myocardial infarction in the rat, a 4–5-fold increase in COX-2 protein occurred within four days in the infarct territory and infarct border zone [13] reflecting the situation in human ischaemic cardiomyopathy where COX-2 expression is abundant within the regions of fibrotic scarring [15]. Sub-lethal episodes of myocardial ischemia also cause COX-2 induction [11, 12]. Thus, in rabbit heart subjected to several short periods of coronary artery occlusion and assessed by immunoblotting 24 hours later, a 2–3-fold increase in COX-2 protein was detectable in the membrane sub-fractions of extracted myocardial risk zone. Corresponding increases in the levels of PGE_2 and 6-keto-PGF_{1a} were also detected, suggesting that the increase in COX-2 protein was associated with an increase in total COX activity. Cell-specific expression of COX-2 in myocardium has not been comprehensively explored but COX-2 induction has been reported in human atrial tissue (cardiac myocytes, microvascular endothelial and smooth muscle cells) following ischemia [16]. There is also evidence that neonatal cardiac myocytes express COX-2 protein at low levels and that oxidative stress up-regulates enzyme expression [18]. Thus the available evidence suggests that COX-2 is induced in myocardium after hypoxic stress but the temporal characteristics and the specific cell types in which expression occurs have not been systemically explored.

The signalling mechanisms regulating COX-2 induction in myocardial tissue have been little studied. Evidence from Bolli's laboratory implies that brief ischaemic stress (preconditioning) induces myocardial COX-2 *via* PKC, tyrosine kinase and NF-κB signalling [12, 21] but mitogen-activated protein kinase (MAPK) signalling has not so far been examined. The p42/44 and p38 families are implicated in the regulation of COX-2 in isolated vascular cell types. Recent data from Wheeler-Jones's laboratory indicate that co-ordinated activation of both p42/p44 MAPK and p38 MAPK is necessary for agonist-stimulated COX-2 expression in endothelial cells. MAPK involvement would be especially relevant to myocardial ischemia since both

MAPK families are known to be differentially activated by a variety of stressful and pharmacological stimuli, including hypoxia-reoxygenation [19, 20]. There is evidence that angiotensin-II-stimulated COX-2 induction in cultured cardiac fibroblasts is dependent on p38 MAPK, but not p42/p44 MAPK, activation [13].

Functional role of cyclooxygenase-2 in acute ischemia

The limited experimental evidence available paints a complex picture of the role of COX-2 in ischaemic myocardium, with evidence supporting a beneficial, deleterious or no role. The complexities of interpretation of these studies relate to (a) acute ischemia *versus* longer-term infarct models, (b) the role of constitutive COX-2 *versus* induced COX-2, (c) *in vitro versus in vivo* models. A number of early studies indicated that PGI_2 and its analogues administered exogenously could protect the myocardium during acute ischemia-reperfusion insult, as assessed by limitation of infarct size and improved functional recovery following ischemia [22–24]. In isolated rat hearts subjected to low-flow ischemia, induction of COX-2 was enhanced by nicotine treatment and this enhancement was associated with deterioration in cardiac contractility and increased creatine kinase release [17]. However, in a less severe low-flow ischemia preparation [25] no clear beneficial effect of a COX-2 inhibitor on cardiac functional recovery was observed. Similarly, selective COX-2 inhibition did not influence functional recovery following low-flow ischemia in guinea pig heart [26]. More recently, Camitta et al. [14] have reported a large series of studies using genetically-targeted mice with deletion of either *cox-1* or *cox-2* genes. In COX-2 knockout mice, functional recovery following ischemia was reduced compared to wild-type control hearts, suggesting that COX-2 serves a protective role. However, somewhat paradoxically, COX-2 protein was not detectable by immunoblotting in wild type hearts. In addition, PGE_2 and 6-keto-$PGF_{1\alpha}$ were present in the hearts of COX-1 knockout mice, albeit at reduced levels, implying that sufficient COX-2 was present to determine basal PG synthesis. Furthermore, administration of exogenous PGI_2 could not substitute for the absence of COX-2. These intriguing data suggest that endogenous COX-2 may be constitutively active and plays an important role in determining outcome from acute ischemia, a role which cannot be substituted by COX-1 or exogenous PGs. Moreover, an intriguing co-operative interaction between COX-2 and nitric oxide synthase has been demonstrated in this form of adaptive cytoprotection, in which NO apparently "drives" COX-2-derived prostanoid formation [27]. A protective role of COX-2 in acute myocardial ischemia is supported by evidence from studies in neonatal cardiac myocytes where COX-2 inhibitors exacerbate damage due to oxidant stress [18]. Other studies reported that myocardial COX-2 induced sub-acutely (24 hours) following preconditioning with brief episodes of ischemia is obligatory for delayed protection against infarction in rabbit and mouse myocardium, yet inhibition of

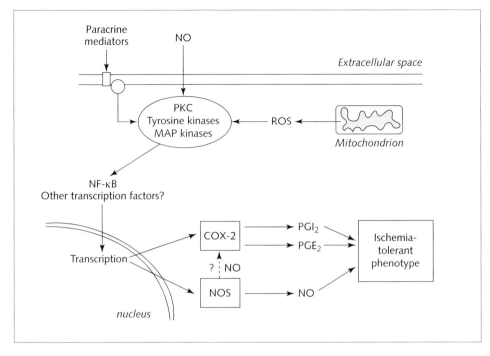

Figure 2

Induction of COX-2 in response to ischemia may result in enhanced tolerance to subsequent ischemia (delayed preconditioning). Paracrine mediators, nitric oxide (NO) and reactive oxygen species (ROS) released in the initial period of ischemia, co-ordinate the activation of major kinase pathways and the activation of nuclear factor-κB (NF-κB). cox-2 gene regulation and inducible nitric oxide synthase (nos-1) are both thought to be NF-κB dependent. Accumulation of the major products of NOS and COX-2 activity confer an ischemia-tolerant phenotype. There is evidence that the cytoprotective activity of COX-2 in myocardium is dependent on the co-expression of NOS.

constitutive COX-2 activity in non-preconditioned hearts did not influence the extent of injury [11, 28].

In addition to COX activity, differential expression of the terminal PG synthases, some of which are inducible, determines the specific profile of PG production in any tissue or cell type. This key aspect of PG synthesis is relatively unexplored in myocardium. Induction of terminal PG synthases in response to hypoxic stress may be critical in determining the fate of PGH_2 generated from COX-2. Thus, information on the regulation of specific PG synthases is germane to interpretation of the role of COX-2 in ischaemic myocardium.

COX-2 and post-infarct remodelling

The possible roles of COX-2 in the post-infarct period have so far been assessed in only two experimental studies. Inhibition of COX-2 during the first two weeks following myocardial infarction in rat heart resulted in improved hemodynamic function [29], supporting the hypothesis that induction of COX-2 during myocardial infarction exerts a deleterious influence on myocardial remodelling processes. Induction of COX-2 4 days after myocardial infarction in rat heart has been reported, but although inhibition of COX-2 during this period was associated with reduced macrophage recruitment and fibroblast proliferation, it was unclear if COX-2 inhibition in this study was beneficial or deleterious [13]. These studies in experimental infarction support evidence in human ischaemic cardiomyopathy that COX-2 induction is associated with functional heart failure classification [15].

Conclusion

In the cardiovascular system, the majority of research on COX-2 has concentrated on its influences on vascular tone, on endothelial-platelet interactions, and in the development of atherosclerosis. So far, relatively little work has been undertaken to characterise COX-2 in myocardium. Such work would be extremely pertinent to our understanding of the molecular pathology of myocardial ischemia and infarction. At present there is conflicting experimental evidence on the role of COX-2 in myocardial ischemia and clinical data from COX-2 inhibitor studies suggest a beneficial role of COX-2 in cardiovascular homeostasis. However, the mechanisms by which COX-2 may be beneficial are unclear. Further studies are warranted to provide a detailed examination of COX-2 regulation in myocardium, especially with repect to its roles in acute ischaemic syndromes, and in longer-term post-infarct remodelling.

Acknowledgement
The authors gratefully acknowledge research funding by the UK National Heart Research Fund and the British Heart Foundation.

References

1   Lopez AD, Murray CCJL (1998) The global burden of disease 1990–2020. *Nat Med* 4: 1241–1243

2   Fitzgerald GA, Austin S, Egan K, Cheng Y, Pratico D (2000) Cyclooxygenase products and atherothrombosis. *Ann Med* 32 (Suppl 1): 21–26

3   Narumiya S, Sugimoto Y, Ushikubi F (1999) Prostanoid receptors: Structures, properties, and functions. *Physiol Rev* 79: 1193–1226

4   Dennis EA (1997) The growing phospholipase A2 superfamily of signal transduction enzymes. *Trends Biochem Sci* 22: 1–2

5   Davidge ST (2001) Prostaglandin H Synthase and vascular function. *Circ Res* 89: 650–660

6   Dean JL, Brook M, Clark AR, Saklatvala J (1999) p38 mitogen-activated protein kinase regulates cyclooxygenase-2 mRNA stability and transcription in lipopolysaccharide-treated human monocytes. *J Biol Chem* 274: 264–269

7   McAdam BF, Catella-Lawson F, Mardini IA, Kapoor S, Lawson JA, FitzGerald GA (1999) Systemic biosynthesis of a prostacyclin by cyclooxygenase (COX)-2: the human pharmacology of a selective inhibitor of COX-2. *Proc Natl Acad Sci USA* 96: 272–277

8   Catella-Lawson F, McAdam B, Morrison BW, Kapoor S, Kujubu D, Antes L, Lasseter KC, Quan H, Gertz BJ, FitzGerald GA (1999) Effects of specific inhibition of cyclooxygenase-2 on sodium balance, hemodynamics and vasoactive eicosanoids. *J Pharmacol Exp Ther* 289: 735–741

9   Mukherjee D, Nissen SE, Topol EJ (2001) Risk of cardiovascular events associated with selective COX-2 inhibitors. *J Am Med Assoc* 286: 954–959

10 Reicin AS, Shapiro D, Sperling RS, Barr E, Yu Q (2002) Comparison of cardiovascular thrombotic events in patients with osteoarthritis treated with rofecoxib *versus* non-selective nonsteroidal anti-inflammatory drugs (ibuprofeb, diclofenac and nabumetone). *Am J Cardiol* 89: 204–209

11 Shinmura K, Tang XL, Wang Y, Xuan YT, Liu SQ, Takano H, Bhatnagar A, Bolli R (2000) Cyclooxygenase-2 mediates the cardio-protective effects of the late phase of ischemic preconditioning in conscious rabbits. *Proc Natl Acad Sci USA* 97: 10197–10202

12 Bolli R, Shinmura K, Tang XL, Kodani E, Xuan YT, Guo Y, Dawn B (2002) Discovery of a new function of cyclooxygenase (COX)-2: COX-2 is a cardioprotective protein that alleviates ischemia/reperfusion injury and mediates the late phase of preconditioning. *Cardiovasc Res* 55: 506–519

13 Scheuren N, Jacobs M, Ertl G, Schorb W (2002) Cyclooxygenase-2 in myocardium, stimulation by angiotensin-II in cultured cardiac fibroblasts and role at acute myocardial infarction. *J Mol Cell Cardiol* 34: 29–37

14 Camitta MG, Gabel SA, Chulada P, Bradbury JA, Langenbach R, Zeldin DC, Murphy E (2001) Cyclooxygenase-1 and -2 knockout mice demonstrate increased cardiac ischemia/reperfusion injury but are protected by acute preconditioning. *Circulation* 104: 2453–2458

15 Wong SC, Fukuchi M, Melnyk P, Rodger I, Giaid A (1998) Induction of cyclooxygenase-2 and activation of nuclear factor-kappa-B in myocardium of patients with congestive heart failure. *Circulation* 98: 100–103

16 Metais C, Bianchi C, Li J, Li J, Simons M, Sellke FW (2001) Serotonin-induced human

coronary micro-vascular contraction during acute myocardial ischemia is blocked by COX-2 inhibition. *Basic Res Cardiol* 96: 59–67

17 Schror K, Zimmermann KC, Tannhauser R (1998) Augmented myocardial ischaemia by nicotine: mechanisms and their possible significance. *Br J Pharmacol* 125: 79–86

18 Adderley SR, Fitzgerald DJ (1999) Oxidative damage of cardiomyocytes is limited by extracellular regulated kinases 1/2-mediated induction of cyclooxygenase-2. *J Biol Chem* 274: 5038–5046

19 Bogoyevitch MA, Gillespie-Brown J, Ketterman AJ, Fuller SJ, Ben-Levy R, Ashworth A, Marshall CJ, Sugden PH (1996) Stimulation of the stress-activated mitogen-activated protein kinase subfamilies in perfused heart. p38/RK mitogen-activated protein kinases and c-Jun N-terminal kinases are activated by ischemia/reperfusion. *Circ Res* 79: 162–173

20 Aikawa R, Komuro I, Yamazaki T, Zou Y, Kudoh S, Tanaka M, Shiojima I, Hiroi Y, Yazaki Y (1997) Oxidative stress activates extracellular signal-regulated kinases through Src and Ras in cultured cardiac myocytes of neonatal rats. *J Clin Invest* 100: 1813–1821

21 Baxter GF, Ferdinandy P (2001) Delayed preconditioning of myocardium: Current perspectives. *Basic Res Cardiol* 96: 329–344

22 Jugdutt BI, Hutchins GM, Bulkley BH, Becker LC (1981) Dissimilar effects of prostacyclin, prostaglandin E1, and prostaglandin E2 on myocardial infarct size after coronary occlusion in conscious dogs. *Circ Res* 49: 685–700

23 Simpson PJ, Mickelson J, Fantone JC, Gallagher KP, Lucchesi BR (1987) Iloprost inhibits neutrophil function *in vitro* and *in vivo* and limits experimental infarct size in canine heart. *Circ Res* 60: 666–673

24 Thiemermann C, Thomas GR, Vane JR (1989) Defibrotide reduces infarct size in a rabbit model of experimental myocardial ischaemia and reperfusion. *Br J Pharmacol* 97: 401–408

25 Bouchard JF, Lamontagne D (1999) Mechanisms of protection afforded by cyclooxygenase inhibitors to endothelial function against ischemic injury in rat isolated hearts. *J Cardiovasc Pharmacol* 34: 755–763

26 Heindl B, Becker BF (2001) Aspirin, but not the more selective cyclooxygenase (COX)-2 inhibitors meloxicam and SC 58125, aggravates postischaemic cardiac dysfunction, independent of COX function. *Naunyn Schmiedebergs Arch Pharmacol* 363: 233–240

27 Shinmura K, Xuan YT, Tang XL, Kodani E, Han H, Zhu Y, Bolli R (2002) Inducible nitric oxide synthase modulates cyclooxygenase-2 activity in the heart of conscious rabbits during the late phase of ischemic preconditioning. *Circ Res* 90: 602–608

28 Guo Y, Bao W, Wu WJ, Shinmura K, Tang XL, Bolli R (2000) Evidence for an essential role of cyclooxygenase-2 as a mediator of the late phase of ischemic preconditioning in mice. *Basic Res Cardiol* 95: 479–484

29 Saito T, Rodger IW, Hu F, Shennib H, Giaid A (2000) Inhibition of cyclooxygenase-2 improves cardiac function in myocardial infarction. *Biochem Biophys Res Commun* 273: 772–775

Inflammation and arrhythmias

Inflammation as a cause and consequence of atrial fibrillation

David R. Van Wagoner and Mina K. Chung

Department of Cardiovascular Medicine, FF-10, Cleveland Clinic Foundation, 9500 Euclid Avenue, Cleveland, OH 44195, USA

Introduction

Atrial fibrillation (AF) is the most prevalent chronic arrhythmia, affecting more than 2 million Americans. Prevalence of AF is strongly age related, with AF afflicting more than 10% of the population over age 80. Currently available antiarrhythmic drugs for treating persistent AF have yielded poor long-term relief from arrhythmia recurrence [1]. AF increases the risk of stroke 5- to 7-fold, and is an independent risk factor (2-fold) for mortality [2]. Thus, while AF is not immediately life threatening, its consequences, particularly in the form of increased stroke risk and stroke severity, can be devastating to the patient. As knowledge about the factors that create a thromboembolic environment in AF are limited, current treatment focuses heavily on adequate anticoagulation therapy as a primary goal. In this chapter, evidence is presented suggesting that inflammatory processes have a crucial role both in the endothelial changes leading to increased stroke risk as well as to the electrophysiological and structural changes that increase the persistence of AF.

Natural history of AF

The early experience of patients with AF is typically characterized by episodes that are transient and self terminating (paroxysmal). With time the duration of episodes tends to increase, sometimes becoming persistent (not stopping unless the patient is treated with an electric shock or antiarrhythmic drug). The progression from paroxysmal AF to persistent and permanent AF involves a combination of structural changes in the atria (with respect to the degree of dilatation, trabeculation, fibrosis, fatty infiltration, etc.), and biochemical changes in the individual atrial myocytes (e.g., hypertrophy, changes in ion channel density or distribution, etc.) [3]. Both the structural and electrical changes can promote the persistence of AF. However, while the electrical changes are generally reversible upon termination of the arrhythmia, structural changes may be irreversible.

Inflammation and Cardiac Diseases, edited by Giora Z. Feuerstein, Peter Libby and Douglas L. Mann
© 2003 Birkhäuser Verlag Basel/Switzerland

AF, risk factors, and the "inflammatory state"

It has become increasingly clear in recent years that many of the risk factors for atrial fibrillation (diabetes, obesity, hypertension) and cardiac co-morbidities (valvular disease, atherosclerosis, stroke, etc.) are characterized by evidence of a systemic inflammatory state, increased activation and migration of blood cells (monocytes, neutrophils and macrophages), and increased production of cytokines (IL-1, IL-6) and acute phase reactants such as C-reactive protein (CRP) [4]. Detection of a systemic inflammatory state has thus far focused primarily on the abundance of CRP in plasma as a risk marker [5]. Elevated plasma CRP levels have been associated with increased risk of atherosclerosis, stroke, and myocardial infarction [5].

The potential role of inflammatory processes in the etiology of atrial fibrillation was first demonstrated in a small study of biopsy specimens from paroxysmal AF patients, published in 1997 [6]. This study showed cellular infiltration, degenerative and fibrotic changes, and some evidence of a myocarditis-like process in about 2/3 of the patient samples evaluated. Histologic and biochemical studies of tissues from patients with persistent atrial fibrillation show signs of apoptotic cell death and subsequent replacement fibrosis [7].

CRP can bind to inner leaflet phospholipids of cell (and bacterial) membranes, and binds to and can activate elements of the complement system [8]. It is thus conceivable that in the fibrillating atria CRP may act as an opsonin and participate in the removal of apoptotic myocytes [9]. Additional evidence supporting an independent role of CRP and low-level inflammatory processes in the etiology of AF was provided in a recent study from our group [10]. Figure 1, from this study, shows that patients with any arrhythmia had higher CRP than the controls, and there was a stepwise increase in CRP with increasing persistence of AF (persistent > paroxysmal > atrial tachycardia > control). This incremental increase in CRP levels suggested to us that low-level inflammatory processes are likely to be involved in structural remodeling (e.g., increased fibrosis) that promotes the stability of AF. It is interesting to note that a second group has confirmed our finding of increased CRP levels in patients with paroxysmal AF [11].

AF in the post-surgical setting

Atrial fibrillation is quite common following cardiac and thoracic surgery, with an incidence of 20–50% depending on the nature of the surgery and the age of the patients. Age is the single most powerful predictor of arrhythmia occurrence. Because AF following surgery can lead to hemodynamic compromise, stroke, and extended length of stay, it is a significant medical issue. Inflammatory changes are prominent in this setting. Whereas we detected an increase in median CRP from 0.96 mg/l in control non-surgical patients to 3.4 mg/l in persistent AF patients (a

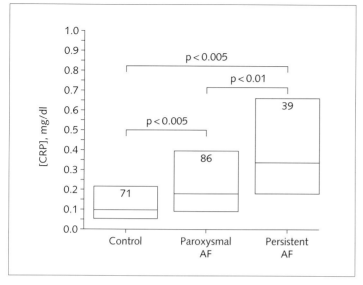

Figure 1
In patients with atrial arrhythmia, CRP levels are increased relative to control patients in normal sinus rhythm. Further, there is a stepwise increase in CRP levels with increasing persistence of arrhythmia. From reference [10], with permission.

3.5-fold increase), peak levels of CRP two to three days following cardiac surgery have been reported to increase up to approximately 60 mg/l ($\sim$200-fold increase) [12]. As mentioned above, CRP can form complexes with components of the complement system (C3b, C4b, C3d, C4d), and participates in complement activation. Following surgery, the increase in C4d-CRP complex formation was correlated with the occurrence of post-operative atrial arrhythmias (predominately AF) [12]. Complement activation can lead to cell lytic activity and neutrophil chemotaxis. Both of these mechanisms may contribute to a significant systemic inflammatory response, myocyte injury and reperfusion arrhythmias [13].

If pericarditis/inflammation is mechanistically important in initiating the arrhythmia, it is intuitive that anti-inflammatory drugs might have antiarrhythmic efficacy. In a pilot study, it has been shown that the anti-inflammatory agent dexamethasone, administered in a single dose to decrease the incidence of post-operative shivering and fever, was associated with a reduction in post-operative AF from 32% to 19% [14]. In another small study thus far presented only in abstract, the non-steroidal drugs ketorolac and ibuprofen were even more effective in decreasing the occurrence of post-operative arrhythmia (from 26% to 4%) [15]. Together, these results suggest that, at least in the perioperative period, anti-inflammatory drugs may have useful antiarrhythmic effects. Studies are ongoing in our laboratory to further evaluate the mechanisms by which the pericarditis promotes arrhythmia initiation. Inflammatory processes could conceivably elicit direct electrophysiological changes in the atrium, alter conduction velocity or pathways, or cause some combination of these effects. Arrhythmias following surgery are typically transient, and likely based primarily on myocyte injury. In contrast, the chronic, low-level inflammatory state associated with non-surgical AF seems more likely to lead to apoptosis, replacement fibrosis and long-term structural remodeling. Studies designed to better elucidate the mechanisms involved in generating these arrhythmias, as well as studies designed to test novel therapeutic approaches with fewer side-effects, are strongly indicated.

AF effects on endocardial / endothelial function: a link to stroke risk

The primary pathologic event linking AF with increased mortality and morbidity is the formation of thrombus in the left atrial appendage followed by stroke or transient ischemic attack (TIA). Clearly, stasis in the fibrillating atrium is one factor that can lead to thrombus formation, however thrombus formation and stroke risk is both age dependent and modified by other factors, broadly classified as the elements of the "metabolic syndrome" [4]. Nitric oxide (NO) is an important modulator of platelet adhesion and activation. Decreased NO availability is strongly associated with impaired endothelial function. In a study using a porcine rapid atrial pacing model [16], detectable NO was decreased in the left but not right atria following a week of high rate pacing. Prothrombotic changes (decreased endocardial NOS expression, increased plasminogen activator inhibitor-1 (PAI-1) expression) were also evident in the left, but not right atria [16]. In post-myocardial infarction patients, AF is strongly associated with increased mortality [17]. In this patient population, elevated PAI-1 levels were strongly associated with the occurrence of atrial arrhythmias. Among patients with AF, we found that CRP levels were strongly correlated with transesophogeal echocardiographic markers of stroke risk. Patients in whom there was visible "smoke" or "sludge" in the left atrial appendage had the highest levels of plasma CRP [18]. Thus, the inflammatory changes in the atria promote a prothrombotic environment in the atrial endocardium and endothelium that leads to increased stroke risk.

Links between oxidative stress, inflammation and AF

In addition to the structural remodeling that accompanies prolonged episodes of AF, electrophysiologic remodeling occurs on a more rapid time scale (minutes to days). Several studies have implicated cellular Ca^{2+} overload in the fibrillating atria as a key factor initiating the electrophysiological remodeling process, however the underlying cellular mechanisms are still unclear. Potential mechanisms include activation of cellular proteases (e.g., calpains [19]), activation of Ca^{2+}-dependent kinases or phosphatases, and increased intracellular oxidative stress [20], resulting from altered mitochondrial function and/or inflammatory mechanisms [10]. We have focused attention on the pathways related to oxidant signaling and inflammatory injury. Activated immune cells produce free radicals (superoxide, hydrogen peroxide, etc.) that are often the mediators of their lethal effects. While such responses are useful and desirable when focused on invading bacteria, oxidants released from these cells can also have direct, deleterious effects on cardiac myocytes. Radicals deplete the antioxidant reserves of the cardiac tissue, and in so doing can significantly modulate the redox state (GSH/GSSG) of the myocardium. The total glutathione levels are decreased, and the ratio of oxidized to reduced glutathione is increased under conditions of oxidative stress. Cellular signaling pathways including NF-κB-mediated transcription, pro-apoptotic enzymes and matrix metalloproteinases that remodel the extracellular matrix (MMP-2 and -9) are sensitive to the redox state of the myocyte and to the effects of oxidants. Thus, inflammation and oxidative stress are two closely related aspects of a common pathological response.

Atrial ion channels, including both the L-type Ca^{2+} current and the transient outward K^+ current, are also quite sensitive to the redox state of the myocyte [21]. To test the hypothesis that oxidant generation is important in the electrophysiological remodeling process, we performed a series of experiments using the canine rapid-atrial pacing model. Pretreatment and daily supplementation of dogs with ascorbate (an antioxidant) was associated with a significant preservation of the effective refractory period (ERP) at 24 and 48 hours of rapid atrial pacing [22]. In tissues from the control animals, the extent of protein nitration was increased with pacing, and ascorbate treatment attenuated this change [22]. Thus, atrial electrophysiologic changes, at least in the short-term, are sensitive to antioxidant intervention. In a pilot study, we also found that pre- and post-surgical treatment of cardiac surgery patients with supplemental ascorbate was associated with a lower incidence of atrial arrhythmias following surgery [22]. It is interesting to note that plasma ascorbate levels are inversely predictive of stroke risk [23]. Thus, it is conceivable that the oxidant-mediated inflammatory processes similarly affect the endothelium, endocardium, and atrial myocytes.

We have also begun to explore the role of oxidative stress in the pathologic structural remodeling associated with AF. In studies of atrial tissue from surgical patients with permanent AF, we have found evidence of significant shifts in atrial myosin isoform expression (from $25 \pm 6\%$ to $63 \pm 5\%$ β-myosin isoform), and reduced creatine kinase activity but not protein expression [20]. Abundance of 3-nitrotyrosine was increased in these tissues, implicating the formation of peroxynitrite as an underlying mechanism in this remodeling. Peroxynitrite formation can occur either *via* the interaction of nitric oxide and superoxide anions, or *via* the enzymatic activity of myeloperoxidase (MPO), using H_2O_2 and nitrite as a substrate. MPO is most prominently contained in and released from neutrophils, the first line of cellular defense in inflammatory responses. In preliminary studies, we have found evidence for increased abundance of MPO-positive cells in atrial specimens from patients with permanent AF (unpublished observation). Our understanding of the role of MPO as a risk factor for inflammatory cardiovascular diseases is evolving [24]. In recent studies, the role of the MPO system, together with PAI-1, has been shown to play a key role in the structural remodeling following myocardial infarction [25]. We suggest that the structural changes that stabilize AF may be quite similar, with characteristic loss of myocytes, increased fibrosis, and altered pathways for excitation.

Summary: a rationale for anti-inflammatory therapeutic intervention in AF

AF is a complex disease with multiple etiologies. Its current prevalence is high, and the numbers of patients suffering from AF will grow sharply with the aging of the "baby boom" generation. Available pharmacologic therapies for AF are only modestly effective and have significant risk of proarrhythmia. Invasive procedures and surgery are frequently effective, but are unlikely to be available to a significant fraction of the patients with AF. Thus, novel therapeutic approaches are urgently needed.

The studies cited above offer intriguing support for the hypothesis that the systemic inflammatory response may be both a cause and consequence of AF. We suggest that selective modulation of components of the systemic inflammatory response may offer novel therapeutic targets for interrupting or preventing atrial arrhythmias, without the confounding proarrhythmic side effects that have plagued many other antiarrhythmic approaches. In the surgical setting, it seems likely that a variety of anti-inflammatory and antioxidant approaches may be effective. In those patients with persistent AF, the efficacy of anti-inflammatory drugs to decrease CRP levels and/or the incidence of AF is currently unevaluated and thus unproven. Statins have been shown to lower CRP [26], to exert anti-inflammatory and antioxidant effects, and are thus logical candidates for further evaluation. Many other pathways are unexplored. Thus, further basic and clinical studies are needed to evaluate the utility of specific anti-inflammatory therapies in either treating or preventing AF.

Acknowledgements
This work was supported in part by NIH grants RO1-HL-65412 and HL-38408 (NHLBI). We gratefully acknowledge the technical assistance of Michelle Lamorgese and Laurie Castel and the collaborative support of John A. Bauer, Ph.D., Cynthia A. Carnes, Pharm.D., Ph.D. Marc A. Gillinov, M.D., Allen Klein, M.D., Patrick M. McCarthy, M.D., and Albert L. Waldo, M.D.

References

1   Naccarelli GV, Wolbrette DL, Khan M, Bhatta L, Hynes J, Samii S, Luck J (2003) Old and new antiarrhythmic drugs for converting and maintaining sinus rhythm in atrial fibrillation: comparative efficacy and results of trials. *Am J Cardiol* 91: 15–26

2   Kannel WB, Wolf PA, Benjamin EJ, Levy D (1998) Prevalence, incidence, prognosis, and predisposing conditions for atrial fibrillation: population-based estimates. *Am J Cardiol* 82: 2N–9N

3   Van Wagoner DR and Nerbonne JM (2000) Molecular basis of electrical remodeling in atrial fibrillation. *J Mol Cell Cardiol* 32: 1101–1117

4   Ridker PM, Buring JE, Cook NR, Rifai N (2003) C-reactive protein, the metabolic syndrome, and risk of incident cardiovascular events: an 8-year follow-up of 14 719 initially healthy American women. *Circulation* 107: 391–397

5   Ridker PM (2003) Clinical application of C-reactive protein for cardiovascular disease detection and prevention. *Circulation* 107: 363–369

6   Frustaci A, Chimenti C, Bellocci F, Morgante E, Russo MA, Maseri A (1997) Histological substrate of atrial biopsies in patients with lone atrial fibrillation. *Circulation* 96: 1180–1184

7   Aime-Sempe C, Folliguet T, Rucker-Martin C, Krajewska M, Krajewska S, Heimburger M, Aubier M, Mercadier JJ, Reed JC, Hatem SN (1999) Myocardial cell death in fibrillating and dilated human right atria. *J Am Coll Cardiol* 34: 1577–1586

8   Ballou SP and Kushner I (1992) C-reactive protein and the acute phase response. *Adv Intern Med* 37: 313–336

9   Mevorach D (2000) Opsonization of apoptotic cells. Implications for uptake and autoimmunity. *Ann NY Acad Sci* 926: 226–235

10 Chung MK, Martin DO, Wazni O, Kanderian A, Sprecher D, Carnes CA, Bauer JA, Tchou PJ, Niebauer M, Natale A, Van Wagoner DR (2001) C-reactive protein elevation in patients with atrial arrhythmias: inflammatory mechanisms and persistence of atrial fibrillation. *Circulation* 104: 2886–2891

11 Dernellis J and Panaretou M (2001) C-reactive protein and paroxysmal atrial fibrillation: evidence of the implication of an inflammatory process in paroxysmal atrial fibrillation. *Acta Cardiol* 56: 375–380

12 Bruins P, Velthuis H., Yazdanbakhsh AP, Jansen PG, van Hardevelt FW, de Beaumont EM, Wildevuur CR, Eijsman L, Trouwborst A, Hack CE (1997) Activation of the complement system during and after cardiopulmonary bypass surgery: postsurgery activation involves C-reactive protein and is associated with postoperative arrhythmia. *Circulation* 96: 3542–3548

13 Ito W, Schafer HJ, Bhakdi S, Klask R, Hansen S, Schaarschmidt S, Schofer J, Hugo F, Hamdoch T, Mathey D (1996) Influence of the terminal complement-complex on reperfusion injury, no-reflow and arrhythmias: a comparison between C6-competent and C6-deficient rabbits. *Cardiovasc Res* 32: 294–305

14 Yared JP, Starr NJ, Torres FK, Bashour CA, Bourdakos G, Piedmonte M, Michener JA,

Davis JA, Rosenberger TE (2000) Effects of single dose, postinduction dexamethasone on recovery after cardiac surgery. *Ann Thorac Surg* 69: 1420–1424

15 Cheruku KK, Ghani A, Ahmad F, Pappas P, Silverman P, Zellinger A, Silver MA (2002) Efficacy of nonsteroidal antiinflammatory medications for prevention of atrial fibrillation following coronary artery bypass surgery. *J Am Coll Cardiol* 39 (Suppl A), 104A

16 Cai H, Li Z, Goette A, Mera F, Honeycutt C, Feterik K, Wilcox JN, Dudley SC Jr, Harrison DG, Langberg JJ (2002) Downregulation of endocardial nitric oxide synthase expression and nitric oxide production in atrial fibrillation: potential mechanisms for atrial thrombosis and stroke. *Circulation* 106: 2854–2858

17 Sinkovic A (2002) Plasminogen activator inhibitor-1 in patients with atrial arrhythmias during acute myocardial infarction, treated with streptokinase. *Blood Coagul Fibrinolysis* 13: 741–747

18 Parakh K, Murray RD, Thambidorai SK, Van Wagoner DR, Klein AL, Chung MK (2002) C-reactive protein is associated with transesophageal echocardiography markers of thromboembolic risk in patients with atrial fibrillation. *Circulation* 106 (Suppl II), II-560

19 Goette A, Arndt M, Rocken C, Staack T, Bechtloff R, Reinhold D, Huth C, Ansorge S, Klein HU, Lendeckel U (2002) Calpains and cytokines in fibrillating human atria. *Am J Physiol Heart Circ Physiol* 283: H264–H272

20 Mihm MJ, Yu F, Carnes CA, Reiser PJ, McCarthy PM, Van Wagoner DR, Bauer JA (2001) Impaired myofibrillar energetics and oxidative injury during human atrial fibrillation. *Circulation* 104: 174–180

21 Van Wagoner DR (2001) Redox modulation of cardiac electrical activity. *J Cardiovasc Electrophysiol* 12: 183–184

22 Carnes CA, Chung MK, Nakayama T, Nakayama H, Baliga RS, Piao S, Kanderian A, Pavia S, Hamlin RL, McCarthy PM, Bauer JA, Van Wagoner DR (2001) Ascorbate attenuates atrial pacing-induced peroxynitrite formation and electrical remodeling and decreases the incidence of postoperative atrial fibrillation. *Circ Res* 89: E32–E38

23 Kurl S, Tuomainen TP, Laukkanen JA, Nyyssonen K, Lakka T, Sivenius J, Salonen JT (2002) Plasma vitamin C modifies the association between hypertension and risk of stroke. *Stroke* 33: 1568–1573

24 Zhang R, Brennan ML, Fu X, Aviles RJ, Pearce GL, Penn MS, Topol EJ, Sprecher DL, Hazen SL (2001) Association between myeloperoxidase levels and risk of coronary artery disease. *JAMA* 286: 2136–2142

25 Askari AT, Brennan ML, Zhou X, Drinko J, Morehead A, Thomas JD, Topol EJ, Hazen SL, Penn MS (2003) Myeloperoxidase and Plasminogen Activator Inhibitor 1 Play a Central Role in Ventricular Remodeling after Myocardial Infarction. *J Exp Med* 197: 615–624

26 Bermudez EA and Ridker PM (2002) C-reactive protein, statins, and the primary prevention of atherosclerotic cardiovascular disease. *Prev Cardiol* 5: 42–46

Summary: Immune and inflammatory modulators as potential therapeutic targets for cardiac diseases

Giora Z. Feuerstein[1], Peter Libby[2] and Douglas L. Mann[3]

[1]Pharmacology Department, WP42-209, Merck Research Laboratories, 770 Sumneytown Pike, West Point, PA 19486, USA; [2]Brigham and Women's Hospital, 221 Longwood Avenue, EBRC 307, Boston, MA 02115, USA; [3]Winters Center for Heart Failure Research, 6565 Fannin, MS 524, Houston, TX 77030, USA

Over the past several years, evidence has been accumulated that the immune and inflammatory systems play a role in diverse diseases. This recognition has been captured in key reviews in a special issue of *Nature*, where the role of inflammation in diseases such as cancer, atherosclerosis, central nervous system and infections has been highlighted [1]. In this perspective, heart diseases are no exceptions. As illustrated in the book *Inflammation and Cardiac Diseases*, immune and inflammatory processes figure prominently in all aspects of human heart diseases – ischemia, heart failure, myocarditis, arrhythmias, and reperfusion injuries. It is, however, important to note that the role of the immune and inflammatory systems in cardiac diseases as discussed in this book focus only on cardiac diseases that are direct outcome of injuries to the heart itself, such as myocardial infarction, myocarditis, arrhythmia or idiopathic disorders of the heart. However, cardiovascular organs may become "casualties" of inflammatory processes associated with other organs. Immune and inflammatory conditions such as gingivitis, rheumatoid arthritis and systemic lupus erythematosus have been associated with increased cardiovascular morbidity and mortality [2–6]. Of particular interest are very recent observations on increased coronary neointima formation in rheumatoid arthritis patients, which could directly explain the increase risk for heart attacks *via* circulatory humoral-mediators of inflammation [7]. These aspects of cardiac disease risk, although beyond the primary focus of the book, are inferred in several chapters such as those dealing with coronary inflammation and systemic inflammatory factors.

The importance of the book *Inflammation and Cardiac Diseases* is that it draws attention to the potential of certain anti-inflammatory strategies to figure prominently in the armamentarium of cardiac protective drugs. Such strategies may include:

A. Immunomodulators such as cytokines with pleiotropic actions or interleukins that have anti-inflammatory action such as interleukin-10.

B. Matrix metalloproteinases that are associated with cardiac remodeling and fibrosis.

C. Nitric oxide synthase inhibitors and certain oxygen radicals.

D. Kinases associated with inflammatory signaling pathways (e.g., MAPK p38 or MEK-1/ERK) that determine cardiomyocyte cell survival or death.

E. Selective macrophage suppressing agents (SMSA) which mitigate macrophage activation and their role in atherosclerosis and cardiac inflammation, e.g., inhibitors of the macrophage alpha 7 nicotinic receptors [8] or MCP-1/CCR-2 chemokine antagonists.

F. Selective nuclear receptors modulators, especially of the alpha and gamma family, could provide diverse opportunities to modulate inflammation as well as myocardial cell resistance to injuries.

These molecular targets are at this time totally un-exploited in cardiac medicine for the simple reason that evidence of the role of these molecules and pathways is incomplete and reagents to decisively explore their potential beneficial roles and adverse effects are incomplete. It is hoped that *via* the book *Inflammation and Cardiac Diseases* more research and pharmaceutical development of novel cardiac drugs will be stimulated.

It is also important to draw attention to the fundamental purpose of the immune and inflammatory systems – the purpose of healing. This Janus face of immune/inflammatory factors in biology and pathology cannot be overemphasized. Adverse manipulation of these systems may prove futile or even harmful. It is therefore imperative that the precise role of targeted mediators is defined vis-à-vis their discrete cellular/spatial and temporal roles. As pointed out in several chapters in the book, recognition of multiplicity of function, contextual function and quantitative aspects of mediators, could be more important then well-advertised function derived in singularity. Moreover, *in vivo* "proof of concepts" on the role of inflammatory mediators in disease processes that represent with greater authenticity the human disease is paramount. The paucity of such information in any research area covered in this book is a "call for arms" to the cardiac research community to invest in proper animal models of heart failure, chronic ischemia, arrhythmias and myocarditis that better represent the respective human disorders. In particular, the almost complete lack of research on cardiac selective, conditioned gene manipulation in heart disease models has a significant impact on the quality of data that assign functional roles for particular genes and proteins in physiological and pathological reactions.

Finally, one needs to recognize that present knowledge on the role of inflammation and immune mediators in heart diseases is rather preliminary in respect to understanding the "big picture" of activation, interaction and regulations of complete pathways over the particular mediators. The genomic and proteomic research in heart diseases is in its infancy; much is left to learn on complete pathways dynamics, and the convergency and divergency of the system at large.

It is hoped that the book *Inflammation and Cardiac Diseases* will help cardiac experimentalists and clinicians to focus attention on key issues in this exciting area of cardiac research.

References

1   Nature insight, inflammation (2002) (Supplement to *Nature Immunology and Nature Medicine*) 420: 845–891

2   Symmons DP, Jones MA, Scott DL, Prior P (1998) Long term mortality outcome in patients with rheumatoid arthritis: early presenters continue to do well. *J Rheumatology* 25: 1072–1077

3   Goodson NJ, Wiles NJ, Lunt M, Barrett EM, Silman AJ, Symmons DPM (2002) Mortality in early inflammatory polyarthritis: cardiovascular mortality is increased in seropositive patients. *Arthritis Rheum* 46: 2010–2019

4   Del Rincon ID, Williams K, Stern MP, Freeman GL, Escalante A (2001) High incidence of cardiovascular events in a rheumatoid arthritis cohort not explained by traditional cardiac risk factors. *Arthritis Rheum* 44: 2737–2745

5   Hurlinmann D, Forster A, Noll G et al (2002) Anti-tumor necrosis factor alpha treatment improves endothelial function, in patients with rheumatoid arthritis. *Circulation* 106: 2184–2187

6   Wallberg-Jonsson S, Csvetkovic, JT, Sundqvist KG, Lefvert AK, Rantapaa- Dahlqvist S (2002) Activation of the immune system and inflammatory activity in relation to markers of atherothrombotic diseases and atherosclerosis in rheumatoid arthritis. *J Rheumatol* 29: 875–882

7   Kumeda Y, Inaba M, Goto H et al (2002) Increased thickness of the arterial intima-media detected by ultrasonography in patients with rheumatoid arthritis. *Arthritis Rheum* 46: 1489–1497

8   Wang H, Yu M, Ochani M et al (2003) Nicotinic acetyl choline receptor alpha 7 subunit is an essential regulator of inflammation. *Nature* 421: 384–388

9   Floto AF, Smith KGC (2003) The vagus nerve, macrophages and nicotine. *Lancet* 361: 1069–1070

Index

The PIR-Series
Progress in Inflammation Research

Homepage: http://www.birkhauser.ch

Up-to-date information on the latest developments in the pathology, mechanisms and therapy of inflammatory disease are provided in this monograph series. Areas covered include vascular responses, skin inflammation, pain, neuroinflammation, arthritis cartilage and bone, airways inflammation and asthma, allergy, cytokines and inflammatory mediators, cell signalling, and recent advances in drug therapy. Each volume is edited by acknowledged experts providing succinct overviews on specific topics intended to inform and explain. The series is of interest to academic and industrial biomedical researchers, drug development personnel and rheumatologists, allergists, pathologists, dermatologists and other clinicians requiring regular scientific updates.

Available volumes:

T Cells in Arthritis, P. Miossec, W. van den Berg, G. Firestein (Editors), 1998
Chemokines and Skin, E. Kownatzki, J. Norgauer (Editors), 1998
Medicinal Fatty Acids, J. Kremer (Editor), 1998
Inducible Enzymes in the Inflammatory Response,
    D.A. Willoughby, A. Tomlinson (Editors), 1999
Cytokines in Severe Sepsis and Septic Shock, H. Redl, G. Schlag (Editors), 1999
Fatty Acids and Inflammatory Skin Diseases, J.-M. Schröder (Editor), 1999
Immunomodulatory Agents from Plants, H. Wagner (Editor), 1999
Cytokines and Pain, L. Watkins, S. Maier (Editors), 1999
In Vivo Models of Inflammation, D. Morgan, L. Marshall (Editors), 1999
Pain and Neurogenic Inflammation, S.D. Brain, P. Moore (Editors), 1999
Anti-Inflammatory Drugs in Asthma, A.P. Sampson, M.K. Church (Editors), 1999
Novel Inhibitors of Leukotrienes, G. Folco, B. Samuelsson, R.C. Murphy (Editors), 1999
Vascular Adhesion Molecules and Inflammation, J.D. Pearson (Editor), 1999
Metalloproteinases as Targets for Anti-Inflammatory Drugs,
    K.M.K. Bottomley, D. Bradshaw, J.S. Nixon (Editors), 1999
Free Radicals and Inflammation, P.G. Winyard, D.R. Blake, C.H. Evans (Editors), 1999
Gene Therapy in Inflammatory Diseases, C.H. Evans, P. Robbins (Editors), 2000
New Cytokines as Potential Drugs, S. K. Narula, R. Coffmann (Editors), 2000
High Throughput Screening for Novel Anti-inflammatories, M. Kahn (Editor), 2000
Immunology and Drug Therapy of Atopic Skin Diseases,
    C.A.F. Bruijnzeel-Komen, E.F. Knol (Editors), 2000
Novel Cytokine Inhibitors, G.A. Higgs, B. Henderson (Editors), 2000
Inflammatory Processes. Molecular Mechanisms and Therapeutic Opportunities,
    L.G. Letts, D.W. Morgan (Editors), 2000

Progress in Inflammation Research
Michael J. Parnham
Series Editor

Inflammation and Stroke

G. Z. Feuerstein

Editor

Birkhäuser

BIOMEDICINE / INFLAMMATION RESEARCH

Feuerstein, G.Z., DuPont Pharmaceuticals Company, Wilmington, USA
(Ed.)

Inflammation and Stroke

2001. 374 pages. Hardcover
ISBN 3-7643-6511-0
PIR - Progress in Inflammation Research

Stroke is a leading cause of death in developed countries. However, current therapeutic strategies for stroke have been largely unsuccessful. One possible explanation is that research and
pharmacological management have focused on very early events in brain ischemia. New research has shown that brain ischemia and trauma elicit strong inflammatory reactions driven by
both external and brain cells. The recognition of inflammation as a fundamental response to
brain ischemia provides novel opportunities for new anti-inflammatory therapies.
For the first time, an international body of researchers presents the latest findings about the
cellular and humoral aspects of immune and inflammatory reactions in the brain. The work may
have an impact on the treatment of neuroinjuries and ancillary brain diseases, and increase the
understanding of the roles infections and immune reactions play in the brain milieu.

For orders originating from all over
the world except USA and Canada:
Birkhäuser Verlag AG
c/o Springer GmbH & Co
Haberstrasse 7
D-69126 Heidelberg
Fax: ++49 / 6221 / 345 4229
e-mail: birkhauser@springer.de

For orders originating in the USA
and Canada:
Birkhäuser
333 Meadowland Parkway
USA-Secaucus
NJ 07094-2491
Fax: +1 201 348 4033
e-mail: orders@birkhauser.com

http://www.birkhauser.ch

Birkhäuser